Internal Medicine Pearls

Second Edition

JOHN E. HEFFNER, MD
Professor and Associate Dean
Department of Medicine
Medical University of South Carolina
Charleston, South Carolina

STEVEN A. SAHN, MD
Professor of Medicine and Director
Division of Pulmonary and
  Critical Care Medicine
Medical University of South Carolina
Charleston, South Carolina

HANLEY & BELFUS, INC./Philadelphia

Publisher: HANLEY & BELFUS, INC.
                Medical Publishers
                210 S. 13th Street
                Philadelphia, PA 19107
                (215) 546-7293, 800-962-1892
                FAX (215) 790-9330
                Website: http://www.hanleyandbelfus.com

Library of Congress Cataloging-in-Publication Data

Internal Medicine Pearls / edited by John E. Heffner, Steven A. Sahn.—2nd ed.
        p. ; cm.—(The Pearls Series®)
    Rev. ed. of: Internal medicine pearls / Clay B. Marsh, Ernest L. Mazzaferri. ©1993.
    Includes bibliographical references and index.
    ISBN 1-56053-404-4 (alk. paper)
    1. Internal medicine—Case studies.   I. Heffner, John E.   II. Sahn, Steven A.
III. Series
    [DNLM: 1. Internal Medicine—Case Report.   WB 115 I608 2000]
    RC66.M277 2001
    616'.09—dc21
                                                                    00-058134

INTERNAL MEDICINE PEARLS, 2nd edition   ISBN 1-56053-404-4

© 2001 by Hanley & Belfus, Inc. All rights reserved. No part of this book may be reproduced, reused, republished, transmitted in any form or by any means, or stored in a database or retrieval system without written permission of the publisher.

Last digit is the print number: 9 8 7 6 5 4 3 2 1

CONTENTS

Patient   **Page**

Patient   **Page**

CONTRIBUTORS

Loutfi S. Aboussouan, MD
Assistant Professor of Medicine, Department of Pulmonary, Critical Care, and Sleep Medicine, Wayne State University, Detroit, Michigan

Nezam H. Afdhal, MD, FRCPI
Associate Professor of Medicine, Harvard Medical School, Boston; Chief, Department of Hepatology, Beth Israel Deaconess Medical Center, Boston, Massachusetts

Selim M. Arcasoy, MD
Assistant Professor, Department of Medicine, Pulmonary, Allergy, and Critical Care Division, University of Pennsylvania, Philadelphia, Pennsylvania

Alejandro C. Arroliga, MD
Head, Section of Critical Care Medicine; Director of Fellowship Program, Department of Pulmonary and Critical Care Medicine, The Cleveland Clinic Foundation, Cleveland, Ohio

John R. Bach, MD
Professor and Vice Chairman, Department of Physical Medicine and Rehabilitation, University of Medicine and Dentistry, Newark, New Jersey

Colleen L. Bailey, MD
Fellow, Pulmonary and Critical Care Division, University of California Medical Center, San Diego, California

Robert A. Balk, MD
Professor, Department of Medicine, Rush Medical College, Chicago; Director, Pulmonary and Critical Care Medicine, Rush Presbyterian–St. Luke's Medical Center, Chicago, Illinois

Alan Barker, MD
Division of Pulmonary and Critical Care Medicine, Oregon Health Sciences University, Portland, Oregon

Helen E. Bateman, MD

Peter Barland, MD
Professor, Division of Rheumatology, Department of Medicine, Montefiore Medical Center, Bronx, New York

Lisa M. Bellini, MD
Assistant Professor, Department of Medicine; Vice Chair for Education, University of Pennsylvania School of Medicine, Philadelphia, Pennsylvania

Tomas Berl, MD
Professor, Department of Medicine, University of Colorado, Denver, Colorado

Dan R. Berlowitz, MD, MPH
Associate Professor, Department of Medicine; Associate Director, Center for Health Quality, Outcomes, and Economic Research, Boston University, Boston, Massachusetts

Richard B. Berry, MD
Professor, Department of Medicine; Medical Director, Sleep Disorders Center, University of Florida, Gainesville, Florida

Stephen J. Bickston, MD
Associate Professor, Division of Gastroenterology, Department of Internal Medicine, University of Virginia, Charlottesville, Virginia

Lewis S. Blevins, Jr., MD
Associate Professor, Departments of Medicine and Neurological Surgery; Director, The Pituitary Center, Vanderbilt University Medical Center, Nashville, Tennessee

Javier E. Bogarin, MD
Fellow, Department of Pulmonary and Critical Care Medicine, Rush Presbyterian–St. Luke's Medical Center, Chicago, Illinois

Michel A. Boivin, MD
Critical Care Fellow, Department of Medicine, University of New Mexico, Albuquerque, New Mexico

Glenn D. Braunstein, MD
Professor of Medicine, University of California School of Medicine, Los Angeles; Chairman, Department of Medicine, Cedars-Sinai Medical Center, Los Angeles, California

Lee K. Brown, MD
Clinical Professor of Medicine, Division of Pulmonary, Critical Care, and Allergy, University of New Mexico School of Medicine; Medical Director, New Mexico Center for Sleep Medicine; Associate Medical Director (Medical Specialties), Lovelace Health Systems, Inc., Albuquerque, New Mexico

Bartolome R. Celli, MD
Professor, Department of Medicine, Tufts University, Boston; Chief, Pulmonary and Critical Care Medicine, St. Elizabeth's Medical Center, Boston, Massachusetts

Anil Chandraker, MD
Instructor, Department of Medicine, Harvard Medical School, Boston; Associate Physician, Brigham and Women's Hospital, Boston, Massachusetts

Stanley W. Chapman, MD
Professor and Director, Division of Infectious Diseases, Department of Medicine, University of Mississippi Medical Center, Jackson, Mississippi

Scott Choi, MD
Department of Gastroenterology, Medical College of Virginia, Richmond, Virginia

Mark Cohen, MD
Senior Fellow, Division of Pulmonary and Critical Care Medicine, Allergy, and Clinical Immunology, Department of Medicine, Medical University of South Carolina, Charleston, South Carolina

Daniel Joseph Combs, MD
Resident Physician, Department of Internal Medicine and Pediatrics, Indiana University, Indianapolis, Indiana

J. Randall Curtis, MD, MPH
Associate Professor of Medicine, Division of Pulmonary and Critical Care Medicine, University of Washington, Seattle, Washington

Kathryn M. Dobmeyer, MD
Senior Fellow, Acting Instructor, Department of Medicine, University of Washington, Seattle, Washington

John W. Doggett, MD
Associate Medical Director, New Mexico Center for Sleep Medicine, Lovelace Health Systems, Albuquerque, New Mexico

Liselle Douyon, MD

Matthew Lingle Esson, MD
Research Fellow, Department of Internal Medicine, Division of Renal Diseases and Hypertension, University of Colorado Health Sciences Center, Denver, Colorado

Ronald M. Fairman, MD
Assistant Professor of Surgery and Radiology, Department of Surgery, University of Pennsylvania, Philadelphia, Pennsylvania

Harrison W. Farber, MD
Professor, Department of Medicine/Pulmonary Center, Boston University School of Medicine, Boston, Massachusetts

Peter F. Fedullo, MD
Professor of Medicine, Pulmonary and Critical Care Division, University of California Medical Center, San Diego, California

Lourdes M. E. Flaminiano, MD

James W. Galbraith, Jr., BS
Research Assistant, Hyperbaric Facility, Marine Biomedical Institute, University of Texas Medical Branch, Galveston, Texas

Peter C. Gazes, MD
Professor of Medicine, Distinguished Clinical University Professor of Cardiology, Medical University of South Carolina, Charleston, South Carolina

James N. George, MD
Professor, Department of Medicine, University of Oklahoma, Oklahoma City, Oklahoma

Thomas A. Golper, MD
Professor, Departments of Nephrology and Medicine, Vanderbilt University, Nashville, Tennessee

Douglas Greene, MD
Professor, Department of Medicine, University of Michigan, Ann Arbor, Michigan

Peter S. Guido, MD
Staff Physician, New Mexico Center for Sleep Medicine, Lovelace Health Systems, Albuquerque, New Mexico

Samir Kumar Gupta, MD
Fellow, Division of Infectious Diseases, Department of Medicine, Indiana University, Indianapolis, Indiana

William D. Haire, MD
Professor, Department of Internal Medicine, University of Nebraska Medical Center, Omaha, Nebraska

John E. Heffner, MD
Professor and Vice Chairman, Department of Medicine, Medical University of South Carolina, Charleston, South Carolina

Katherine P. Hendra, MD
Assistant Clinical Professor, Department of Medicine, Tufts University School of Medicine, Boston; Director of Fellowship Program– Pulmonary/Critical Care Medicine, St. Elizabeth's Medical Center, Boston, Massachusetts

Nicholas S. Hill, MD
Professor, Department of Pulmonary and Critical Care Medicine, Brown University School of Medicine, Providence; Director, Critical Services, Rhode Island Hospital, Providence, Rhode Island

Gary S. Hoffman, MD
Professor of Medicine; Chairman, Rheumatic and Immunologic Diseases; Harold C. Schott Chair for Rheumatic and Immunologic Diseases, Cleveland Clinic Foundation, Cleveland, Ohio

Jean L. Holley, MD
Professor, Department of Medicine–Nephrology Unit, University of Rochester, Rochester, New York

Russell D. Hull, MBBS, MSc
Professor of General Internal Medicine, Department of Medicine, University of Calgary, Calgary, Alberta, Canada

David H. Ingbar, MD
Professor, Departments of Medicine and Pediatrics, University of Minnesota, Minneapolis, Minnesota

Richard S. Irwin, MD
Professor, Department of Medicine, University of Massachusetts Medical School, Worcester; Director, Division of Pulmonary, Allergy, and Critical Care Medicine, UMASS Memorial Healthcare, Worcester, Massachusetts

Allan S. Jaffe, MD
Professor of Medicine and Consultant, Department of Cardiology, Mayo Clinic and Medical School, Rochester, Minnesota

Shubhada M. Jagasia, MD
Clinical Fellow, Department of Endocrinology and Metabolism, Vanderbilt University, Nashville, Tennessee

Amal Jubran, MD
Associate Professor, Division of Pulmonary and Critical Care Medicine, Loyola University of Chicago, Stritch School of Medicine, Maywood, Illinois

Peter J. Kahrilas, MD
Gilbert H. Marquardt Professor of Medicine; Chief, Division of Gastroenterology and Hepatology, Department of Internal Medicine, Northwestern University School of Medicine, Chicago, Illinois

Wayne Katon, MD
Professor and Vice Chair, Department of Psychiatry and Behavioral Sciences; Director, Division of Health Services and Epidemiology, University of Washington Medical School, Seattle, Washington

Steven Mark Kawut, MD
Fellow, Department of Medicine, Pulmonary, Allergy, and Critical Care Division, University of Pennsylvania, Philadelphia, Pennsylvania

Thomas J. Kayani, MD
Clinical Fellow in Nephrology, Department of Medicine, Vanderbilt University Medical Center, Nashville, Tennessee

Andrew P. Keaveny, MB, MRCPI
Fellow in Gastroenterology, Boston Medical Center, Boston, Massachusetts

Reshma Kewalramani, MD
Senior Medical Resident, Department of Medicine, Massachusetts General Hospital, Boston, Massachusetts

Kiarash Kojouri, MD
Postdoctoral Fellow, University of Oklahoma, Oklahoma City, Oklahoma

Kris V. Kowdley, MD
Associate Professor of Medicine, Division of Gastroenterology, University of Washington School of Medicine, Seattle, Washington

Robert A. Kyle, MD
Professor of Medicine and Laboratory Medicine, Department of Hematology, Mayo Clinic, Rochester, Minnesota

Roberto M. Lang, MD
Professor, Department of Medicine, University of Chicago, Chicago, Illinois

Robert A. Larson, MD
Vascular Surgery Fellow, Department of Surgery, University of Pennsylvania Medical Center, Philadelphia, Pennsylvania

Clarence W. Legerton, III, MD
Associate Professor, Department of Medicine, Medical University of South Carolina, Charleston, South Carolina

Timothy M. Lenardo, MD
Fellow, Department of Rheumatology, Cleveland Clinic Foundation, Cleveland, Ohio

Howard Levy, MD, PhD
Associate Chief of Critical Care Medicine; Professor, Department of Medicine, University of New Mexico, Albuquerque, New Mexico

Richard W. Light, MD
Professor, Department of Medicine, Vanderbilt University, Nashville; Director, Pulmonary Diseases, Saint Thomas Hospital, Nashville, Tennessee

George F. Longstreth, MD
Chief, Department of Gastroenterology, Kaiser Permanente Medical Care Program, San Diego, California

Navid Madani, MD
Fellow, Department of Medicine, Section of Gastroenterology, Boston University, Boston, Massachusetts

Jon T. Mader, MD
Professor, Department of Internal Medicine and Pathology, University of Texas Medical Branch, Galveston, Texas

Peter F. Malet, MD
Associate Professor, Department of Internal Medicine, Liver Unit, University of Texas Southwestern Medical School, Dallas; Attending Physician, Parkland Memorial Hospital, Dallas, Texas

Stephanie Marglin, MD
Department of Medicine, Jordan Hospital, Plymouth, Massachusetts

Catherine J. Markin, MD
Fellow, Department of Medicine, Division of Pulmonary and Critical Care Medicine, Oregon Health Sciences University, Portland, Oregon

Richard J. Martin, MD
Professor, Department of Medicine, University of Colorado, Denver; Head, Pulmonary Division, and Vice Chair, Department of Medicine, National Jewish Medical and Research Center, Denver, Colorado

David K. McCulloch, MD, FRCP
Clinical Associate Professor of Medicine, Department of Endocrinology and Metabolism, University of Washington, Seattle; Diabetologist, Group Health Cooperative of Puget Sound, Seattle, Washington

C. Crawford Mechem, MD
Assistant Professor, Department of Emergency Medicine, Hospital of the University of Pennsylvania, Philadelphia, Pennsylvania

Marc L. Miller, MD
Clinical Assistant Professor, Department of Medicine, University of Vermont School of Medicine, Burlington, Vermont; Attending Physician, Maine Medical Center, Portland, Maine

Omar A. Minai, MD
Clinical Associate, Department of Pulmonary and Critical Care Medicine, Cleveland Clinic Foundation, Cleveland, Ohio

Emile R. Mohler III, MD
Assistant Professor, Department of Medicine, Cardiovascular Division, University of Pennsylvania School of Medicine, Philadelphia, Pennsylvania

Mahesh S. Mokhashi, MD, MRCP (UK)
Assistant Professor, Division of Gastroenterology and Hepatology, Medical University of South Carolina, Charleston, South Carolina

Liza C. O'Dowd, MD
Instructor, Department of Pulmonary, Allergy, and Critical Care Medicine, University of Pennsylvania Health System, Philadelphia, Pennsylvania

John Erik Pandolfino, MD
Fellow, Department of Gastroenterology, Northwestern University Medical School, Chicago, Illinois

Richard V. Paul, MD
Associate Professor, Department of Medicine, Medical University of South Carolina, Charleston, South Carolina

Robert S. Pinals, MD
Professor and Vice Chairman, Department of Medicine, University of Medicine and Dentistry–Robert Wood Johnson Medical School, New Brunswick, New Jersey

Graham Pineo, MD, FACP
Professor of Medicine and Oncology, Department of Medicine, University of Calgary, Calgary, Alberta, Canada

Chaim Putterman, MD
Assistant Professor, Division of Rheumatology, Department of Medicine, Albert Einstein College of Medicine, Bronx, New York

Muredach P. Reilly, MB
Instructor, Department of Medicine, University of Pennsylvania School of Medicine, Philadelphia, Pennsylvania

Robert S. Rosenson, MD
Associate Professor, Departments of Medicine and Pathology; Director, Preventive Cardiology Center; Director, Lipoprotein and Hemorheology Research Facility; Director, Cardiac Rehabilitation Program, Rush-Presbyterian-St. Luke's Medical Center, Chicago, Illinois

Alan L. Rothman, MD
Associate Professor, Department of Medicine, University of Massachusetts Medical School, Worcester; Active Medical Staff, UMASS Memorial Medical Center, Worcester, Massachusetts

Gordon D. Rubenfeld, MD, MSc
Assistant Professor of Medicine, Division of Pulmonary and Critical Care Medicine, Harborview Medical Center, University of Washington, Seattle, Washington

Lewis J. Rubin, MD
Professor, Department of Medicine, University of California School of Medicine, San Diego; Director, Pulmonary and Critical Care Medicine, UCSD Medical Center, San Diego, California

Bruce A. Runyon, MD
Chief, Liver Unit, Department of Internal Medicine, Rancho Los Amigos, University of Southern California, Downey, California

Julius Sagel, MB, ChB
Professor, Department of Medicine; Vice Chair for Education, Medical University of South Carolina, Charleston, South Carolina

Arun J. Sanyal, MD
Associate Professor and Chairman, Department of Gastroenterology, Medical College of Virginia, Richmond, Virginia

George A. Sarosi, MD
Professor, Department of Internal Medicine, Indiana University, Indianapolis, Indiana

Mohamed H. Sayegh, MD
Associate Professor, Department of Medicine, Harvard Medical School, Boston; Associate Physician, Brigham and Women's Hospital, Boston Massachusetts

Paul C. Schroy III, MD, MPH
Associate Professor, Section of Gastroenterology, Department of Medicine, Boston University School of Medicine, Boston; Associate Visiting Physician, Director of Clinical Research, Boston Medical Center, Boston, Massachusetts

Marvin I. Schwarz, MD
Chief, Department of Pulmonary and Critical Care Medicine, University of Colorado Health Sciences Center, Denver, Colorado

Winston Sequeira, MD
Associate Professor, Department of Medicine, Section of Rheumatology, Rush Medical College, Chicago; Attending Physician, Rush-Presbyterian-St. Luke's Hospital, Chicago; Chairman, Rheumatology, Cook County Hospital, Chicago, Illinois

Marie-Florence Shadlen, MD
Assistant Professor, Department of Medicine, University of Washington, Seattle, Washington

Om Prakash Sharma, MD
Professor, Department of Medicine, The Keck School of Medicine, University of Southern California, Los Angeles; Senior Physician, USC Medical Center, Los Angeles, California

Mark E. Shirtliff, PhD
Research Director, Hyperbaric Facility, Department of Microbiology and Immunology, Marine Biomedical Institute, University of Texas Medical Branch, Galveston, Texas

Leonard H. Sigal, MD
Professor and Chief, Division of Rheumatology, Medicine, and Pediatrics, University of Medicine and Dentistry of New Jersey–Robert Wood Johnson Medical School, New Brunswick, New Jersey

Nicholas A. Smyrnios, MD
Associate Professor, Department of Medicine, University of Massachusetts Medical School, Worcester; Director, Medical Intensive Care Unit, UMASS Memorial Healthcare, Worcester, Massachusetts

James K. Stoller, MD
Vice Chairman, Division of Medicine Head, Section of Respiratory Therapy; Professor, Department of Pulmonary and Critical Care Medicine, Cleveland Clinic Foundation, Cleveland, Ohio

Ayalew Tefferi, MD
Consultant, Division of Hematology and Internal Medicine, Mayo Clinic and Mayo Foundation, Rochester; Associate Professor of Medicine, Mayo Medical School, Rochester, Minnesota

Saul G. Trevino, MD
Professor, Department of Orthopedic Surgery and Rehabilitation, University of Texas Medical Branch, Galveston, Texas

Elbert P. Trulock, MD
Professor of Medicine, Pulmonary Division, Department of Internal Medicine, Washington University School of Medicine, St. Louis; Medical Director, Lung Transplant Program, Barnes-Jewish Hospital, St. Louis, Missouri

Bruce Y. Tung, MD
Assistant Professor of Medicine, Division of Gastroenterology, University of Washington School of Medicine, Seattle, Washington

Michael B. Wallace, MD, MPH
Assistant Professor, Department of Medicine, Division of Gastroenterology and Hepatology, Medical University of South Carolina, Charleston, South Carolina

R. Parker Ward, MD
Department of Medicine, University of Chicago, Chicago, Illinois

Idelle M. Weisman, MD
Associate Professor, Department of Internal Medicine, Texas Tech University Health Sciences Center, El Paso; Chief, Department of Clinical Investigation, William Beaumont Army Medical Center, El Paso, Texas

Anne B. Whitehurst, MD
Assistant Professor, Infectious Diseases Division, Department of Medicine, University of Mississippi Medical Center, Jackson, Mississippi

Spencer Van B. Wilking, MBBS, MPH, FACP
Associate Professor, Section of Geriatric Medicine, Boston University School of Medicine, Boston, Massachusetts

Arthur P. Wolinsky, MD
Associate Professor, Department of Internal Medicine, Medical University of South Carolina, Charleston; Staff Physician, Ralph H. Johnson VA Medical Center, Charleston, South Carolina

Richard G. Wunderink, MD
Director of Clinical Research, Physicians Research Network, Methodist Healthcare Foundation, Memphis; Clinical Associate Professor, Department of Medicine, University of Tennessee, Memphis, Tennessee

R. Jorge Zeballos, MD
Associate Professor, Departments of Anesthesiology and Internal Medicine, Texas Tech University Health Sciences Center, El Paso; Department of Clinical Investigation, William Beaumont Army Medical Center, El Paso, Texas

Dedication

To

the patients who have shared with us their clinical stories

and who have entrusted us with their care

PREFACE

Observe, record, tabulate, communicate.

~ William Osler

Osler continuously admonished that the practice of medicine could only be learned through clinical experience. He was fond of saying, "The whole art of medicine is in observation."

In this second edition of *Internal Medicine Pearls*, we have collected the personal observations gained through clinical practice of recognized master clinicians in their fields of expertise. These patient-centered case summaries—or what we like to call "patient stories"—provide descriptive observations of the presentation of disease, use of diagnostic tests, implementation of therapeutic interventions, and clinical outcome. They also examine the human experience of disease, capturing the impact of illness on patients' lives and sometimes touching on the unfolding of death through end-of-life decision making.

Authors were encouraged to present state-of-the-art content and to offer readers sound clinical approaches to the clinical problems discussed. No other source of case studies is as up-to-date on these clinical topics. The authors also were reminded, however, to entwine their patients into the discussions—respecting that the most effective lessons are learned through contact with real patients.

We have followed the format of other books in the Pearls Series®, wherein important lessons learned from patients are captured at the end of the discussion in the form of Clinical Pearls. These succinct summaries of teaching points assist readers in retaining and applying the wisdom of the master clinicians who contributed to this book.

Internal Medicine Pearls, 2nd edition is intended to stimulate the self-learning of clinicians at all levels of experience. The case summaries and patient-centered discussions aptly demonstrate that our expert authors themselves followed Osler's self-learning advice to "record and tabulate" their experiences, which is the most direct route toward gaining clinical expertise. We also hope that this book, by its effort to convey our clinical experiences, will encourage readers to follow the last element of Osler's admonition to "communicate" to their colleagues lessons learned from patient care, so as to contribute to the ongoing progress of medical science.

We thank Marianne Grac and Jacqueline Mahon for their dedicated and expert assistance with this project. We also acknowledge the mentors and teachers who shared their clinical observations and devotion to the art of medicine with the contributors to this book.

John E. Heffner, MD
Steven A. Sahn, MD

Samir K. Gupta, MD
Daniel J. Combs, MD
George A. Sarosi, MD

PATIENT 1

A 40-year-old HIV-positive man with dyspnea, fever, and weight loss

A 40-year-old man, diagnosed with the human immunodeficiency virus (HIV) 14 years ago, presents to the emergency department with a 3-day history of progressive dyspnea at rest. He has had nausea, vomiting, vague right-sided abdominal pain, 15-pound weight loss, and non-bloody diarrhea over the previous 2 weeks. The patient notes subjective fevers, rigors, night sweats, and a nonproductive cough for the past 10 days. He was recently treated with trimethoprim/sulfamethoxazole and levofloxacin by his primary physician, with no improvement in his symptoms.

Physical Examination: Temperature 37.1; pulse 126; respirations 22; blood pressure 120/74. General: pale, thin, mildly labored respirations. HEENT: oral thrush. Cardiac: tachycardia, without murmur. Chest: scattered bibasilar crackles with good air exchange. Abdomen: liver edge palpable 3 cm below right costal margin, spleen tip palpable in left upper quadrant, no tenderness. Extremities: normal. Skin: no rash.

Laboratory Findings: WBC 1200/µl with 4% bands, 90% neutrophils. Sodium 124 mEq/L, potassium 3.3 mEq/L, chloride 94 mEq/L, bicarbonate 22 mEq/L, BUN 16 mg/dl, creatinine 0.8 mg/dl, SGOT 237 U/L. Arterial blood gas (room air): pH 7.59, pCO$_2$ 23 mmHg, pO$_2$ 55 mmHg. Chest radiograph: see below left. Peripheral smear: see below right.

Question: What clinical syndrome accounts for these features?

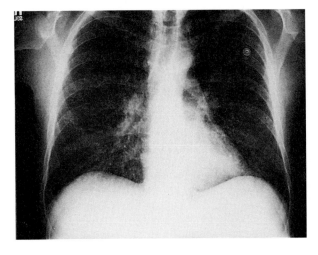
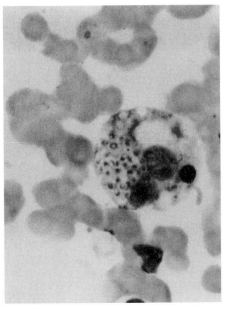

Diagnosis: Progressive disseminated histoplasmosis (PDH).

Discussion: *Histoplasma capsulatum* is an endemic, thermal, dimorphic fungus seen throughout the world, but the areas of heaviest concentration are in North, Central, and South America. Within the United States, it is found primarily along the Ohio and Mississippi River valleys. The mycelial form is seen in soil, while the yeast form (which grows only at temperatures over 35°C) exclusively causes human infection.

Microconidia sprout from the mold form of *H. capsulatum*. These infectious particles are then inhaled into the lungs, where the host's immune system responds by containing the infection with neutrophils and macrophages. However, the yeast form can infect macrophages without being destroyed, thereby allowing dissemination of the organism throughout the reticuloendothelial system (lungs, liver, spleen, bone marrow, lymph nodes). To eliminate the infection, T-cell mediated immunity is crucial. Therefore, immunocompromised patients, especially those diagnosed with the acquired immunodeficiency syndrome (AIDS), are most susceptible to progressive disseminated disease. In fact, PDH is frequently the AIDS-defining illness in those with HIV infection. PDH is usually seen when CD4 counts are depressed below 100.

Patients with AIDS and PDH usually present

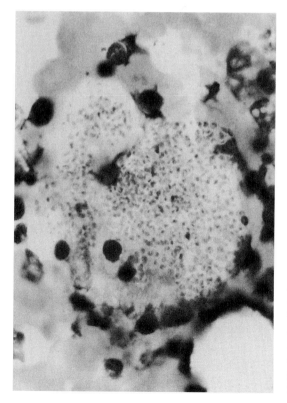

with fever and weight loss. Other common symptoms are cough, dyspnea, and diarrhea (as seen in the present patient). Clinical signs include hepatosplenomegaly, lymphadenopathy, and oral or mucosal lesions. Surprisingly, many patients may have no abnormalities on physical examination, whereas others present in a toxic state suggestive of bacterial sepsis.

Laboratory abnormalities include cytopenias, coagulopathies, and elevations in lactate dehydrogenase, alkaline phosphatase, and ferritin. In the septic form, evidence of multiorgan failure is seen, such as elevations in serum aminotransferases and creatinine. Chest radiography may be normal at presentation, but it usually shows **diffuse reticulonodular markings**, with 1- to 2-ml nodules visible throughout the lung fields (see present patient's chest radiograph).

Diagnosis depends on actual visualization of the organism in tissue or positive results from culture. Because of the reticuloendothelial nature of PDH, there usually is evidence of infection in the blood smear, the bone marrow, or in pulmonary specimens (bronchoalveolar biopsy, brushings, or lavage). Tissue obtained from liver or skin biopsy also may be helpful if lesions are present in those organs. Blood cultures are positive in over 80% of PDH cases, especially if lysis-centrifugation is performed, but may require 2–4 weeks of growth. If *H. capsulatum* is not seen within peripheral smear leukocytes, or if corroborating evidence is required, bone marrow biopsy usually provides the safest means to definitive diagnosis. Detection of *Histoplasma* antigen in the blood or urine is 80–98% sensitive in PDH.

The treatment for disseminated histoplasmosis in a patient with immunosuppression is **amphotericin B** at doses of 50 mg/day or 0.7 mg/kg/day for patients weighing less than 50 kilograms. Relapse rates are high in AIDS patients; therefore, maintenance suppression therapy is required. Amphotericin B can be given at maintenance doses of 50 mg weekly or biweekly, but this regimen may not be well tolerated. The alternative is 200–400 mg of itraconazole, but this may cause significant drug-drug interactions.

The present patient initially was treated for *Pneumocystis carinii* pneumonia based on a poor-quality, portable chest radiograph. However, once the diffuse reticulonodular pattern was appreciated on an upright posterior-anterior film, PDH was considered. His peripheral blood smear showed leukocytes loaded with *Histoplasma* organisms. The patient's hepatosplenomegaly and peripheral smear findings supported the diagnosis. Bone marrow biopsy (see figure at left) showed a macrophage filled with yeast, thereby firmly establishing the diagnosis of progressive disseminated histoplasmosis. Urine *Histoplasma* antigen also was positive.

The patient responded quickly to amphotericin B and is currently being treated with itraconazole suppression and highly active antiretroviral therapy. There has been no evidence of relapse.

CLINICAL PEARLS

1. Progressive disseminated histoplasmosis (PDH) affects the organs of the reticuloendothelial system.

2. PDH may be the presenting syndrome in HIV patients, especially if the CD4 count is < 100.

3. Clues to diagnosis include a diffuse reticulonodular pattern seen on chest radiography, hepatosplenomegaly, and evidence of infection on peripheral blood smear.

REFERENCES

1. Sarosi GA, Johnson PC: Disseminated histoplasmosis in patients infected with HIV. Clin Infec Dis 1992;14(Suppl 1):S60–66.
2. Wheat J: Histoplasmosis: Recognition and treatment. Clin Infec Dis 1994;19(Suppl 1):S19–27.
3. Wheat J: Histoplasmosis: Experience during outbreaks in Indianapolis and review of the literature. Medicine 1997;76:339–354.
4. Goldman M, Johnson PC, Sarosi GA: Fungal pneumonias: The endemic mycoses. Clin Chest Med 1999;20:507–519.

Peter C. Gazes, MD

PATIENT 2

A 52-year-old man with exertional chest pain

A 52-year-old man experienced mid-substernal squeezing discomfort while rushing in the airport 1 year ago. The pain was relieved immediately by rest. Since then, he has noted this discomfort whenever he walks fast. It never occurs at rest or at night. He has smoked approximately 1½ packages of cigarettes daily for at least 30 years. There is no history of diabetes or hypertension, and he has never had a lipid analysis. Both parents died of coronary artery disease in their mid 50s.

Physical Examination: Vital signs: pulse 80, blood pressure 120/70. Chest: clear. Cardiac: no murmurs or extra sounds. Peripheral pulses: normal.

Laboratory Findings: CBC: normal. Cholesterol: 260 mg/dl, HDL 40 mg/dl, triglycerides 180 mg/dl, LDL 174 mg/dl. Resting EKG: normal. Bruce stress test: after 3 minutes of exercise with a heart rate of 122 per min, EKG changes developed.

Question: What is your diagnosis? How would you manage this patient?

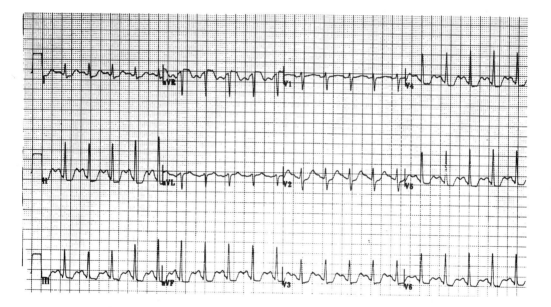

Answer: Stable angina. Perform nuclear exercise perfusion study and then individualize management depending on the extent of disease, ischemia, and left ventricular function.

Discussion: Angina is considered stable when it has been present for several months without change in duration or frequency; is usually precipitated by a known amount of exercise and anxiety; and is relieved by rest and nitroglycerin. Over the last two decades, management of coronary artery disease has evolved significantly. The challenge today is whether **revascularization or medical therapy** should be offered to the patient with stable angina. Options for revascularization include coronary bypass surgery (CABG), angioplasty, and placement of stents. Patients require an individualized approach and appropriate therapy based on the extent of coronary artery disease, severity and extent of ischemia, and the presence of left ventricular dysfunction.

Perform coronary arteriography if a nuclear or echocardiographic stress study shows significant ischemia or left ventricular dysfunction. Also consider it in those with stable angina who have significant EKG ST depression with exercise during the first 3 minutes of a Bruce protocol, and a heart rate less than 70% of predicted maximal heart rate that persists for 6 minutes or more. Optimal medical therapy includes nitroglycerin, beta-blocker, calcium blocker, aspirin, and management of risk factors such as hyperlipidemia, exercise, smoking, blood pressure, and weight loss.

The approach to the patient with stable angina evolves around these factors: the presence of three-vessel disease, or two-vessel disease that includes proximal left anterior descending artery (LAD) disease, significant ischemia detected by noninvasive testing, and left ventricular dysfunction. If two of these three are present, patients do better with revascularization, and when only one factor is present, medical therapy may be sufficient. Many studies and meta-analyses of randomized trials show that patients with three-vessel disease, especially with a decreased ejection fraction, or left main vessel coronary artery disease have less mortality with **CABG** than with medical therapy. No survival benefit was noted in patients with one- or two-vessel disease unless there was two-vessel disease with significant proximal LAD disease.

Several studies have compared surgery with **angioplasty** in patients with multivessel disease (ERACI, RITA, EAST, BARI, GABI Trials). Death or nonfatal myocardial infarctions were no different in the two groups after 5 years, but the rate of repeat revascularization was greater for the angioplasty group and, after the first year, angina was more frequent in the angioplasty group. A sub-group with diabetes did better with CABG. Stents were not used in these studies.

The use of **intracoronary stents** reduces the restenosis rate compared to percutaneous transluminal coronary angioplasty (PTCA) by one quarter to one third, and may show, in the future, better results than surgery for multi-vessel disease. In addition, restenosis has been reduced with the use of clopidogrel (Plavix) and abciximab (Reopro) administered with PTCA and stents. Patients with single-vessel disease and suitable lesions should be considered for PTCA with stenting if the thallium stress test shows a large area of decreased perfusion with good redistribution or a decrease in left ventricular function either at rest or with stress.

Most of the studies comparing CABG with medical therapy, or CABG with angioplasty, or medical therapy with angioplasty, were done prior to stents and drugs such as the GP IIb/IIIa inhibitors being available. In addition, medical therapy has advanced especially since the introduction of the statin drugs that lower cholesterol, LDL, and triglycerides, increase HDL, and stabilize plaques. In fact, the AVERT trial compared **atorvastatin** to angioplasty in patients with stable coronary artery disease with single or double-vessel disease and preserved left ventricular function. Atorvastatin subjects had less angina, reduction in nonfatal myocardial infarction, less revascularization, and shorter hospitalization compared to angioplasty. In the study, 80 mg of atorvastatin was administered. This AVERT trial supports an extremely aggressive approach to cholesterol lowering in patients with established coronary artery disease.

The HIT trial with **gemfibrozil**, with a follow-up of 7 years, showed a significant decrease in coronary artery disease death and nonfatal infarction compared to placebo. Aggressive medical therapy in the future may change the natural history of coronary artery disease and reduce the need for CABG and noninvasive interventions.

Some patients with persistent chronic stable angina who have not been helped by aggressive medical therapy are not considered for revascularization procedures. Transmyocardial laser revascularization, enhanced external counter pulsation, and spinal cord stimulation warrant consideration in such cases. Each of these claim benefits, but also limitations.

The present patient demonstrated significant ST depression during exercise (EKG, previous page). He had a 95% proximal LAD lesion that showed a large area of decreased perfusion involving the lateral wall and septum, with good redistribution by nuclear stress test. The vessel was stented with good results, and aggressive risk factor management was begun. A statin drug was given for the lipid abnormality, and he was advised to stop smoking. Six months later, a repeat thallium test was normal.

Clinical Pearls

1. Patients with stable angina should have a thallium-Sestimibi or echocardiographic stress test. If extensive ischemia or left ventricular dysfunction is present, perform coronary arteriography.

2. Those with one-vessel, two-vessel, or three-vessel disease should be individualized for medical therapy, PTCA, stents, surgery, or combinations depending on the severity of symptoms, coronary artery pathology, extent of ischemic, and left ventricular function.

3. Patients with three-vessel disease and decreased left ventricular ejection fraction or left main disease should receive CABG.

REFERENCES

1. Serruys PW, de Jaegere P, Kiemeneij F, et al.: A comparison of balloon-expandable-stent implantation with balloon angioplasty in patients with coronary artery disease. Benestent Study Group. N Engl J Med 1994;331:489–495.
2. Gutstein DE, Fuster V: Management of stable coronary artery disease. Am Fam Phys 1997;56:99–106.
3. ACC/AHA Guidelines for Coronary Angiography: Executive Summary and Recommendations. A report of the American College of Cardiology/American Heart Association Task Force on Practice Guidelines. Circulation 1999;99:2345–2357.
4. Whitlow PL, Dimas AP, Bashore TM, et al.: Relationship of extent of revascularization with angina at one year in the Bypass Angioplasty Revascularization Investigation (BARI). J Am Col Cardiol 1999;34:1744–1749.

Jean L. Holley, MD

PATIENT 3

A 62 year-old man with diabetic nephropathy on hemodialysis with questions about vaccinations

A 62 year-old man with diabetes mellitus for 12 years recently started hemodialysis. Despite the repeated efforts of his internist and nephrologist, he had been reluctant to accept the inevitability of his kidney failure and would participate in recommended pre-dialysis medical care only to a limited degree. He had undergone placement of an arteriovenous fistula 4 months before the initiation of hemodialysis, but he had refused to begin pre-dialysis recombinant human erythropoietin or to undergo the recommended series of hepatitis B vaccination. He is now resigned to the fact that his kidneys have failed, is tolerating hemodialysis without difficulty, and is in the process of completing his medical evaluation to be listed for a cadaveric renal transplant. He has no allergies.

Physical Examination: Vital signs normal. General: well-appearing. HEENT, Cardiac, Chest, Abdomen: unremarkable. Extremities: left forearm fistula with good thrill and bruit; trace pretibial edema bilaterally.

Laboratory Findings: BUN 72 mg/dl, creatinine 10.3 mg/dl. Hepatitis B surface antigen and antibody: negative. Transplant evaluation: positive varicella antibody.

Question: What vaccinations do you recommend for this gentleman?

Answer: This patient should be given the influenza vaccine and also started on the hepatitis B vaccine series.

Discussion: When planning the appropriate immunization strategy for patients with end-stage renal disease, consider the likelihood of reduced antibody response, the risk of contracting illnesses that are potentially preventable through immunization, and the patient's candidacy as a renal transplant recipient. For unclear reasons, patients with renal failure often are relatively immune suppressed. Evidence for this includes the reduced antibody response to vaccination occurring in end-stage renal failure patients.

Only 50–60% of dialysis patients who receive hepatitis B vaccine produce protective antibodies. Moreover, the hepatitis B surface antibody titres achieved are lower and the duration of the immunity is shorter in dialysis patients compared with healthy controls. Efforts to improve the antibody response to hepatitis B vaccination in dialysis patients include increasing the vaccine dose (40 μg vs. the usual 20 μg dose in non-renal failure patients) and the number of doses given (4 vs the standard three). The route of administration (intradermal vs. intramuscular) also is a factor.

Although the overall incidence of hepatitis B infection is low, outbreaks in hemodialysis units have occurred. A recent study showed that the risk of hepatitis B infection was 70% lower among hemodialysis patients who had been vaccinated. Thus, the recommendation continues to be that all dialysis patients receive the hepatitis B vaccination series. Since this patient has not received the vaccine and is neither surface antigen or antibody positive, he should be vaccinated (Engerix 40 μg IM at 0, 1, 2, and 6 months or Heptavax 40 μg IM at 0, 1, and 6 months). Antibody titre should be checked 1 month after the last dose, and if he remains antibody negative, one additional booster dose may be given.

Some suggest that the degree of renal failure influences the antibody response to vaccination. Therefore, patients with early renal failure who are likely to progress to end-stage renal disease should undergo the vaccination series once it is determined that chronic renal failure is present.

As with hepatitis B vaccine, reduced antibody response and duration also are likely with other vaccines given to dialysis patients. However, additional vaccines that should be given to dialysis patients are yearly influenza, and tetanus and pneumovax per the usual adult protocol. Patients who are awaiting renal transplantation probably also should receive the varicella vaccine if varicella antibody is not present. Like dialysis patients, patients with functioning renal transplants are more likely to exhibit reduced response to vaccines, but such patients should also receive the influenza, tetanus, pneumococcal, diphtheria, and hepatitis B vaccines. Live vaccines should *not* be given to transplant recipients, because their immunosuppressed state may predispose them to infection from injected virus.

The present patient was offered the hepatitis B vaccine series, pneumococcal vaccine (because he had not received it in the previous 5 years), tetanus toxoid per routine care, and the influenza vaccine.

Clinical Pearls

1. Patients with renal failure exhibit reduced peak and duration of antibody response to vaccines; generally only 50-70% of dialysis patients will develop antibodies after vaccination.

2. An improved antibody response may be seen in the early stages of renal failure so it is useful to initiate vaccination protocols as soon as chronic renal failure is diagnosed rather than waiting until the patient is on dialysis.

3. All patients with renal failure should receive hepatitis B, pneumococcal, and yearly influenza vaccines in the absence of a specific contraindication.

4. Patients who have a functional renal transplant should also receive routine vaccinations but live vaccines should not be given to transplanted patients.

REFERENCES

1. Stevens CE, Alter HJ, Taylor PE, et al.: Hepatitis B vaccine in patients receiving hemodialysis: Immunogenicity and efficacy. N Engl J Med 1984;311:496–501.
2. Rodby RA, Trenholme GM: Vaccination of the dialysis patient. Semin Dial 1991;4:102–105.
3. Dukes CS, Street AC, Starling JF, Hamilton JD: Hepatitis B vaccination and booster in predialysis patients: A 4-year analysis. Vaccine 1993;11:1229–1232.
4. Girndt M, Pietsch M, Kohler H: Tetanus immunization and its association to hepatitis B vaccination in patients with chronic renal failure. Am J Kidney Dis 1995;26:454–460.
5. Favero MS, Alter MJ: The reemergence of hepatitis B virus infection in hemodialysis centers. Semin Dial 1996;9:373–374.
6. Fuchshuber A, Kuhnemund O, Keuth B, et al: Pneumococcal vaccine in children and young adults with chronic renal disease. Nephrol Dial Transpl 1996;11:468–473.
7. Huzly D, Neifer S. Reinke P, et al.: Routine immunizations in adult renal transplant recipients. Transpl 1997;63:839–845.
8. Propst T, Propst A, Lhotta K, et al: Reinforced intradermal hepatitis B vaccination in hemodialysis patients is superior in antibody response to intramuscular or subcutaneous vaccination. Am J Kidney Dis 1998;32:1041–1045.
9. Miller ER, Alter MJ, Tokars JI: Protective effect of hepatitis B vaccine in chronic hemodialysis patients. Am J Kidney Dis 1999;33:356–360.

R. Parker Ward, MD
Roberto M. Lang, MD

PATIENT 4

A 32-year-old woman with post-partum dyspnea

A 32-year-old African-American woman is admitted with dyspnea and bilateral lower extremity swelling 2 weeks after vaginal delivery of her third child. All three of her pregnancies were uncomplicated and resulted in full-term, healthy children. She denies chest pain, fever, or recent viral illness, and has no history of hypertension, or alcohol or drug use.

Physical Examination: Vital signs: afebrile, BP 105/60 mm/Hg, pulse 120, RR 32. General: mildly obese; moderate respiratory distress. Neck: JVP to 10 cm. Chest: rales to mid lung field bilaterally. Cardiac: tachycardia with regular rhythm, diffuse laterally displaced PMI, II/VI holosystolic murmur at apex, S3 gallop. Extremities: 2+ pitting edema to knee. Neurological: normal.

Laboratory Findings: CBC and chemistries: normal. Chest x-ray: bilateral alveolar infiltrates. EKG: sinus tachycardia, nonspecific T-wave flattening in the lateral leads. Echocardiogram: see below.

Question: What is the likely diagnosis?

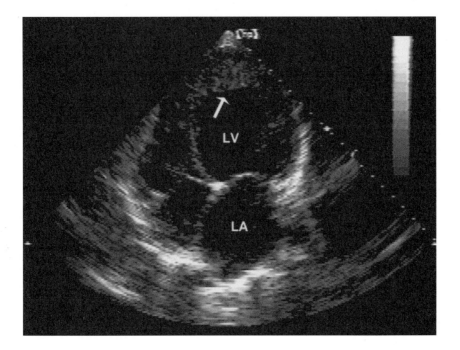

Diagnosis: Peripartum cardiomyopathy with left ventricular apical thrombus.

Discussion: Peripartum cardiomyopathy (PPCM) is a rare form of dilated cardiomyopathy of unclear etiology that affects women in their reproductive years. The diagnosis should be considered in patients with: (**1**) cardiac failure at any time during pregnancy or within 6 months of delivery, (**2**) evidence of impaired left ventricular systolic function on echocardiogram, and (**3**) absence of prior heart disease or a determinable cause for cardiac failure. Although the majority of patients with PPCM are diagnosed in the last antepartal or the first postpartal month, the diagnosis has been reported as early as the third gestational month, and many cases are reported in the second and third trimester. Diagnosis can be complicated by a number of conditions that mimic clinical systolic heart failure (e.g., diastolic left ventricular dysfunction, infections, pulmonary or amniotic fluid embolus) or other causes of left ventricular dysfunction that become clinically manifest with the increasing hemodynamic burden imposed by pregnancy. Therefore, cardiomyopathies due to infections, toxins, metabolic disorders, or ischemic or valvular disease must be carefully excluded.

The incidence of PPCM has been estimated between 1:1300 and 1:15,000 live births in the U.S. In regions of Africa, the incidence has been reported as high as 1:100, though many of these cases may represent pure volume overload caused by the tradition of ingesting a dried lake salt in the postpartum period.

Although PPCM is most common in **multiparous women of African descent**, it has been documented in primiparous women and women of Caucasian and Asian heritage. Other reported risk factors include advance age, preeclampsia/eclampsia, maternal cocaine abuse, selenium deficiency, and long-term (>4 weeks) oral tocolytic therapy.

The etiology of PPCM is unknown. Many potential etiologies have been investigated and remain unproven. Myocarditis has been suggested as a mechanism, but the most recent studies report a low incidence of myocarditis in PPCM. Trials of immunosuppressive agents have shown no benefit. Endomyocardial biopsy in patients with PPCM are no longer routinely performed because of the failure to yield diagnostic or clinically useful information.

Patients presenting with PPCM most commonly complain of **dyspnea**, but also may report cough orthopnea, paroxysmal nocturnal dyspnea, palpitations, hemoptysis, and lower extremity edema. The physical exam generally reveals the typical **findings of congestive heart failure**, including cardiomegaly, tachycardia, third heart sound, pulmonary rales, elevated jugular veins and peripheral edema.

The EKG usually demonstrates **sinus tachycardia**. Nonspecific ST-T wave changes, anteroseptal Q waves, and conduction defects also may be found. Chest radiograms invariably reveal cardiomegaly often with pulmonary congestion and small bilateral pleural effusions. As seen in the present patient, the echocardiogram (see figure) reveals a dilated left ventricle, marked impairment of systolic function, and right ventricular and bi-atrial enlargement. Dilated cardiac chambers and decreased systolic function, along with the hypercoagulable state of the peripartum period, predispose patients to atrial or ventricular thrombi. A large apical left ventricular thrombus is demonstrated in the present patient (*arrow*).

The treatment of PPCM is similar to that for other forms of dilated cardiomyopathy. Thus, diuretics, digoxin, afterload-reducing agents, and salt restriction are the mainstays of treatment. The timing of this condition in the peripartum period does raise the additional concerns of using medicines that may have adverse consequences to the fetus. Digoxin and diuretics generally are considered safe for use in pregnancy and mothers who are breastfeeding, although rare adverse effects have been reported. Ace inhibitors are contraindicated in pregnancy due to a high incidence of complications, including severe adverse neonatal renal effects and increased neonatal mortality. Hydralazine has proven to be safe in pregnancy after decades of use for treatment of gestational hypertension; it is the vasodilator of choice in PPCM. Warfarin is contraindicated in pregnancy, but is not secreted in breast milk. Use heparin for anticoagulation prior to delivery.

The prognosis for patients with PPCM is variable. Mortality estimates in the U.S. have been as high as 25–48%, with the majority of deaths due to progressive pump failure, arrhythmia, or thromboembolic complications. In contrast, approximately 50% of patients have marked improvement in clinical symptoms and left ventricular function, with recovery generally complete within 6 months of the diagnosis. Cardiac transplantation has been performed with favorable outcome and should be strongly considered for patients with persistent severe left ventricular dysfunction more than 6 months after diagnosis.

Patients with PPCM with or without persistent left ventricular dysfunction are at high risk for further complications or recurrence should they become pregnant again. Therefore, strongly discourage subsequent pregnancies.

The present patient received 6 months of treatment with standard heart failure therapy and warfarin.

She is doing well, with minimal symptoms despite an active lifestyle. A repeat echocardiogram revealed resolution of the thrombus and improved left ventricular function.

Clinical Pearls

1. Consider the diagnosis of PPCM in patients with: (1) cardiac failure at any time during pregnancy or within 6 months of delivery, (2) evidence of impaired left ventricular systolic function on echocardiogram, and (3) absence of prior heart disease or a determinable cause for cardiac failure.

2. Peripartum cardiomyopathy has a high early mortality, but approximately 50% of patients demonstrate significant improvement occurring in the first 6 months after diagnosis.

3. Patients with PPCM are at high risk for recurrence with subsequent pregnancies.

REFERENCES

1. Lang RM, Borow KM: Medical disorders during pregnancy. In Barron WM, Lindheimer MD (eds): Heart Disease. St. Louis, Mosby-Year Book, 1991,pp 184–188.
2. Rickenbacher PR, Rizeq MN, Hunt SA, et al: Long-term outcome after heart transplantation for peripartum cardiomyopathy. Am Heart J 127(5):1318–1323, 1994.
3. Lampert MB, Lang RM: Peripartum cardiomyopathy. Am Heart J 130:860–870, 1995.
4. Lang RM, Lampert MB, Poppas A, et al: Peripartal cardiomyopathy. Cardiac Problems in Pregnancy 87–100, 1998.
5. Hibbard, JU, Lindheimer, M., and Lang, RM: A modified definition for peripartum cardiomyopathy and prognosis based on echocardiography. Obstet Gynecol 94:311–316, 1999.

Marvin I. Schwarz, MD

PATIENT 5

A 35-year-old man with fatigue, mild cough, and severe dyspnea

A 35-year-old previously healthy man reports fatigue and mild, nonproductive cough of 2-week duration. Three days before admission he noted progressive and eventually severe dyspnea. Review of symptoms, not including myalgias, is negative. He has smoked for 20 pack years, is taking no prescribed or illicit drugs, and denies HIV risk factors.

Physical Examination: Vital signs: afebrile, BP 136/90 mm Hg, pulse 110 beats/min, respiratory rate 32 breaths/min. Pulse oximetry (6 L/min O_2 nasal cannula): 87%. Extremities: petechiae and several pupuric areas. Ophthalmologic: normal; sclera clear. Chest: diffuse crackles without wheezing. Cardiac: tachycardia and a grade II/IV systolic flow murmur. Abdomen: normal.

Laboratory Examination: WBC: 10,500/μl, hematocrit 31%, platelets 256,000/μl, ESR 85 mm/hr. Serum electrolytes, creatinine, and glucose: normal. Prothrombin time and partial thromboplastin time: normal. Urinalysis: 3+ protein, red blood cells, and several red blood cell casts. Chest x-ray: diffuse and patchy alveolar infiltrates without cardiomegaly, septal lines, or pleural effusion.

Clinical Course: Within 3 hours after admission, his respiratory status worsened. He was admitted to the ICU, intubated, and ventilated.

Question: What procedure should be performed to establish the nature of the pulmonary infiltrates?

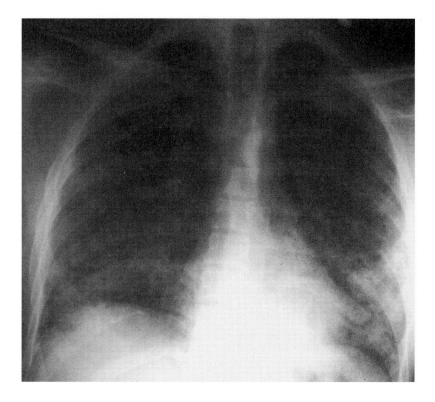

Answer: Bronchoalveolar lavage.

Discussion: This patient has a pulmonary renal syndrome secondary to a systemic vasculitis known as microscopic polyangiitis (MPA). This is a small-vessel variant of periarteritis nodosa. The underlying lung disease is diffuse alveolar hemorrhage (DAH), resulting from a small-vessel vasculitis of the lung referred to as pulmonary capillaritis. The clues to systemic vasculitis in this patient are the **petechiae and purpura** due to a dermatologic leukocytoclastic vasculitis, the **elevated sedimentation rate**, and the abnormal urinalysis indicating **red blood cell casts**. The renal disease common to all systemic vasculitis syndromes and collagen vascular diseases, as well as Goodpasture's syndrome, is a focal segmental necrotizing glomerulonephritis. This is a rapidly progressive form of glomerulonephritis.

Approximately 25–33% of of patients with DAH regardless of etiology do not report hemoptysis. As a general rule, unexplained pulmonary infiltrates in the face of a low and/or falling hematocrit should raise the suspicion of underlying DAH. The indicated procedure for this patient is bronchoalveolar lavage, in which sequential aliquots are likely to show persistent and often more intense hemorrhagic return. DAH in this patient is due to pulmonary capillaritis, and lung biopsy is not necessarily indicated. Note, however, that other systemic vasculitis syndromes (e.g., Wegener's granulomatosis, Henoch-Schönlein purpura, Behçet's syndrome, IgA nephropathy, and cryoblobulinemia); collagen vascular diseases (systemic lupus erythematosis [SLE], rheumatoid arthritis [RA], scleroderma, and mixed connective tissue disease [MCTD]); and some cases of Goodpasture's syndrome and drug-induced hypersensitivity vasculitis (e.g., due to propylthiouracil, diphenylhydantoin, or pencillamine) may have an identical clinical-radiographic-pathologic presentation.

Distinction between the aforementioned entities usually is accomplished by history and serologic testing. In the present patient, an antibody (p-ANCA) directed against neutrophil cytoplasmic myeloperoxidase was found in the serum; it is diagnostic of MPA. As in the other systemic vasculitides, there may be nonspecific increases in serum rheumatoid factors and antinuclear antibodies. In Wegener's granulomatosis, 5–10% of patients initially present with DAH and underlying pulmonary capillaritis, glomerulonephritis, and possibly other signs of a systemic vasculitis (i.e., eye, skin, upper respiratory tract, and joint involvement), as opposed to the typical necrotizing granulomatous vasculitis of small- and medium-sized vessels, which results in cavitating lung masses. An antibody to a neutrophil cytoplasmic serine protease, proteinase 3 or c-ANC,

present in the serum establishes the diagnosis of the pulmonary-renal syndrome in Wegener's granulomatosis. Henoch-Schönlein purpura is an uncommon vasculitis cause of the pulmonary-renal syndrome in adults. The presence of IgA circulating and/or tissue bound immune complexes establishes the diagnosis. The same is true for IgA nephropathy, which is the most common cause of glomerulonephritis, but is rarely associated with DAH. Cryoglobulinemia, often associated with evidence of prior hepatitis B and C infection, is identified by the demonstration of serum cryoglobulins. DAH also is uncommon in this condition.

A pulmonary-renal syndrome often complicates a collagen vascular disease, particularly SLE. The pathology in the lungs, kidney, skin, and other organs is identical to that seen in systemic vasculitis. The major difference is that MPA and Wegener's granulomatosis are pauci-immune (no tissue-bound immune complexes), and the collagen vascular disease often exhibits evidence of immune complex disposition. In 90% of patients with DAH and SLE, it occurs in an established case, and almost all have accompanying glomerulonephritis. In SLE patients presenting with a pulmonary-renal syndrome as the initial disease event, serum antinuclear factors, antibodies against double-stranded DNA, and low serum complement are helpful in establishing the diagnosis. With other forms of collagen vascular disease (e.g., RA, MCTD, scleroderma), a pulmonary-renal syndrome is an unusual complication and always occurs in an established case.

Goodpasture's syndrome, a disease more common in young men, is another important cause of the pulmonary renal syndrome. It usually presents with the simultaneous onset of lung and renal disease (60–80%), but can present with just DAH (5–10%) or glomerulonephritis (30%, particularly in older individuals). In smokers with Goodpasture's syndrome there is an 100% incidence of DAH; in non-smokers, 20%. The presence of a dermatologic leucocytoclastic vasculitis makes this diagnosis unlikely in the present patient. As opposed to the other causes of pulmonary-renal syndrome, only the lung and kidney are involved. Goodpasture's syndrome is thought to be caused by the development of an antibody to type 4 collagen, the principle collagen of basement membranes. This antibody (antibasement membrane antibody) can be detected in the serum or demonstrated in tissue as an interrupted immunofluorescence linear deposit when stained with antibodies to IgG or complement.

Occasionally, DAH is an isolated finding and not a component of a systemic disease. Unless the

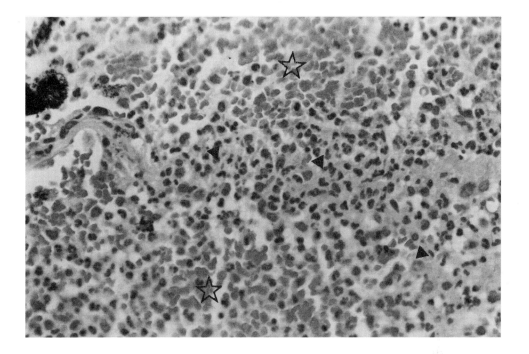

cause is apparent, thoracoscopic open lung biopsy is recommended. There are instances of Goodpasture's syndrome without renal disease both with and without pulmonary capillaritis. Immunoflourescent studies of the lungs can establish the diagnosis. There are reports of isolated DAH due to capillaritis in RA and MCTD. Patients with the primary antiphospholipid syndrome, in addition to thrombotic complications, can develop isolated DAH due to capillaritis.

In isolated forms of pulmonary capillaritis causing DAH, all serologic studies are negative. In one series, this isolated small-vessel vasculitis of the lung was the most common cause of DAH. Pulmonary capillaritis and also DAH occur in patients who have received allogeneic lungs transplants.

DAH also can be bland (no capillaritis or inflammation). This occasionally occurs in SLE and Goodpasture's syndrome. Any problem with clotting, either due to anticoagulation or thrombocytopenic states, can result in DAH. Crack cocaine inhalation

can result in DAH. Patients with previously unrecognized mitral stenosis can first present with DAH.

For most pulmonary-renal syndromes, treatment consists of a corticosteroid preparation and cyclophosphamide. In patients with Goodpasture's syndrome, plasmapheresis also is recommended. An important point is to initiate treatment as soon as possible, since progression to irreversible renal failure can occur rapidly. The lung disease is much more responsive to therapy, even with severe respiratory failure.

In the present patient, bronchoalveolar lavage revealed, pulmonary capillaritis and DAH (H and E × 40) (see figure above). Red blood cells and some neutrophils fill the alveolar spaces (*stars*). The alveolar wall (interstititium) is broadened due to edema, fibrin deposition, and fibrinoid necrosis (*triangles*). The predominant cell type infiltrating the alveolar wall is neutrophils, many of which are fragmented (leucocytoclasis). The darker-staining nuclei are pyknotic (apoptotic).

Clinical Pearls

1. Diffuse alveolar hemorrhage can exist without hemoptysis. Diffuse chest radiographic infiltrates, a falling hematocrit, and hemorrhagic bronchoalveolar lavage establish the diagnosis of DAH.

2. Rapid diagnosis and institution of therapy are mandated in the pulmonary-renal syndromes because of the potential for irreversible or only partially reversible renal disease due to the rapidly progressive glomerulonephritis.

3. In a patient with pulmonary-renal syndrome, but with other systemic manifestations, perform tissue biopsy (lung or kidney) with routine histology and immunofluorescent staining.

REFERENCES

1. Leatherman JW, Davies SF, Hoidal JR: Alveolar hemorrhage syndromes: Diffuse microvascular lung hemorrhage in immune and idiopathic disorders. Medicine 1984;63:343–361.
2. Savage COS, Winearls CG, Evans DV, et al: Microscopic polyarteritis: Presentation, pathology, and prognosis. A J Med 1985; 56:467–483.
3. Hudson BG, Wieslander J, Widsom BJ, Woelken ME: Goodpasture's syndrome: Molecular architecture and function of basement membrane antibody. Lab Invest 1989;61:256–269.
4. Travis WD, Colby TV, Lombard C, Carpenter HA: A clinicopathologic study of 34 cases of diffuse pulmonary hemorrhage with lung biopsy conformation. Am J Surg 1990;14:1112–1125.
5. Goeken JA: Antineutrophil cytoplasmic antibody: A useful serologic marker for vasculitis. J Clin Immunol 1991;2:161–174.
6. Savige JA, Gallicchio M, Change L, Parkin JD: Autoantibodies in systemic vasculitis. Aust N Z J Med 1991;21:433–437.
7. Travis WD, Hoffman GS, Leavitt RV, et al: Surgical pathology of the lung in Wegener's granulomatosis: A review of 87 open lung biopsies from 67 patients. Am J Surg Pathol 1991;15:315–333.
8. Kelly PT, Haponik EF: Goodpasture's syndrome: Molecular and clinical advances. Medicine 1994;73:171–185.
9. Jennings CA, King TE Jr, Tuder R, et al: Diffuse alveolar hemorrhage with underlying isolated pauci-immune pulmonary capillaritis. Am J Respir Crit Care Med 1997;155:1101–1109.
10. Zamora MR, Warner ML, Tuder R, Schwarz MI: Diffuse alveolar hemorrhage and systemic lupus erythematosus: Clinical presentation, histology, survival, and outcome. Medicine 1997;76:192–202.
11. Schwarz MI: Diffuse alveolar hemorrhage. In Schwarz MI, King TE (eds): Interstitial Lung Disease, 3rd ed. BC Decker, Hamilton, pp 535–558.

Elbert P. Trulock, MD

PATIENT 6

A 32-year-old woman with cough and declining lung function after lung transplantation

A 32-year-old woman with cystic fibrosis underwent bilateral lung transplantation for end-stage bronchiectasis 5 months ago. She now presents with a 1-week history of a nonproductive cough. She denies fever and dyspnea, but her exercise tolerance has been below par for a few days.

Both the patient and her organ donor were seropositive for cytomegalovirus (CMV) before transplantation. The immediate postoperative course was uncomplicated except for *Pseudomonas aeruginosa* bronchitis that responded well to antibiotic treatment, and the patient was discharged 12 days after surgery. She had recuperated without major problems, except for an episode of CMV viremia 7 weeks after transplantation that resolved with ganciclovir therapy. The maintenance immunosuppressive drug regimen included cyclosporine, azathioprine, and prednisone. Other maintenance medications were trimethoprim-sulfamethoxazole, acyclovir, and famotidine.

Physical Examination: Temperature 37.3° C; pulse 94; respirations 12; blood pressure 106/74 mmHg. General appearance: nontoxic; no respiratory distress. HEENT: unremarkable. Chest: scattered crackles at both bases. Cardiac: regular rhythm; no murmur or rub. Abdomen: nontender; liver and spleen not palpable. Extremities: trace symmetrical ankle edema.

Laboratory Findings: Hgb 9.8 g/dl; WBC 3800/μl. Chest radiograph: unchanged from baseline post-transplantation study, with blunting of the right costophrenic angle and focal, linear scar versus atelectasis at left base. Spirometry: FVC 2.52 L (77%), FEV$_1$ 2.18 L (78%); one month earlier FVC 2.63 L, FEV$_1$ 2.42 L.

Hospital Course: The patient underwent fiberoptic bronchoscopy with transbronchial biopsy. Tissue sample: hematoxyllin-eosin stain, magnification 50× (see below).

Question: What is the best management strategy in this situation?

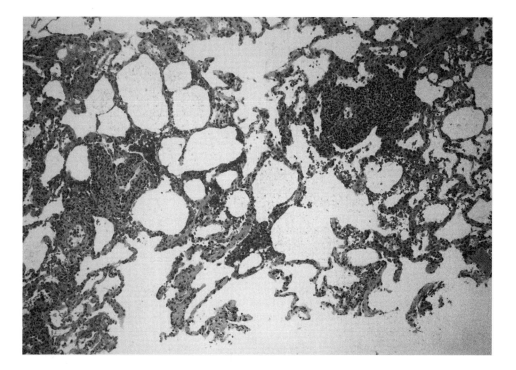

Answer: A 3-day course of methylprednisolone, with follow-up biopsy 3–6 weeks later.

Discussion: Rejection is the alloimmune response to a transplanted organ. When rejection occurs after a transplanted solid organ, it is classified as acute or chronic. **Acute rejection** is common in the first 6–12 months after lung transplantation, regardless of the immunosuppressive protocol used. Fortunately, it usually responds to adjustments of the immunosuppressive regimen and is rarely fatal. Acute rejection of transplanted lungs is characterized by **lymphocytic inflammation** around arterioles, although bronchioles also may be affected (see figure).

Chronic rejection, which also is termed **bronchiolitis obliterans syndrome**, affects 50% of patients by the third year after lung transplantation. It is characterized by airway inflammation and fibrosis. Unlike acute rejection, chronic rejection does not respond well to any treatment modality. Patients usually experience progressive airflow limitation and deterioration in lung function. Chronic rejection is the primary source of morbidity and mortality beyond the first year after transplantation.

Acute rejection produces nonspecific clinical manifestations. Episodes of mild acute rejection may be asymptomatic, but most patients experience symptoms suggestive of bronchitis, such as cough, dyspnea, and low-grade fever. The chest examination demonstrates crackles. The chest radiograph usually is normal or unchanged from baseline when acute rejection occurs after the first post-transplantation month. When abnormal, chest radiographs typically demonstrate interstitial infiltrates.

Monitoring **spirometric parameters** is an important approach for detecting acute rejection. Most patients without complications experience a stabilization of their spirometric values during the first 3 to 6 months after lung transplantation. Spirometric values usually normalize after bilateral lung transplantation. After unilateral transplantations, pulmonary function improves, but does not normalize because of functional abnormalities of the remaining native lung. Once lung function stabilizes, test results are reproducible with a small coefficient of variation for FVC and FEV_1. A decrement of 15% or more during the first post-transplantation year and 10% or more thereafter signifies that significant respiratory deterioration has occurred compatible with acute rejection. Unfortunately, spirometric abnormalities are not specific for rejection.

Because clinical, radiographic, and physiologic findings do not differentiate rejection from infection or other respiratory disorders, transbronchial biopsy is the preferred approach for evaluating patients for acute rejection. Transbronchial biopsy yields a specific diagnosis in 60–70% of patients when acute rejection or infection are suspected. The Lung Rejection Study Group recommends obtaining at least five pieces of lung parenchyma that contain alveolated specimens, which have a sensitivity of 70–90% in patients with acute rejection.

Bronchoalveolar lavage (BAL) is a useful adjunct to transbronchial biopsy for the diagnosis of infection. Analysis of BAL cell counts and lymphocyte subsets, however, does not distinguish rejection from infection.

Cytomegalovirus pneumonitis is the primary alternative diagnosis in patients with suspected acute rejection. The prevalence of CMV infection is high during the first year after lung transplantation. The clinical spectrum of CMV infection ranges from a mild viral syndrome with constitutional symptoms to overt disease, which includes pneumonia, hepatitis, and gastroenteritis. Chest radiographic abnormalities of CMV pneumonia may be subtle or absent, but a diffuse interstitial infiltrate is the characteristic pattern. A positive blood test for CMV viremia confirms the presence of CMV pneumonitis, but does not exclude acute rejection because the two disorders can occur together. Also, a negative test does not exclude CMV infection because pneumonitis can develop before viremia becomes detectable.

The standard treatment for the first episode of acute rejection is a 3-day course of high-dose methylprednisolone (10–20 mg/kg IV qd). If the maintenance prednisone dosage has been tapered, it can be increased to 0.5–1.0 mg/kg/d with a gradual taper to the maintenance dose over 7 to 21 days. Other components of the maintenance immunosuppressive regimen should be optimized. A follow-up transbronchial biopsy should be considered 3 to 6 weeks after treatment to assess the effect of therapy.

Persistent or recurrent acute rejection mandates a change in the maintenance immunosuppressive drugs. Options include substituting tacrolimus for cyclosporine and/or mycophenolate mofetil for azathioprine. Acute rejection that is refractory to these approaches is rare, but should be treated aggressively with antilymphocyte antibody treatment (antilymphocyte globulin or OKT3 monoclonal antibody) or total lymphoid irradiation. Other antirejection drugs, such as sirolimus (rapamycin), are undergoing evaluation and will be integrated into the management of lung allograft rejection in the next few years.

In the present patient, the diagnosis of acute rejection was made by transbronchial lung biopsy, which showed perivascular and parabronchiolar infiltration of lymphocytes. A 3-day course of methylprednisolone was given. The patient's cough resolved, and her lung function improved but did not return to baseline. A follow-up biopsy 3 weeks later showed less intense, but persistent rejection. Another course of methylprednisolone was prescribed, and her maintenance regimen was adjusted by replacing cyclosporine with tacrolimus. One month later, a transbronchial biopsy specimen showed no residual rejection.

Clinical Pearls

1. Acute rejection is common during the first year after lung transplantation, regardless of the immunosuppressive drug regimen.

2. The signs and symptoms of acute rejection are nonspecific, and the clinical picture of acute rejection is difficult to distinguish from CMV pneumonia.

3. Documentation of CMV viremia does not exclude acute rejection because rejection and CMV pneumonitis can occur together.

4. Bronchoscopy with transbronchial lung biopsy is the best approach to suspected acute rejection or infection after lung transplantation.

REFERENCES

1. Tazelaar HD: Perivascular inflammation in pulmonary infections: Implications for the diagnosis of lung rejection. J Heart Lung Transplant 1991;10:437–441.
2. Guilinger RA, Paradis IL, Dauber JH, et al: The importance of bronchoscopy with transbronchial lung biopsy and bronchoalveolar lavage in the management of lung transplant recipients. Am J Respir Crit Care Med 1995;152:2037–2043.
3. Yousem SA, Berry GJ, Cagle PT, et al: Revision of the 1990 working formulation for the classification of pulmonary allograft rejection: Lung Rejection Study Group. J Heart Lung Transplant 1996;15:1–15.
4. Chaparro C, Kesten S: Infections in lung transplant recipients. Clin Chest Med 1997;18:339–351.
5. King-Biggs MB: Acute pulmonary allograft rejection. Mechanisms, diagnosis, and management. Clin Chest Med 1997; 18:301–310.
6. Trulock EP: State of the art: Lung transplantation. Am J Respir Crit Care Med 1997;155:789–818.
7. Trulock EP: Flexible bronchoscopy in lung transplantation. Clin Chest Med 1999;20:77–87.

James N. George, MD
Kiarash Kojouri, MD

PATIENT 7

A 24-year-old woman with asymptomatic thrombocytopenia
at 38 weeks of pregnancy

A 24-year-old woman previously in good health is evaluated at a routine prenatal visit during the 38th week of her first pregnancy. The pregnancy has been uncomplicated, and she has no complaints. Review of systems demonstrates no neurologic abnormalities and, specifically, no visual symptoms.

Physical Examination: Temperature, pulse, and respirations normal; blood pressure 112/72. Remainder of physical examination: normal. Fetal movement and heart tones: normal. Extremities: no peripheral edema.

Laboratory Findings: Hemoglobin 11.2 g/dl, WBC normal, platelets 74,000/µl. Urinalysis: normal, without albuminuria. Serum creatinine: 0.5 mg/dl. Previous platelet counts: reviewed in her medical record (see below).

Question: What is the etiology of the thrombocytopenia? How will it impact management of the delivery and the health of the newborn infant?

Platelet Counts

Date	Clinical Setting	Platelet Count
November 1992	Appendectomy	126,000/µl
October 1999	Initial prenatal visit, 10 weeks' gestation	152,000/µl
May 2000	Current visit, 38 weeks' gestation	74,000/µl

Diagnosis: Idiopathic (immune) thrombocytopenic purpura (ITP).

Discussion: Mild thrombocytopenia occurs commonly near term during normal pregnancies. The principal diagnostic considerations include **ITP** and **gestational thrombocytopenia**, also known as incidental thrombocytopenia of pregnancy. Preeclampsia and disseminated intravascular coagulation (DIC) due to fetal demise are additional possible diagnoses.

Gestational thrombocytopenia represents the most common cause of thrombocytopenia late in the third trimester of normal pregnancy. It is defined by the presence of: (**1**) asymptomatic, mild thrombocytopenia, with a platelet count typically > 70,000/μl, (**2**) onset in late gestation, (**3**) absence of a history of thrombocytopenia (except possibly during a previous pregnancy), (**4**) the absence of fetal thrombocytopenia, and (**5**) spontaneous resolution after delivery. Gestational thrombocytopenia is estimated to occur in 5% of normal pregnancies and is not associated with maternal or neonatal morbidity.

The etiology of gestational thrombocytopenia is unknown, but it may represent a mild form of ITP. In support of this concept, it cannot be distinguished from ITP with anti-platelet antibody tests, which are abnormal in both conditions. Also, ITP, as well as other autoimmune disorders such as autoimmune hemolytic anemia, often exacerbate near the end of pregnancy, with remission following delivery.

Preeclampsia is another common obstetrical disorder that is associated with thrombocytopenia. Occurring in approximately 10% of women near term during their first pregnancy, preeclampsia is associated with hypertension, proteinuria, and edema.

Gestational thrombocytopenia presents important considerations for the management of the mother and infant. Most patients have sufficient platelets, as demonstrated by the present patient, to promote normal hemostasis with a vaginal delivery or a caesarean section. The presence of even mild thrombocytopenia, however, may **alter plans for anesthesia**; a minimum platelet count of 100,000/μl is required for epidural anesthesia. Patients with thrombocytopenia can be managed with alternative anesthesia avoiding an epidural approach. Platelet transfusions or initiation of therapy with glucocorticoids or intravenous IgG to correct thrombocytopenia solely to allow epidural anesthesia is *not* warranted. Although the new observation of thrombocytopenia during pregnancy may be alarming, it is a common event and does not require more than routine obstetrical care in otherwise healthy women.

Fetuses of mothers with ITP are at risk for **intrauterine thrombocytopenia**, because antiplatelet antibodies cross the placenta. Even in women with severe and symptomatic thrombocytopenia, however, intrauterine fetal hemorrhage has never been reported. This contrasts with fetal alloimmune thrombocytopenia due to platelet alloantigen incompatibility; these infants are at risk for severe intrauterine hemorrhage.

It is estimated that 4% of infants born to mothers with ITP have **platelet counts** less than 20,000/μl after birth. Infants with this degree of thrombocytopenia are at risk for bleeding—the most critical manifestation is intracranial hemorrhage related to head trauma sustained during delivery. However, clinically important episodes of neonatal bleeding are rare, and elective cesarean section is not routinely indicated. Platelet counts in neonates correlate with the severity of maternal thrombocytopenia. Consequently, the infant born to the present patient, who had a platelet count of 74,000/μl, would be unlikely to have a clinically important degree of thrombocytopenia. Note, however, that splenic function is minimal at birth, but rapidly acquires its normal ability to destroy sensitized platelets. Therefore, it is important to monitor infants for several days following birth, because platelet counts may decrease substantially during this time in neonates born to mothers with ITP.

The present patient's course was most compatible with mild ITP. The key diagnostic information was the slightly low platelet count 8 years earlier after the patient had an appendectomy—a higher-than-normal platelet count is expected with any acute illness. This finding suggests ITP. Preeclampsia was excluded by the absence of hypertension and proteinuria, and DIC was not considered because the fetus was viable. The patient's platelet count improved several days after delivery. No further diagnostic studies were indicated, although the patient underwent periodic measurement of her platelet count during her routine medical care.

Clinical Pearls

1. Mild thrombocytopenia is common near term in normal pregnancies.
2. When thrombocytopenia is mild and there are no previous platelet counts, gestational thrombocytopenia cannot be distinguished from ITP, but neither diagnosis requires further diagnostic or treatment intervention.
3. The risk for thrombocytopenia in infants born to mothers with ITP is related to the severity of maternal thrombocytopenia.
4. Monitor platelet counts in newborn infants of mothers with ITP for several days after delivery, since their platelet count may fall as splenic function matures.

REFERENCES

1. Burrows RF, Kelton JG: Low fetal risks in pregnancies associated with idiopathic thrombocytopenic purpura. Am J Obstet Gynecol 1990;163:1147–1150.
2. Burrows RF, Kelton JG: Fetal thrombocytopenia and its relation to maternal thrombocytopenia. N Engl J Med 1993;329:1463–1466.
3. George JN, Woolf SH, Raskob GE, et al: Idiopathic thrombocytopenic purpura: A practice guideline developed by explicit methods for the American Society of Hematology. Blood 1996;88:3–40.
4. Lescale KB, Eddleman KA, Cines DB, et al: Antiplatelet antibody testing in thrombocytopenic pregnant women. Am J Obstet Gynecol 1996;174:1014-1018.
5. Valat AS, Caulier MT, Devos P, et al: Relationships between severe neonatal thrombocytopenia and maternal characteristics in pregnancies associated with autoimmune thrombocytopenia. Br J Haematol 1998;103:397–401.

Om P. Sharma, MD

PATIENT 8

A 57-year-old woman with sarcoidosis and intermittent nausea, vomiting, and diarrhea

A 57-year-old woman presents with a several-month history of intermittent nausea, vomiting, and diarrhea. Her health has been otherwise excellent recently, although she does report that 24 years earlier she experienced dyspnea, enlargement of both parotid glands, skin rash, and pulmonary opacities. At that time, transbronchial lung biopsy showed noncaseating granulomas, and special stains and cultures of bronchoscopic specimens were negative for acid fast bacilli and fungi. She was treated with prednisone for a diagnosis of sarcoidosis. The patient continued her prednisone until 12 years ago when her sarcoid symptoms remitted.

Physical Examination: Temperature 98.8°, pulse 76, respirations 14, blood pressure 160/90. General: no respiratory distress. HEENT: unremarkable, with normal parotid glands. Chest: clear. Cardiac: no murmurs, normal S1 and S2. Abdomen: no organomegaly.

Laboratory Findings: CBC, electrolytes, and renal indices: normal. Calcium: 10.5 mEq/L. Urinalysis: normal.

Clinical Course: Gastroscopy: erythematous, infiltrative plaques on the gastric mucosa (see figure, *top*). Biopsy of one of lesions: see figure, *bottom*.

Question: What is the etiology of the patient's symptoms? How should she be managed?

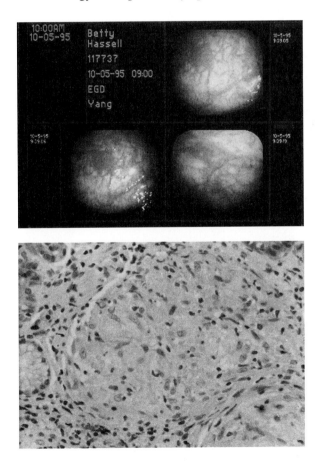

Diagnosis: Gastric sarcoidosis.

Discussion: Sarcoidosis is an idiopathic, multisystem disorder characterized by granulomatous inflammation. Although sarcoidosis most commonly involves the lungs, lymph nodes, liver, and spleen, any tissue can be affected. The stomach is a relatively uncommon site of involvement, although 10% of patients with sarcoidosis who undergo screening gastroscopy have evidence of granuloma formation in gastric mucosa. In most instances, gastric involvement is silent.

When symptoms of gastric involvement do occur in sarcoidosis, **epigastric pain** is the predominant manifestation. Pain occurs most often after eating and is described as dull, burning, or cramping in nature. Weight loss also occurs and can amount to 20–25 pounds within 2 to 3 months. Patients with pain and weight loss mimic the clinical presentation of gastric lymphoma. Nausea and vomiting due to gastric obstruction, impaired peristalsis, or gastrointestinal bleeding can be the initial clinical presentation, as in the present patient. Additional symptoms include heartburn, abdominal discomfort, and diarrhea.

The radiographic features of gastric sarcoidosis vary. Mucosal irregularities, nodular lesions, and indurated plaques with irregular borders resemble a gastric malignancy. Segmental linitis plastica, deformity of the pyloric antrum, and mucosal polyps also are observed.

The diagnosis of gastric sarcoidosis rests on biopsy demonstration of **noncaseating granulomas** in the gastric mucosa. Adequate tissue must be obtained to exclude alternative diagnoses, such as infiltrating carcinomas and lymphomas associated with nonspecific granulomatous tissue reactions. Crohn's disease, tuberculosis, fungal infections, syphilis, and foreign body granulomas may resemble the histologic appearance of sarcoidosis and require diagnostic evaluation in appropriate settings. In patients with isolated gastric sarcoidosis without multisystem involvement, the diagnosis is difficult to confirm. Such patients require close monitoring to exclude a clinically silent, alternative underlying diagnosis as the cause of the gastric granulomas.

Treatment of gastric sarcoidosis depends on the severity of symptoms and the extent of the granulomatous reaction in the gastric mucosa. Systemic **corticosteroids** are the treatment of choice. Some patients with mild manifestations of disease may benefit from antacids or metoclopramide. Hydroxychloroquine or methotrexate is indicated for patients who cannot tolerate prednisone or who have failed to respond to a corticosteroid trial.

The present patient's endoscopy demonstrated indurated, erythematous lesions on the gastric mucosa. Gastric biopsy specimens demonstrated granulomatous inflammation compatible with sarcoidosis. In view of the patient's history of sarcoidosis and the absence of clinical manifestations of another diagnosis, she was treated with corticosteroids for a diagnosis of gastric sarcoidosis. She did not tolerate prednisone, but responded to hydroxychloroquine with resolution of her symptoms.

Clinical Pearls

1. The presence of nausea, vomiting, anorexia, and weight loss in a patient with sarcoidosis suggests the diagnosis of gastric sarcoid.

2. Endoscopic biopsy of gastric mucosa is indicated to confirm the presence of granulomatous inflammation and exclude alternative diagnoses, such as gastric carcinoma, lymphoma, and tuberculosis.

3. The primary therapy for gastric sarcoidosis is corticosteroids. Patients who fail to respond to prednisone or develop intolerable corticosteroid reactions may respond to hydroxychloroquine or methotrexate.

REFERENCES:
1. Palmer ED: A note on silent sarcoidosis of stomach. J Lab Clin Med 1968;52:231–234.
2. Sharma A, Kadakia J, Sharma O. Gastrointestinal sarcoidosis. Sem Respir Med 1992;13:442–446.
3. American Thoracic Society/European Respiratory Society/World Association of Sarcoidosis and Other Granulomatous Disorders statement on sarcoidosis: Sarcoidosis, vasculitis, and diffuse lung diseases 1999;16: 149–173.

Gordon D. Rubenfeld, MD, MSc

PATIENT 9

A 67-year-old man with respiratory failure and a living will

A 67-year-old man is being maintained on mechanical ventilation for respiratory failure and aspiration pneumonia. He had been admitted after he fell during a 5-kilometer run and sustained an intertrochanteric fracture. The patient underwent surgical repair of his hip, but vomited and aspirated in the recovery room, which required intubation and mechanical ventilation. His subsequent course has been complicated by agitated delirium and an inferior myocardial infarction; during brief intervals the patient responds to voice commands, but otherwise requires heavy sedation. Now on the seventh day of hospitalization, the patient's wife and daughter request that mechanical ventilation be withdrawn, stating that the patient would not want prolonged life support. They bring in the patient's living will to demonstrate his previous wishes.

In a family meeting, the physicians state their belief that the patient has an excellent probability of experiencing a complete recovery, and they would like to maintain him on the ventilator with full support. The family refuses the physicians' request.

Question: What is the best course of action?

Diagnosis: Aspiration pneumonia with respiratory failure in a patient without neurologic injury.

Discussion: The right of competent adults to refuse any medical treatment is a cornerstone of modern medical ethics. As long as patients are competent and the decision is informed, diabetics can refuse insulin, patients with gangrenous legs can refuse amputation, and ventilator-dependent patients can request removal from life support—even if such actions will lead to their deaths. Ethical decisions become more complex, however, when we try to extend this right of autonomy to patients with impaired decision-making capacity who cannot provide informed consent.

To assist decision-making in such circumstances, instruments of advance directives and surrogate decision-makers allow patients to maintain their autonomy. In most instances, a consensus emerges between families and clinicians regarding the continuation or withdrawal of life-supportive care for patients with dismal hopes of recovery. When disagreements do occur, surrogate decision-makers most often request continuation of life-supportive care when physicians consider further care futile. In some instances, however, families may believe that withdrawal of life-supportive care is in the best interests of a patient when physician estimates of recovery are good. Although these disagreements are not common, the first legal judgments that supported the right of surrogates to substitute their decisions for incompetent patients derived from cases wherein physicians refused to accommodate families' requests to stop treatment.

Case law and most state jurisdictions support the rights of patient surrogates to participate in decisions that promote patients' end-of-life wishes. However, physicians do not have an absolute duty to fulfill surrogate requests. Physicians must balance the burdens and benefits of the proposed treatment with an analysis of the surrogates' decision (see figure). Requests to stop life support are most difficult when the intervention or level of care does not seem burdensome to the patient, the prognosis with continued treatment appears excellent, and the ability of the surrogate to speak for the patient is in question.

In emergency situations, always initiate life-sustaining care when the validity of the surrogate's decisions cannot be assessed, the patient cannot participate in informed consent, and the prognosis is uncertain. Life-supportive care can be later withdrawn after the prognosis is ascertained and the surrogate is found to be acting in the patient's best interests.

Patient-caregiver disagreements are more complex in nonemergency situations and require more thoughtful deliberations. In such circumstances, a series of meetings with the attending physician and surrogate decision-makers can assist a negotiated settlement that meets the patients' needs. Physicians have several responsibilities in these meetings. They must inform the surrogate of the diagnosis, prognosis, and burdens of the proposed treatment. They must elicit from the surrogate the rationale and justification for his or her decision. Sometimes surrogates have had no relevant discussions with the patient, and project their own values, rather than the patient's, into treatment decisions. Pointing out to surrogates the assumptions upon which their decisions are made sometimes helps. Physicians must remind the surrogate that the goal of decision-making is to identify what the *patient's*—not the *surrogate's*—wishes would be in the existing situation. In rare occasions, the surrogate may not be competent to make decisions for the patient, and legal proceedings may be necessary to replace the surrogate with a guardian.

Physicians should be wary of several pitfalls in these conferences. The mere fact that the surrogate makes a decision that seems irrational to the physician is not sufficient grounds for questioning the surrogate's competence or the validity of his or her decisions. Physicians should be cautious of being over-confident in their convictions about the best interests of the patient. There are ample data to show that different physicians arrive at different judgments regarding prognosis and the use of life support when presented with identical clinical information. When clinicians disagree with surrogates, they should avoid losing the surrogates' trust or breaking the lines of communication. Without trust, there is little hope for agreement; once trust is lost during a hostile or impatient interaction, it is rarely regained.

Some disagreements may prove insoluable despite clinicians' best efforts. Contrary to some perceptions, civil lawsuits arising from end-of-life decisions in critical care are rare, and concern over legal liability should not be the physician's primary concern. Ethics committees, ombudsmen, consultations with respected colleagues, and assistance from a social worker can all help move the discussions toward resolution.

The physicians caring for the present patient met with the family to better understand their concerns. The patient's father had died of emphysema on a ventilator after a prolonged illness, and the patient had expressed fear about having the same death. The family also wanted to carry out the requests of the living will. In the meeting, the physicians reassured the family members that the living will only applied when the patient was permanently unconscious or terminally ill. They also explained that the patient, a nonsmoker, did not have emphysema and was unlikely to suffer the same outcome as his father. Despite these reassurances the patient's wife was reluctant to continue life support; however, she was willing to agree to a limited trial of life-supportive care. After 2 days the patient improved, and he underwent successful extubation 4 days later.

Evidence that the surrogates' choice is
• Competent—the surrogate must be capable of making decisions
• Informed—the surrogate must understand the implications of the decision
• Accurate—the surrogate should have some knowledge of the patient's wishes
• Unbiased—the surrogate should have no secondary financial or emotional gain from the decision

Evidence that:
• Medical treatment is not burdensome
• Good prognosis with treatment

Clinical Pearls

1. In emergency situations when there is doubt about the patient's preferences always provide life sustaining treatment. Life support can be withdrawn ethically and compassionately when the circumstances become clearer.

2. Always question your personal biases about prognosis and burdens of care when contemplating the decision to over-ride the wishes of a family member.

3. Only consider replacing the surrogate decision-makers with a court-appointed guardian when all attempts at negotiation have failed and colleagues and members of the ethics committee have attempted to assist in a resolution.

REFERENCES

1. Asch DA, Hansen F-J, Lanken PN: Decisions to limit or continue life-sustaining treatment by critical care physicians in the United States: Conflicts between physicians' practices and patients' wishes. Am J Respir Crit Care Med 1995;151(2 Pt 1):288–292.
2. Gawande A: Whose body is it, anyway? What doctors should do when patients make bad decisions. The New Yorker 1999;75:84–92.
3. Plows CW, Tenery RM, Hartford A, et al. Medical futility in end-of-life care: Report of the Council on Ethical and Judicial Affairs. JAMA 1999;281:937–941.

James K. Stoller, MD

PATIENT 10

A 45-year-old nonsmoking man with obstructive lung disease

A 45-year-old man who never smoked presents to your office with a several-year history of progressive breathlessness. He denies a history of wheezing, cough, or regular phlegm production and has never carried a diagnosis of asthma. He also denies a history of skin or liver disease, although an older brother has cirrhosis, which remains of unknown etiology after evaluation with hepatitis serologies and iron studies.

Physical Examination: Temperature 98.6°, blood pressure 135/74, respirations 18, pulse 87. General: comfortable at rest, but tachypnic after walking into the examination room. HEENT: unremarkable. Chest: slightly increased anterior-posterior diameter, with dimpling of intercostal space at the level of diaphragm insertion (i.e., positive Hoover's sign); no wheezing or crackles. Cardiac: regular rate without murmur. Abdomen: soft, no organomegaly or ascites. Extremities: no cyanosis, clubbing, or edema. Skin: normal.

Laboratory Findings: Complete blood count: normal. Liver function tests: normal. Spirometry: moderately severe airflow obstruction characterized by an FEV_1 of 45% predicted, FVC 85% predicted, FEV_1/FVC 0.40; no significant post-bronchodilator response in FEV_1. Resting ABG (room air): pH 7.43, PCO_2 39 mmHg, PaO_2 75 mmHg. Chest radiographs: see below.

Question: What diagnosis accounts for this patient's condition?

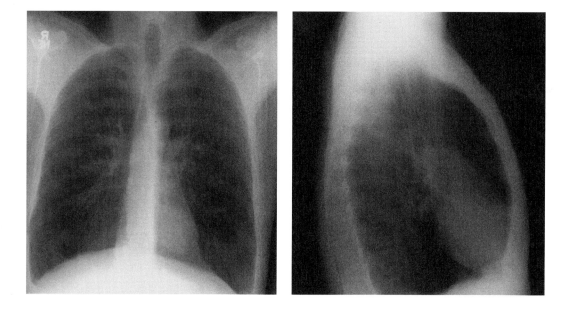

Diagnosis: Severe alpha 1-antitrypsin deficiency (likely PI*ZZ phenotype) with fixed airflow obstruction.

Discussion: Severe alpha 1-antitrypsin deficiency, characterized by serum levels of alpha 1-antitrypsin < 80 mg/dl or 11 μM, is an under-recognized cause of **early-onset emphysema**. This disease is inherited as an autosomal, codominant condition in which the abnormal Z allele causes a structural abnormality of the protein, which is synthesized within the liver. The single amino acid substitution that characterizes the Z-type protein prevents secretion of the normal alpha 1-antitrypsin molecule (termed M-type protein) from the hepatocyte, causing intrahepatocyte accumulation and decreased antitrypsin levels in the serum. The serum level below which the risk of emphysema rises is 80 mg/dl, or 11 μM, which is approximately one-third of the lower limit of the normal serum value.

Alpha 1-antitrypsin deficiency is present in approximately 3% of all patients with emphysema, but often goes unrecognized by health care providers. Population studies suggest a PI*ZZ prevalence of one per 3500 to 5000 Americans, which predicts that approximately 100,000 Americans are currently affected. Yet, fewer than 10,000 have been clinically recognized as having PI*ZZ alpha 1-antitrypsin deficiency. In some instances, individuals with severe deficiency (such as the PI*ZZ phenotype) have no clinical sequelae, though available data suggest that individuals with early-onset emphysema due to alpha 1-antitrypsin deficiency often escape clinical detection and experience long diagnostic delays. For example, in one series, the interval between the first onset of dyspnea (in a population of mean age 45 years) and the initial detection of alpha 1-antitrypsin deficiency was 7.2 years. Furthermore, at least 40% of these young, dyspneic individuals with airflow obstruction reported seeing at least three different physicians before the initial diagnosis of alpha 1-antitrypsin deficiency was made. Although at least 75 abnormal alleles for the alpha 1-antitrypsin protein have been identified to date, the homozygous PI*ZZ phenotype is responsible for over 95% of clinical cases.

Although nonsmokers with PI*ZZ alpha 1-antitrypsin deficiency can sometimes remain free of disease, the hallmark of severe alpha 1-antitrypsin deficiency is early-onset emphysema. Functional abnormalities are classically characterized by diminished FEV1, decreased FEV1/FVC, concomitant reduction in the diffusing capacity for carbon monoxide (DLCO), and the absence of a sufficient post-bronchodilator response to normalize the FEV1. In addition, liver disease, characterized by neonatal jaundice, or cryptogenic cirrhosis in childhood or adulthood complicates PI*ZZ alpha

1-antitrypsin deficiency in approximately 15% of individuals. Panniculitis, characterized by weeping skin ulcers, is a rare complication. Finally, an association between alpha 1-antitrypsin deficiency and Wegener's granulomatosis has been made recently, such that the number of deficient individuals among patients with established Wegener's granulomatosis has increased.

Clinical features that should prompt the clinician to suspect alpha 1-antitrypsin deficiency include: (**1**) emphysema of early chronologic onset, i.e., before age 50 vs. the usual time of onset "smoking-related" emphysema (in alpha 1-antitrypsin–replete individuals) at age 65–75 years, (**2**) emphysema in association with a family history of liver disease, obstructive lung disease, and/or panniculitis, (**3**) emphysema characterized by basilar hyperlucency on the chest x-ray (in contrast to the usual chest x-ray picture of increased lucency at the lung apices in alpha 1-antitrypsin–replete emphysema), and (**4**) emphysema occurring in a never- or trivial smoker (as in the current case).

The diagnosis of alpha 1-antitrypsin deficiency requires initial clinical suspicion. Once suspected, a serum level identifies whether severe deficiency exists. Although the range of normal values varies in different laboratories, serum levels of < 100 mg (or approximately 12–13 μM) should prompt further testing with serum phenotyping, performed by isoelectric focusing.

In addition to pulmonary function tests, full clinical evaluation of the individual with alpha 1-antitrypsin deficiency should include liver function tests, a thorough skin examination, and a careful family history regarding the presence of liver, lung, or skin disease in first-degree relatives (i.e., children, siblings, and parents), as well as inquiry regarding the smoking status of relatives. Because the disease is inherited as an autosomal codominant condition, clinicians should consider phenotype testing family members, but only after a careful discussion with them of the risks and the benefits of such genetic testing.

General treatment of alpha 1-antitrypsin deficiency resembles that of "usual" emphysema. Specifically, preventive strategies include smoking cessation counseling and vaccination for influenza and pneumococcal pneumonia. To optimize airflow, bronchodilators often are prescribed, sometimes with a brief (8- to 10-day) course of prednisone, with plans to re-evaluate spirometry after completion. Ascertainment of a significant rise to the FEV1 after such a brief course of prednisone may justify long-term use of inhaled corticosteroids, which would otherwise not be indicated in patients with emphysema. In patients with severe airflow obstruction (i.e., FEV1 < 20% predicted), arterial blood gases often are assessed to evaluate the possibility of hypercapnea. Supplemental oxygen should be prescribed on a 24-hour basis when the resting room air PaO2 is ≤ 55 mmHg on optimal bronchodilatory therapy. Participation in a pulmonary rehabilitation program can enhance functional status. Lung transplantation is a consideration for patients with far-advanced disease. The role of lung volume reduction surgery for patients with alpha 1-antitrypsin deficiency is still being clarified.

Currently, the only specific therapy for severe alpha 1-antitrypsin deficiency is **intravenous augmentation therapy** with purified, pooled human plasma alpha 1-antitrypsin. The rationale for such therapy is that by increasing serum levels of alpha 1-antitrypsin above the "protective threshold" value, the risk of progressive airflow obstruction is diminished. Intravenous augmentation therapy has no effect on the natural history of liver disease due to alpha 1-antitrypsin deficiency.

Although proof from randomized clinical trials that intravenous augmentation therapy has clinical efficacy is not currently available, the weight of available evidence does support clinical efficacy, at least for individuals who have established moderately severe emphysema (e.g., FEV1 35–49% predicted). Finally, a serum IgA level should be measured before initiating intravenous augmentation therapy to minimize the risk of anaphylaxis following administration of this pooled human plasma preparation.

The present patient's chest radiograph demonstrated hyperinflated lung fields. He was found to have alpha 1-antitrypsin deficiency of the PI*ZZ type, with low alpha 1-antitrypsin serum levels. First-degree relatives were tested, and his older brother (with cirrhosis) was also found to have PI*ZZ alpha 1-antitrypsin deficiency. Weekly intravenous augmentation therapy was begun.

Clinical Pearls

1. PI*ZZ alpha 1-antitrypsin deficiency may cause early-onset emphysema, even in never-smokers.

2. A plain chest radiograph showing disproportionate hyperlucency at the lung bases suggests alpha 1-antitrypsin deficiency.

3. Identification of an individual with severe deficiency of alpha 1-antitrypsin should prompt testing first-degree relatives for alpha 1-antitrypsin deficiency.

4. Recent observations suggest an association between alpha 1-antitrypsin deficiency and Wegener's granulomatosis.

REFERENCES

1. Gadek JE, Crystal RG: Alpha 1-antitrypsin deficiency. In Stanbury JB, Wyngaarden JB, Frederickson DS, et al (eds): The Metabolic Basis of Inherited Disease, 5th ed. New York, McGraw-Hill, 1983, pp 1450–1467.
2. Stoller JK, Smith P, Yang P, et al: Physical and social impact of alpha 1-antitrypsin deficiency: Results of a 1-antitrypsin deficiency: Results of a mail survey of the readership of a national newsletter. Cleve Clin J Med 1994;61:461–467.
3. Stoller JK: Clinical features and natural history of severe alpha 1-antitrypsin deficiency. Chest 1997;111:123S–128S.
4. Dirksen A, Kijkman JH, Madsen F, et al: A randomized clinical trial of alpha 1-antitrypsin augmentation therapy. Am J Respir Crit Care Med 1999;160:1468–1472.

George F. Longstreth, MD

PATIENT 11

A 42-year-old man with upper abdominal discomfort

A 42-year-old man complains of "aching" in the upper abdomen for the last year. The discomfort is sometimes "sharp" and comes and goes for several minutes at a time throughout the day. It does not awaken him from sleep. It initially was episodic, but now has occurred nearly every day for 1 month. The discomfort is sometimes partly relieved by food or antacid use, but is unrelated to bowel function, which has remained normal. He also has occasional nausea and insomnia. The patient denies heartburn, regurgitation, vomiting, dysphagia, and weight loss. He drinks 8 cups of coffee and smokes 1 pack of cigarettes daily, but denies use of alcohol and prescription or over-the-counter drugs. He is a computer software engineer, and he recently has had to work much overtime; he is fearful of losing his job. Recent upper gastrointestinal barium radiography was normal. He had failed to respond to cimetidine therapy, and a previous physician had found him to have a positive *Helicobacter pylori* serologic test, but the symptoms persisted after a course of eradication therapy.

Physical Examination: Temperature 37.1°; pulse 80; respirations 16; blood pressure 132/78. General: mildly overweight; anxious-appearing. HEENT: normal. Cardiac: normal. Chest: unremarkable. Abdomen: mild epigastric tenderness without organomegaly. Extremities: normal.

Laboratory Findings: Complete blood count, ESR, routine blood chemistry determinations, TSH level, and urinalysis: normal.

Question: What test should be done next?

Answer: Endoscopy to confirm functional dyspepsia.

Discussion: "Dyspepsia," which derives from Greek ("bad digestion"), is a symptom of many disorders rather than a disease in itself. In the past, physicians variously defined dyspepsia and included such symptoms as eructation, abdominal fullness, heartburn, regurgitation, and nausea. A multinational group of experts, however, has recommended the term dyspepsia for "persistent or recurrent abdominal pain or discomfort centered in the upper abdomen." Other symptoms such as nausea and anorexia may be associated with dyspepsia.

The clinical history of a patient with dyspepsia lacks typical features of gastroesophageal reflux disease, irritable bowel syndrome (IBS), and biliary pain, which are important diagnoses to consider before planning further diagnostic testing and therapy. Characteristic symptoms of reflux, such as ascending, substernal discomfort; regurgitation; and an association of symptoms with recumbency, are absent in dyspepsia. IBS cannot be diagnosed in the absence of bowel habit alterations. Gallstone pain is usually severe, lasts at least 1 hour, and is less frequent than in the present patient. The differential diagnosis also includes a variety of other disorders. The most common diagnostic problem, however, is in distinguishing between peptic ulcer disease, gastric malignancy, and functional dyspepsia.

Differential Diagnosis of Dyspepsia

Functional dyspepsia	Chronic pancreatitis
Peptic ulcer disease	Drug-induced
Malignancy (gastro-	dyspepsia
intestinal, pancreatic	Diabetic gastroparesis
hepatobiliary)	Metabolic disorders
Gastroesophageal	(e.g., hypercalcemia)
reflux disease	Ischemic heart pain
Irritable bowel syndrome	Abdominal wall pain
Symptomatic	Eosinophilic
cholelithiasis	gastroenteritis

The history alone, such as relief with food, usually does not reliably discriminate peptic ulcer disease from functional dyspepsia. Warning ("alarm") features, such as weight loss and anemia point toward an organic etiology, most notably cancer. Most patients without warning features who are similar to the present patient in age and fail to respond to *H. pylori* eradication therapy have functional (nonulcer) dyspepsia.

The diagnosis of functional dyspepsia is made from a characteristic history and exclusion of organic causes of dyspepsia. The disorder typically has a chronic or recurrent course, and may alternate or overlap with other functional disorders, such as IBS. Functional dyspepsia is best considered as a

result of an interaction between physiologic and psychosocial factors. Specifically, the pathophysiologic factors can include **gastric motor dysfunction** (delayed emptying, antral hypomotility, and impaired gastric accommodation), **enhanced visceral sensitivity** to gastric distension or duodenal acid infusion (visceral hyperalgesia), **psychosocial factors** (anxiety, neuroticism, depression, and childhood abuse), and ***H. pylori* infection**. The latter factor is the most controversial. Although *H. pylori* infection causes chronic gastritis, there is no consistent relationship between gastritis and symptoms. Furthermore, the infection is not consistently linked with gastric motor dysfunction and enhanced visceral sensitivity.

The controversial role of *H. pylori* in functional dyspepsia and hence, the value of testing and empirical eradication therapy, is further underscored by the mixed results reported from placebo-controlled studies on the benefit of *H. pylori* eradication in patients with functional dyspepsia. At best, few patients have responded in these trials; research results do not provide convincing evidence of long-term benefit. However, multiple consensus recommendations have agreed that in young patients in primary care practice who lack warning features, testing followed by empirical *H. pylori* treatment may be cost effective. In older patients (i.e., > 45 to 50 years) or those with warning signs, **upper gastrointestinal endoscopy** is the strategy of choice.

Endoscopy is more accurate than barium radiography. Although initial costs are higher for gastroenterology consultation with endoscopy than barium radiography, long-term costs may be lower, partly due to the tendency for radiography-negative patients to undergo endoscopy for persisting dyspepsia, as in this patient. In addition, patient satisfaction is higher. No endoscopy guideline should be used universally; rather, the best decision is a clinical judgement that considers the patient's age, dyspepsia duration, other symptoms, past history, drug use, endoscopy availability and cost, and patient preference. Gallbladder sonography generally is not useful for patients whose pain is atypical for gallstones, because cholecystectomy usually is not indicated in such cases.

The most important aspects of treatment are explanation, reassurance, modification of dietary factors, and an attempt to ameliorate psychosocial factors. No drug therapy has proven to be consistently beneficial over the long term, but some patients may respond to acid inhibitors, gastrokinetic agents, or low-dose antidepressant drugs (alleviation of insomnia also is a potential benefit). Use of the latter is supported mainly by more extensive experience with them in other functional pain disorders.

The present patient's physician referred him to a gastroenterologist, who reported a normal endoscopy, explained the diagnosis of functional dyspepsia, and prescribed amitriptyline, 25 mg at bedtime. The patient initiated a regular exercise program, stopped smoking, and reduced coffee ingestion. His job became less stressful. He continued to have episodic dyspepsia, but it became less bothersome.

Clinical Pearls

1. Symptomatic gastroesophageal reflux and biliary pain usually can be distinguished from dyspepsia with the clinical history.

2. The role of *H. pylori* in the pathogenesis of functional dyspepsia is uncertain, and few, if any, patients have long-term benefit from eradication therapy.

3. In dyspepsia patients who are older than 45 to 50 years or those with warning signs, initial upper gastrointestinal endoscopy is preferred over *H. pylori* testing.

4. No drug is of proven benefit for functional dyspepsia over the long term.

REFERENCES

1. Longstreth GF: Long-term costs after gastroenterology consultation with endoscopy versus radiography in dyspepsia. Gastro Endosc 1992;38:23–26.
2. Rabinek L, Wray NP, Graham DY: Managing dyspepsia: What do we know and what do we need to know? Am J Gastroenterol 1995;20:182–183.
3. Talley NJ: Editorial: Gallstones and upper abdominal discomfort. Innocent bystander or a cause of dyspepsia? J Clin Gastroenterol 1995;20:182–183.
4. American Gastroenterological Association Medical Position Statement: Evaluation of dyspepsia. Gastroenterology 1998;114:582–595.
5. Mertz H, Fass A, Kodner F, et al: Effect of amitryptiline on symptoms, sleep, and visceral perception in patients with functional dyspepsia. Am J Gastroenterol 1998;93:160–165.
6. Wiklund I, Glise H, Jerndal P, et al: Does endoscopy have a positive impact on quality of life in dyspepsia? Gastrointest Endosc 1998;47:449.
7. Ofman JJ, Rabeneck L: The effectiveness of endoscopy in the management of dyspepsia: A qualitative systemic review. Am J Med 1999;106:335–346.
8. Talley NJ, Axon A, Bytzer P, et al: Management of uninvestigated and functional dyspepsia: A working party report for the World Congresses of Gastroenterology 1998. Aliment Pharmacol Ther 1999;13:1135–1148.
9. Talley NJ, Stranghellini V, Heading KL, et al: Functional gastroduodenal disorders. Gut 1999;45(Suppl II):II37–42.
10. Talley NJ, Vakil N, Ballard ED, Fennerty MB: Absence of benefit of eradicating *Helicobacter pylori* in patients with nonulcer dyspepsia. N Engl J Med 1999;341:1106–1111.

Robert S. Rosenson, MD

PATIENT 12

A 57-year-old man seeking cardiovascular risk assessment

A 57-year-old man has had known hypercholesterolemia for 10 years. He reports a total cholesterol level of 240 mg/dl, and is on statin (3-hydroxy-3-methylglutaryl coenzyme A reductase inhibitor) therapy. He has had known coronary artery disease since age 49 years, and has undergone multiple angioplasties of the left circumflex coronary artery. At age 56 years, he had an angioplasty procedure of a 95% left anterior descending coronary lesion and subsequent stent placement. He experienced recurrent angina 3 months later, and the repeat coronary arteriogram revealed a left anterior descending stent stenosis of 90–95%, a mid left circumflex narrowing of 50%, and a proximal right coronary lesion of 80%.

Physical Examination: Height 71 inches; weight 262 pounds; body mass index 37 kg/m². Blood pressure (seated): 130/92 mmHg right arm, 126/92 mmHg left arm. Pulse 64. Skin: xanthelasmas affecting both upper eyelids. Cardiac: soft S_1 and normal A_2P_2; no gallops or murmurs; carotid and peripheral pulsations normal. Remainder of examination: normal.

Medications: Aspirin 325 mg q am; clopidrogrel 75 mg q am; warfarin 10 mg/d; allopurinol 300 mg/d; atorvastastin 20 mg/d (see table); dilitiazem CD 180 mg q am; atenolol 50 mg q am; ramipril 5 mg q am.

Laboratory Findings: Glucose 99 mg/dl; creatinine 1.1 mg/dl; alanine aminotransferase 69 U/L (3-50); homocysteine 7.2 μmol/L; TSH 2.83 μIU/ml.

Plasma lipids and lipoproteins on atorvastatin 20 mg daily

TC (mg/dl)	LDL-C (mg/dl)	HDL-C (mg/dl)	TG (mg/dl)	LDL Particle Conc. (nmol/L)	LDL Particle Size (nm)	Large HDL-C (mg/dl)	Large VLDL-TG (mg/dl)
179	109	33	208	1460	19.6	13	87

Question: What other therapeutic options may potentially lower his CHD risk?

Diagnosis: Atherogenic dyslipidemia (combined hyperlipidemia with predominant small LDL size and hypoalphalipoproteinemia).

Discussion: In CHD patients, secondary preventive therapies have emphasized a reduction in LDL cholesterol to a "desirable" level below 100 mg/dl. On statin (atorvastatin) therapy, the present patient's LDL cholesterol was less than 130 mg/dl. The event reduction analyses from the Cholesterol and Recurrent Events (CARE) and Long-term Intervention (LIPID) studies suggest an attenuation of the therapeutic benefit when the LDL cholesterol level is less than 125 mg/dl. Whether more aggressive LDL cholesterol reduction equates with more clinical benefit remains unanswered, and this issue is the topic of ongoing clinical trials of low- versus high-dose statin therapy. In addition, this man's triglycerides exceed the 90th percentile, and his HDL cholesterol falls below the 10th percentile for his age and gender.

Further characterization of the lipoproteins reveals a small LDL size, borderline-high LDL cholesterol concentration, predominantly large VLDL size, and reduced concentration of large HDL particles (see table, previous page). This combination of lipoprotein abnormalities often is referred to as "atherogenic dyslipidemia," and it typically is associated with central obesity, hypertension, and hyperglycemia.

In a cross-sectional study of 158 men, large VLDL size and small HDL size were associated with severe coronary stenoses. Small LDL size is associated with a 3- to 4-fold increased CHD event rate as compared to subjects with predominantly large LDL. The atherogenicity of small LDL particles is multi-factorial.

Small LDL particle size and atherosclerosis

Facilitated LDL endothelial transport

Increased LDL oxidation

Endothelial dysfunction

Enhanced LDL trapping in intima

The importance of lipoprotein subclass distribution on the progression of coronary stenoses was recently highlighted from a post hoc analysis of the Pravastatin Limitation of Atherosclerosis in the Coronaries (PLAC I). CHD subjects with predominantly small LDL particles had more rapid coronary progression than observed in subjects with predominantly large LDL particles. Statin therapy retards coronary progression in all subjects with hypercholesterolemia; however, the relative benefits may be greater for those with small average LDL size.

Several possible therapeutic options for this patient's dyslipidemia may reduce his risk. These choices include increasing the atorvastatin dose to further lower the LDL cholesterol and LDL particle concentration, or targeting the small LDL particle size, elevated triglycerides, and low HDL cholesterol concentrations through combined therapy with either nicotinic acid or a fibric acid derivative (see table, page bottom).

The Veterans Administration HDL Intervention Trial (VA HIT) randomized men with CHD who had an HDL cholesterol < 40 mg/dl, LDL cholesterol ≤ 140 mg/dl and triglycerides ≤ 300 mg/dL to either gemfibrozil (600 mg twice daily) or placebo. The baseline lipid profile revealed an LDL cholesterol of 111 mg/dl, HDL cholesterol of 32 mg/dl, and a triglyceride of 161 mg/dl. After 5.1 years, CHD patients treated with gemfibrozil had 22 % fewer cardiac events (CHD death/nonfatal myocardial infarctions). In a post hoc analysis, HDL cholesterol was the most important CHD predictor.

Although VA HIT did not include statin-treated patients and then add a fibrate, this trial provides insight into the management of CHD patients with hypercholesterolemic, low HDL cholesterol levels and high-normal triglycerides. The implications from VA HIT are that CHD subjects with LDL cholesterol levels in the borderline-high range, according to NCEP II guidelines, who have low HDL cholesterol levels may benefit from therapy directed toward increasing low levels of HDL cholesterol. Clearly, this combined approach to secondary prevention needs evaluation in an outcomes-based study, and the use of a hydrophilic statin (e.g., pravastatin) that may be more safely combined with a fibric acid derivative than a lipophilic agent.

In summary, CHD risk in hypercholesterolemic subjects may be more accurately characterized by direct measurements of LDL and measurement of total LDL particles or apolipoprotein B concentrations. Low levels of HDL cholesterol and reduced concentrations of the cardioprotective large HDL subclasses contribute to CHD risk.

The present patient was placed on gemfibrozil to lower his triglycerides and increase his HDL cholesterol (see table next page). Due to the potential risk of myopathy with lipophilic statins (e.g., atorvastatin) and fibrates (e.g., gemfibrozil), atorvastatin was discontinued. He was placed on a hydrophilic statin (pravastatin) due to the long-term safety of combined pravastatin and gemfibrozil therapy. On gemfibrozil and pravastatin, the LDL cholesterol remained unchanged, but the LDL particle size increased from small to large. The triglycerides were reduced by 38%, and the HDL cholesterol increased by 15%.

Plasma lipids and lipoproteins on pravastatin 20 mg nightly, gemfibrozil 600 mg twice daily

TC (mg/dL)	LDL-C (mg/dL)	HDL-C (mg/dL)	TG (mg/dL)	LDL Particle Conc. (nmol/L)	LDL Particle Size (nm)	Large HDL-C (mg/dL)	Large VLDL-TG (mg/dL)
167	110	38	128	1206	20.8	10	64

Clinical Pearls

1. LDL cholesterol reduction is the prime focus of secondary preventive therapies.
2. LDL subclass distribution is an important predictor of coronary progression rates.
3. Low HDL cholesterol levels remain an important risk factor in CHD patients who receive statin therapy.

REFERENCES

1. The Expert Panel on detection, evaluation, and treatment of high blood cholesterol in adults: Summary of the second report of the National Cholesterol Education Program (NCEP) Expert Panel on detection, evaluation, and treatment of high blood cholesterol in adults (Adult Treatment Panel II). JAMA 1993;269:3015–3023.
2. Lamarche B, Tchernof A, Moorjani S, et al: Small, dense low-density lipoprotein particles as a predictor of the risk of ischemic heart disease in men. Circulation 1997;95:69–75.
3. Freedman DS, Otvos JD, Jeyarajah EJ, et al: Relation of lipoprotein subclasses as measured by proton nuclear magnetic resonance spectroscopy to coronary artery disease. Arterioscler Thromb Vasc Biol 1998;18:1046-53.
4. Iliades L, Rosenson RS: Long-term safety of pravastatin-gemfibrozil therapy in mixed hyperlipidemia. Clin Cardiol 1999;22:25–28.
5. Rubins HB, Robins SJ, Collins D, et al. for the Veterans Affairs High-Density Lipoprotein Cholesterol Intervention Trial Study Group: Gemfibrozil for the secondary prevention of coronary heart disease in men with low levels of high-density lipoprotein cholesterol. N Engl J Med 1999;341:410–418.
6. Sacks FM, Braunwald E, Simes RJ, et al. Pretreatment lipid concentrations and coronary event reduction with pravastatin: The Prava-3 Pooling Project. Circulation 1999;100:I-739.
7. Rosenson RS, Shalaurova I, Otvos JD: Relations of lipoprotein subclass levels and LDL size to reduction in coronary atherosclerosis in the PLAC-I trial. J Am Coll Cardiol 2000;35(Suppl A):299A. Abstract.

Lourdes M. E. Flaminiano, MD
Bartolome R. Celli, MD

PATIENT 13

A 76-year-old woman with post-operative respiratory failure
and prolonged weaning from mechanical ventilation

A 76-year-old woman with a 50 pack-year cigarette-smoking history was treated for breast cancer with radical mastectomy and radiation therapy 5 years prior to admission. Subsequently she had multiple excisions for recurrence, and required two rib resections and a skin flap in the left anterior hemithorax. Aortic and mitral valve damage developed from the radiation, and she underwent replacement via a right thoracotomy. Post-operatively, she failed to wean from the ventilator and required a tracheostomy. She eventually was transferred to a chronic rehabilitation facility. After 3 months, she was discharged home with nighttime mechanical ventilation and capping of the tracheostomy during the day. At home she requires assistance in activities of daily living and experiences fatigue with minimal exertion.

Physical Examination: Vital signs: pulse 98 respirations 28, blood pressure 140/60 mmHg. Oxygen saturation: 91% on room air. General: well developed, mildly tachypneic; tracheostomy present. Chest: visible precordial impulses at rib resection and skin flap, and palpable heart beats; decreased breath sounds on left; bronchial breath sounds and crackles on right. Abdomen: soft; slightly tender liver. Extremities: +2 leg edema above ankles.

Laboratory Findings: ABGs (room air): pH 7.36, pCO_2 48 mmHg, PaO_2 63 mmHg; other lab values normal.

Pulmonary Function Tests:

	Predicted	Observed	% Predicted
PI max, cmH_2O	66	22	30%
PE max, cmH_2O	95	38	40%

Question: What therapeutic intervention is likely to benefit this patient?

Answer: Comprehensive pulmonary rehabilitation and respiratory muscle training.

Discussion: We hypothesized that ventilatory muscle training, as part of a comprehensive pulmonary rehabilitation program, could help this patient wean from mechanical ventilation and improve her quality of life. This approach would likely reduce dyspnea, increase exercise tolerance, enhance the ability to perform activities of daily living, improve psychological function, and increase feelings of hope, control, and self-esteem.

Inspiratory resistive training is achieved with a device that offers constant inspiratory resistance. The device can be used independently or can be connected to the inspiratory limb of the ventilator. Belman et al. reported two patients that underwent ventilatory muscle training while on the ventilator. After training, they showed improvement in maximal ventilatory capacity and arterial $PaCO_2$, and marked resolution in dyspnea.

Aldrich et al. reported similar findings in 27 patients with respiratory failure who failed weaning attempts. Inspiratory resistive muscle training resulted in an improvement in maximal inspiratory pressures and vital capacity and shortened time of weaning from mechanical ventilation.

As a complement to inspiratory muscle training, other breathing retraining techniques such as diaphragmatic and pursed-lips breathing may improve the ventilatory pattern, prevent dynamic airway obstruction, and improve abdominal and thoracic muscle synchrony and gas exchange. Breathlessness may be relieved by leaning forward with arms resting on the patient's thighs or on a table. The patient also learns how to coordinate expansion of the abdominal wall with inspiration. Improvement in clinical symptoms, more than any other measurable physiologic parameter, is a consistent observation. An improvement in tidal volume and decrease in respiratory rate are changes that may be observed. The patient should engage in aerobic lower-extremity endurance exercises to enhance performance of daily activities and reduce dyspnea.

The oldest, simplest, and most useful tests of respiratory muscle strength are the **maximal inspiratory (PI max)** and **expiratory (PE max) pressures**. Serial evaluation of PI max over time can provide information on the progression or regression of muscle strength. Patients with maximal inspiratory pressures less than 25 cm H_2O, as our patient had, are at high risk of developing ventilatory failure. Maximal expiratory force of less than 30 cm H_2O at functional reserve capacity is seen in patients with ineffective cough. This leads to accumulation of secretions, atelectasis, pneumonia, and ventilatory failure. The **maximal diaphragmatic pressure (PDI max)** measures the strength of the diaphragm. A value higher than 100 cm H_2O effectively rules out weakness as the cause of ventilatory failure.

Other tests that may help assess respiratory muscle function include the measurement of **forced vital capacity** (FVC) and **maximal voluntary ventilation** (MVV). The measurement of FVC is a practical means to evaluate and follow patients suspected of ventilatory muscle dysfunction. In acute situations such as Guillain-Barré syndrome, close routine monitoring of FVC has proved to be useful. In bilateral diaphragmatic muscle paralysis, FVC decreases significantly in the supine position (between 30–50%). MVV also may be a helpful test in assessing respiratory muscle function and provides an indirect evaluation of respiratory muscle endurance.

In the present patient, inspiratory muscle training was initiated as part of a comprehensive pulmonary rehabilitation program. This helped her eventually wean from mechanical ventilation. She was decannulated after several months of intense pulmonary rehabilitation. Her PI max improved to 45 cm H_2O, and her PE max increased to 62 cmH_2O. She continues to maintain good gas exchange with a normal $PaCO_2$. Her functional status has improved, and she is now independent in all of her activities of daily living.

Clinical Pearls

1. Respiratory muscle weakness is a common cause of respiratory failure and failure to wean from mechanical ventilation.

2. Measurements of vital capacity and inspiratory and expiratory pressures are helpful in assessing respiratory muscle strength.

3. Respiratory muscle training as part of a comprehensive rehabilitation program may facilitate successful weaning.

REFERENCES

1. Belman MJ: Respiratory failure treated by ventilatory muscle training. Eur J Respir Dis 1981;62:391–395.
2. Aldrich TK, et al: Weaning from mechanical ventilation: Adjunctive use of inspiratory muscle resistive training. Crit Care Med 1989;17(2):143–147.
3. Celli BR, Snider, et al: Standards for diagnosis and care of patients with chronic obstructive pulmonary disease. Am J Respir Crit Care Med 1995;152:s77–s120.
4. Celli BR, Grassino A: Respiratory muscles: Functional evaluation. Semin Respir Crit Care Med 1998;19(4):367–381.

Marc L. Miller, MD

PATIENT 14

A 21-year-old woman with severe myalgias and dark urine

A 21-year-old woman was in good health until 1 week before admission when she developed malaise, fever, and a nonproductive cough. She was treated with erythromycin for presumed bronchitis. Two days before admission, severe myalgias developed, and she began to pass dark, tea-colored urine. There is no history of similar episodes of myalgias or pigmenturia. The patient is a college student and denies recent trauma, unusual physical activity, drug use, or a family history of muscle disease. She is taking no medications.

Physical Examination: Temperature 37°; pulse 100; blood pressure 100/60. General: well developed, alert, uncomfortable due to muscle pain. HEENT: dry mucous membranes. Chest: clear. Cardiac: no murmur or rub. Abdomen: soft, no hepatosplenomegaly or tenderness. Skin: no rash. Musculoskeletal: diffuse muscular tenderness of all extremities and of abdominal wall muscles; unable to walk because of leg pain, and unable to sit up without assistance because of abdominal wall pain.

Laboratory Findings: WBC 4700/μl, Hct 41%, ESR 12 mm/hr. Na^+ 140 mEq/L, K^+ 4.2 mEq/L, creatinine 0.9 mg/dl, CK 640,000 IU/L, AST 2715 IU/L, LDH 43,165 IU/L. Urinalysis: urine dark brown; hematest positive; 0–2 RBCs/hpf, no casts. EKG: normal. Blood cultures, viral throat culture, toxic drug screen, and acute viral serologies for influenza A and B: all negative.

Question: What laboratory test would help confirm the etiology of this patient's myopathy?

Answer: Convalescent influenza A titer showed a fourfold rise from the baseline level.

Discussion: The clinical spectrum of muscle involvement in viral infections includes: (**1**) commonly experienced diffuse myalgias that occur in the prodromal or early phase of the infection, (**2**) an intermediate syndrome affecting mostly children and characterized by localized calf myalgias and elevated muscle enzymes, and (**3**) severe, diffuse myositis with rhabdomyolysis, as occurred in this patient. The intermediate and severe syndromes tend to develop as the acute viral illness is resolving.

Severe myositis has been reported with a variety of viral infections (see table below). Patients present with a history of a preceding upper respiratory or gastrointestinal tract infection, followed by high fever, diffuse myalgias, and weakness. Medical attention is sought because of the development of severe muscle pain that interferes with normal function or because of the development of pigmenturia. In some cases, patients present with complications of rhabdomyolysis, including life-threatening arrhythmias or altered mental status. Both upper and lower extremities as well as trunk muscles may be involved. Muscles are tender and may be boggy or edematous, especially in children. In severe cases, a compartment syndrome may occur. Weakness parallels the severity of muscle involvement. CK levels vary widely, ranging from less than 10,000 IU/L to more than 500,000 IU/L. The course of acute viral myositis is generally one of full recovery within 1–2 weeks of onset of the myalgias, although the course may be prolonged by the complications of rhabdomyolysis, including renal failure, fluid and electrolyte abnormalities, and cardiac arrhythmias.

Viral Causes of Myositis with Rhabdomyolysis

Influenza A and B	Adenovirus
Coxsackievirus	Echovirus
Epstein-Barr	Cytomegalovirus
Herpes simplex	Measles
Varciella-zoster	Human immunodeficiency
Parainfluenza	virus

The diagnosis of acute viral myositis with rhabdomyolysis is first suspected on a clinical basis. The history of a preceding viral infection or the presence of other manifestations of acute viral infections such as aseptic meningitis, myocarditis, or an exanthem in the absence of another explanation for muscle necrosis may be all that is necessary or possible to establish the diagnosis. Acute viral infection may be confirmed by isolation of the virus during the acute phase of the illness, but negative cultures are common. More often the diagnosis is supported in retrospect with the demonstration of at least a fourfold increase in viral antibody titer between paired acute and convalescent titers. Muscle biopsy does not provide specific diagnostic information in viral myositis, and is performed only to evaluate other diagnostic possibilities. Virus has not been directly cultured from muscle in cases of acute viral myositis with rhabdomyolysis.

Acute viral myositis with rhabdomyolysis must be distinguished from other causes of rhabdomyolysis (see table below). Trauma or crush injuries, coma, seizures, environmental heat illness, and extreme physical exertion may be obvious or can be excluded by history. Both prescribed and illicit drugs can cause rhabdomyolysis. Electrolyte abnormalities, disturbances of serum osmolality, and thyroid myopathy should be evaluated by appropriate laboratory testing. Pyomyositis due to bacterial infections tends to cause more localized muscle tenderness and swelling, and is diagnosed by isolation of the organism from the blood or involved muscle. The inflammatory myopathies, polymyositis and dermatomyositis, rarely cause rhabdomyolysis. Persistence of weakness and elevated muscle enzymes for more than 1 or 2 weeks after the onset of rhabdomyolysis should lead to the consideration of a chronic inflammatory myopathy. The inherited metabolic myopathies are very rare and typically cause recurrent episodes of myoglobinuria following exertion. Carnitine palmityltransferase (CPT) deficiency most closely resembles acute viral myositis because it can cause rhabdomyolysis in the absence of exertion, often in the setting of an acute bacterial or viral infection. Muscle biopsy with special stains for CPT is necessary if there is a strong clinical suspicion of CPT deficiency based on family history or the presence of repeated episodes of nonexertional rhabdomyolysis.

Differential Diagnosis of Rhabdomyolysis

Massive trauma/crush injuries	Electrolyte abnormalities
Prolonged coma	Inherited metabolic myopathies
Seizures	
Environmental heat illness/extreme physical exertion	Pyomyositis
	Bacterial sepsis
	Thyroid myopathy
Drug- and toxin-induced myopathies	Inflammatory myopathy

Treatment of acute viral myositis with rhabdomyolysis is supportive and directed at preventing or managing the complications of rhabdomyolysis with vigorous hydration, correction of electrolyte abnormalities, and management of renal insufficiency as needed.

The present patient was treated with aggressive intravenous hydration. The myalgias gradually resolved during the 10-day hospitalization. Urine output and renal function remained normal. CK levels decreased to 2915 IU/L at discharge. Four weeks after discharge the patient felt entirely well, with no muscle tenderness or weakness, and the CK had returned to normal. Myositis has not recurred over the subsequent 8 years.

Clinical Pearls

1. Acute viral myositis typically presents as the viral illness is resolving.
2. Influenza A is the most common viral etiology of acute myositis.
3. Rhabdomyolysis due to CPT deficiency most closely resembles acute viral myositis, but is much less common and typically is recurrent.

REFERENCES

1. Gabow PA, Kaehny WD, Kelleher SP: The spectrum of rhabdomyolysis. Medicine 1982;61:141–152.
2. Kelly KJ, Garland JS, Tang TT, et al: Fatal rhabdomyolysis following influenza infection in a girl with familial carnitine palmityl transferase deficiency. Pediatrics 1989; 84:312–316.
3. Pesik NT, Otten EJ: Severe rhabdomyolysis following a viral illness: A case report and review of the literature. J Emerg Med 1996; 14:425–428.
4. Singh U, Scheld WM: Infectious etiologies of rhabdomyolysis: Three case reports and review. Clin Infect Dis 1996;22:642–649.
5. Annerstedt M, Herlitz H, Molne J, et al: Rhabdomyolysis and acute renal failure associated with influenza virus type A. Scand J Urol Nephrol 1999;33:260–264.

Colleen Bailey, MD
Peter F. Fedullo, MD

PATIENT 15

**A 48-year-old man with dyspnea, fever, leukocytosis, and syncope
following umbilical hernia repair**

A 48-year-old man is transferred from his home to the emergency department after abrupt onset of chest pain, dyspnea, and diaphoresis, followed by syncope. He underwent an uncomplicated elective umbilical hernia repair under general anesthesia 1 week earlier. In the emergency department, he is awake and alert. On further questioning, he admits to intermittent chest pain and dyspnea for 3 days.

Physical Examination: Temperature 38.4°; pulse 112; respirations 22; blood pressure 90/50. General: obese; tachypneic, but in no obvious respiratory distress. HEENT: unremarkable. Cardiac: regular rate, without murmur or gallop. Chest: bilateral lower lobe crackles. Abdomen: healing incision, without tenderness. Extremities: no edema. Neurologic: awake, alert, without focal findings.

Laboratory Findings: WBC 13,700/µl with 80% neutrophils, 20% lymphocytes. Chest radiograph: patchy infiltrates both lower lobes, small right pleural effusion. Arterial blood gas (room air): pH 7.49, PO_2 62 mmHg, PCO_2 30 mmHg. Echocardiogram: dilated right atrium and right ventricle, estimated pulmonary artery systolic pressure 55 mmHg. Lower extremity duplex examination: technically inadequate due to the patient's obesity. Ventilation/perfusion scan: indeterminate.

Question: What diagnostic and/or therapeutic procedures are indicated?

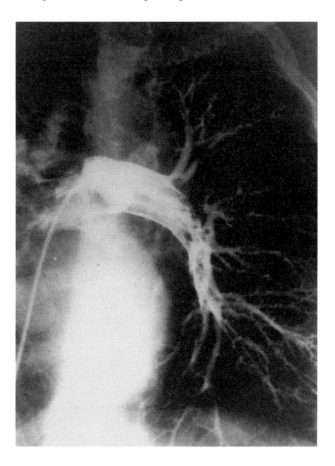

Answer: Pulmonary angiography to confirm diagnosis of pulmonary embolism, followed by IVC filter placement and anticoagulant therapy.

Discussion: Syncope occurs as the initial presentation of pulmonary embolism (PE) in approximately 10% of patients. The diagnosis of embolism following syncope may be hampered by a focus on primary cardiac or neurologic conditions known to result in transient loss of consciousness. The mechanism underlying syncope with PE has not been clearly established, although it is likely related to an abrupt decrease in cardiac output related to the pulmonary vascular obstruction; transient sinus bradycardia and AV block during recurrent embolism have been described, and may account for the mechanism in certain patients. Fever and leukocytosis also may occur in the setting of pulmonary embolism. When combined with pulmonary infiltrates, also a known accompaniment of embolism, the clinician may be misled into considering a pneumonic process and overlooking this potentially fatal disorder.

Available information suggests that the majority of the 50,000 to 100,000 deaths resulting from PE annually in the United States are due to either single massive embolic events or to those that are recurrent and undiagnosed. The outcome from PE, once the diagnosis has been established and effective therapy instituted, is quite good. The one exception to this rule involves patients with embolism associated with hemodynamic compromise. Irrespective of the degree of pulmonary vascular obstruction, patients with PE who present with shock have a mortality at least three- to four-fold greater than those without shock. Therefore, the significant mortality risk associated with hemodynamically massive PE justifies a more aggressive therapeutic approach than that utilized in uncomplicated venous thromboembolism.

The central goal of therapy in massive PE is to **support hemodynamic function** until the degree of pulmonary vascular obstruction is relieved by thrombolysis, either through intrinsic or extrinsic mechanisms. The severely compromised nature of the pulmonary vascular bed and its effect on right ventricular function makes **prevention of recurrence** an important secondary consideration. Therefore, assuming the requisite expertise in inferior vena caval (IVC) filter placement is available, and that placement of a filter will not interfere with the primary management of the patient, filter placement should be considered in all patients with PE associated with hemodynamic compromise.

The utilization of IVC filters has rapidly increased with the advent of improved delivery techniques, although many of the proposed indications remain controversial. Well-accepted indications for the placement of an IVC filter with proximal deep vein thrombosis or PE include: (**1**) contraindication to anticoagulant therapy (recent surgery or trauma, hemorrhagic stroke, active bleeding, or serious complication of heparin therapy including hemorrhage or thrombocytopenia); (**2**) recurrence of embolism despite adequate anticoagulation; and, (**3**) anatomically or hemodynamically massive embolism when a recurrent PE may be fatal.

Carefully controlled trials demonstrating the impact of IVC filters on recurrence rates and mortality from embolism have not been performed. While anecdotal data suggest that recurrent embolism and death from embolism are unusual following filter insertion, strong scientific evidence that IVC filters prevent death is lacking.

The largest controlled clinical trial to date examining the effectiveness of IVC filters involved 400 anticoagulant-treated patients with proximal venous thrombosis randomized to IVC filter placement or no filter. In the group randomized to filter placement, there was a significant reduction in the risk of PE at 12 days. This initial benefit, however, was mitigated by an increased venous thrombosis recurrence rate at 2 years. There were no significant differences in survival or symptomatic embolism between the two groups.

Mortality from filter complications is rare, occurring in only 4 of 3256 patients (0.12%) in one report. Numerous nonfatal complications of IVC filters have been reported, including technical difficulties during placement, venous thrombosis at the insertion site, filter migration, filter erosion through the IVC wall, and IVC obstruction. The majority of clinically significant complications involve insertion site thrombosis and IVC obstruction. When studied carefully, early insertion site thrombosis can be detected in as many as 25% of patients undergoing filter placement irrespective of filter type.

Anticoagulant therapy is critical following placement of an IVC filter in the setting of active thrombosis. While filter insertion may protect the pulmonary vascular bed, it does not affect the growth characteristics of the existing thrombus, the underlying thrombotic diathesis, or the long-term symptomatic outcome of the disease. Patients with active venous thromboembolism in whom IVC filters are placed and who are *not* anticoagulated are at risk, in the short term, for proximal extension of the existing thrombus, recurrent pulmonary embolism, or insertion site thrombosis, and, in the long term, for the development of IVC obstruction, recurrent venous thrombosis, or postphlebitic syndrome. Recent data have confirmed that an initial episode of venous thrombosis is associated with an increased risk for recurrent thromboembolic events that may persist for years, and that such episodes of recurrence are strongly associated with the subsequent risk of postphlebitic syndrome. Therefore, even when a filter has been placed for anticoagulant-related bleeding complications, every effort should be made to identify and correct the source of bleeding and to reinstitute anticoagulant therapy when clinically prudent to do so. The need for anticoagulation when filters are placed for purely prophylactic indications has not been established. However, given the incidence of early insertion site thrombosis, sequential noninvasive testing should be considered if anticoagulation is not provided. IVC filter placement can be a lifesaving procedure under appropriate circumstances. However, physicians should be aware that the decision to do so is irrevocable, and, given the absence of long-term follow-up studies, one that should be made with due consideration.

In the present patient, pulmonary angiography (see figure) demonstrated intraluminal filling defects involving the main, lobar, and segmental arteries, consistent with pulmonary embolism. Anticoagulation with intravenous, unfractionated heparin was initiated, maintaining the activated partial thromboplastin time at 1.5–2.5 times control, and an IVC filter was placed *without* interruption of the anticoagulation. The recent surgical procedure in this patient contraindicated the use of thrombolytic agents. Normalization of the blood pressure and pulse rate occurred within 48 hours of admission. Intravenous heparin therapy was continued for 7 days and the patient was discharged on the 9th hospital day on oral warfarin. Perfusion scan obtained 6 weeks following the acute event revealed two left lower lobe subsegmental defects. Repeat echocardiogram at that time demonstrated normalization of the right atrial and right ventricular chamber size and an estimated pulmonary artery pressure within normal range. Given that the embolic event occurred in the setting of a well-defined predisposition (surgery under general anesthesia), anticoagulation will be discontinued after the patient has completed a full 6-month course.

Clinical Pearls

1. Patients with pulmonary embolism who present with shock have a mortality at least three- to four-fold greater than those without shock.

2. Accepted indications for placement of an IVC filter in patients with proximal venous thrombosis or pulmonary embolism include: (1) contraindication to anticoagulant therapy (recent surgery or trauma, hemorrhagic stroke, active bleeding, or serious complication of heparin therapy including hemorrhage or thrombocytopenia); (2) recurrence of embolism despite adequate anticoagulation; and, (3) anatomically or hemodynamically massive embolism when a recurrent PE may be fatal.

3. IVC filter placement should *not* be considered as an adequate, solitary form of therapy in patients with active venous thromboembolism unless an absolute and irreversible contraindication to anticoagulation exists.

REFERENCES

1. Dalen JE, Alpert JS: Natural history of pulmonary embolism. Prog Cardiovasc Dis 17: 259–270,1975.
2. Stein PD, Terrin ML, Hales CA, et al: Clinical, laboratory, roentgenographic, and electrocardiographic findings in patients with acute pulmonary embolism and no pre-existing cardiac or pulmonary disease. Chest 100:598–603, 1991.
3. Becker DM, Philbrick JT, Selby JB: Inferior vena caval filters: Indications, safety, effectiveness. Arch Intern Med 1992; 152: 1985–1994.
4. Carson JL, Kelley MA, Duff, et al: The clinical course of pulmonary embolism. N Engl J Med 1992; 326: 1240–1245.
5. Prandoni P, Lensing AW, Cogo A, et al: The long-term clinical course of acute deep venous thrombosis. Ann Intern Med 1996; 125: 1–7.
6. Decousus H, Leizorovicz A, Parent F, et al. A clinical trial of vena caval filters in the prevention of pulmonary embolism in patients with proximal deep-vein thrombosis. N Engl J Med 1998; 338: 409-415.
7. Afzal A, Noor HA, Shazia AG, et al: Leukocytosis in acute pulmonary embolism. Chest 1999; 115: 1329–1332.
8. Koutkia P, Wachtel TJ: Pulmonary embolism presenting as syncope: Case report and review of the literature. Heart Lung 1999; 28: 342–347.
9. Stein PD, Afzal A, Henry JW, Villareal CG: Fever in acute pulmonary embolism. Chest 2000; 117: 39–42.

Michel A. Boivin, MD
Howard Levy, MD, PhD

PATIENT 16

A 21-year-old woman with worsening asthma, cough, and sputum production

A 21-year-old woman with a history of asthma presents to the emergency department (ED) with a 2-day history of worsening shortness of breath. She complains of new, greenish sputum production and an increasing cough with wheezing. Her medications include inhaled triamcinolone, albuterol, montelukast, and fluoxetine. She has not visited the ED in the past year for asthma, and has never been mechanically ventilated. The patient is treated for worsening asthma, but does not improve despite repeated treatment with β_2-agonists, so she is intubated for worsening respiratory distress. A subclavian venous catheter and radial arterial line are placed. The patient is paralyzed with vecuronium to improve patient-ventilator synchrony. She becomes hypotensive 1 hour after admission, and dopamine is started. Tachycardia worsens over the next hour, with continued hypotension. The patient abruptly develops pulseless electrical activity. Review of a chest x-ray discloses a tension pneumothorax. Needle decompression and chest tube insertion are performed, and blood pressure returns 2 minutes after its loss. Subsequently, her respiratory function gradually improves. Oliguric renal failure and shock liver develop over the next day. In light of her multi-organ dysfunction, a CT scan of the head is performed to assess if she has sustained any injury.

Physical Examination: Pulse 110, blood pressure 130/70, temperature 37.5° C. General: obese, chemically paralyzed, and intubated. Neurological: pupils 2 mm and reactive. HEENT: unremarkable. Chest: diffuse bilateral wheezes. Cardiac: regular rhythm; no murmurs, rubs, or gallops. Abdomen: no masses felt. Extremities: 2+ pedal edema; otherwise unremarkable.

Laboratory Examination: WBC 23,000/μl, Hct 33%, platelets 154. BUN 48 mg/dl, creatinine 4.5 mg/dl (renal function normal on admission). Remainder of electrolytes: normal. ALT 2568, total bilirubin 0.5 mg/dl. CT scan of the head (see figures): wedge-shaped infarctions in the left frontal and left parieto-occipital areas (*arrowheads*); not shown is an additional right cerebellar infarct.

Question: What caused the patient's cerebral and cerebellar infarctions?

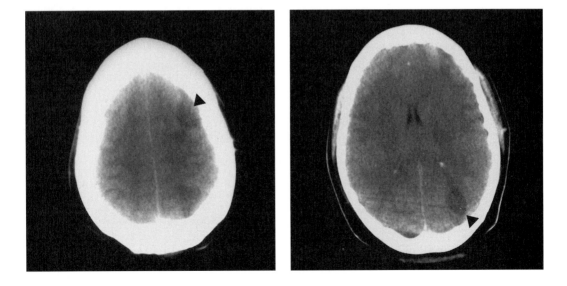

Answer: Arterial air embolism.

Discussion: Gas embolism can occur in various circumstances, including surgery (particularly head-up neurosurgery or cardiopulmonary bypass), cesarean section or vaginal delivery, insertion or removal of central venous catheters, mechanical ventilation, diving accidents, transthoracic needle biopsy, and pulmonary barotrauma. The present patient had three of these risk factors. In addition, gases other than air can embolize, including nitrogen, carbon dioxide, and argon. Physiologically, air embolism has different effects depending on whether air enters the venous or arterial tree.

Venous gas embolism can occur anytime a non-collapsible vein is exposed to the atmosphere, and the atmospheric pressure is greater than the venous pressure. Air bubbles gradually occlude the pulmonary circulation, causing pulmonary hypertension, hypoxia, increased dead-space, and, eventually, cor pulmonale and right ventricular collapse. Larger volumes (50 ml or greater) can cause immediate cardiovascular collapse. Diagnosis is made by clinical suspicion in an appropriate setting, auscultating a mill-wheel murmur (splashing sound), and signs of right ventricular strain on EKG, hemodynamic monitoring, or cardiac ultrasonography. Treatment consists of removal of the cause, intravascular volume loading (to decrease gradient for air entry) and inotropes and pressors to maintain hemodynamic stability, and 100% oxygen to increase the gradient for nitrogen egress from the bubbles. Numerous methods and positions for removal of right ventricular air using catheters are described.

Arterial air embolism occurs under different circumstances, for example when pulmonary veins are opened to the atmosphere, such as during pneumothorax, or when catheters are placed directly in the heart, such as during cardiac bypass. Furthermore, arterial air embolism can occur after venous embolism if a right-to-left shunt occurs (especially a patent foramen ovale, which may open due to elevated right-sided pressures). In addition, massive venous air embolism can cause air to "overflow" into the arterial circulation, even in the absence of right-to-left shunting. The symptoms of arterial air embolism are mostly cerebral and include headache, confusion, weakness, and generalized seizure or coma, as well as any focal deficit. Other organ systems are affected, although the primary symptomatology is usually cerebral.

Diagnosis typically is clinical, based on an appropriate setting and elimination of other causes. CT of the head reveals infarctions and or diffuse edema. Occasionally, air can be visualized within the arterial tree. Treatment involves removal of the offending cause, intravascular volume loading, 100% oxygen, and, if available, hyperbaric oxygen. This latter therapy greatly increases the partial pressure of oxygen in the bloodstream, causing a much greater gradient for the exit of nitrogen and reducing bubble size. The greater ambient pressures also physically shrink the bubbles.

While not all causes are preventable in patients in intensive care, the most important measure is to *pay close attention to vascular devices*, always having patients in a head-down position (or leg-down with lower extremity lines) when inserting *or removing* central venous catheters. Catheter lumens should never be open to the atmosphere during the procedure. Pulmonary barotrauma should be avoided whenever possible.

In the present patient, the diagnosis of arterial air embolism was determined by the multiple territories of the cerebral infarctions, without other cause. A transesophageal echocardiogram demonstrated no patent foramen ovale or valve lesions. The diagnosis was delayed due to confounding factors (paralysis), and it was too late to institute hyperbaric therapy. After a long hospital stay and rehabilitation, she eventually made a good recovery.

Clinical Pearls

1. Suspect venous embolism when sudden cardio-pulmonary deterioration occurs shortly after central line placement or at-risk surgical procedures.

2. Suspect arterial embolism in a patient with cerebral impairment after pulmonary barotrauma, mechanical ventilation or cardio-pulmonary bypass.

3. Suspect arterial embolism in the patient who survives a venous embolic event but has cerebral impairment.

REFERENCES

1. Palmon SC, Moore LE, Lundberg J, et.al. Venous Air Embolism: a Review. J of Clin Anaes 1997: 9; 251-257.
2. Ibrahim AE, Stanwood PL, Freund PR. Pneumothorax and Systemic Air Embolism during Positive-Pressure Ventilation. Anaesthesiology 1999: 90(5); 1479-1481.
3. Muth CM, Shank ES. Gas Embolism. NEJM 2000; 342(7): 476-482.

Matthew Esson, MD
Tomas Berl, MD

PATIENT 17

A 68-year-old diabetic woman with chronic renal failure, a COPD exacerbation, and an acid-base disturbance

A 68-year-old woman with a history of type II diabetes mellitus, chronic renal failure (serum creatinine 1.8–2.0 mg/dl), and hypertension is admitted to the hospital with a COPD exacerbation. Medications on admission include glyburide, nifedipine, theophylline, and beclomethasone inhaler. She is placed on bronchodilators and systemic steroids. While hemodynamically stable, progressive hypercapnea and marked acidosis develop. Her chest x-ray demonstrates cardiomegaly and hyperinflation, but no infiltrates. Due to her refusal of intubation, she is treated conservatively.

Physical Examination: Blood pressure: 150/98. Fundi: proliferative retinopathy. Neck: no jugular venous distention. Chest: diffuse wheezing. Cardiac: S4. Abdomen: normal. Extremities: no edema.

Laboratory Findings:

	Hospital Day				
Serum	1	3	5	7	9
Glucose, mg/dl	142	147	152	155	160
Creatinine, mg/dl	1.9	1.8	1.9	1.9	2.1
Sodium, mEq/L	140	144	142	142	145
Potassium, mEq/L	5.8	6.0	5.9	3.9	4.2
Chloride, mEq/L	112	114	113	109	105
HCO_3^-, mEq/L	19	20	20	23	30
Arterial blood					
pH	7.34	7.20	7.20	7.24	7.34
$PaCO_2$	35	55	54	56	55
PaO_2	75	82	84	88	90
Urine					
pH	5.2	5.1	5.2	5.3	5.2
Sodium, mEq/L	95	75	78	72	82
Potassium, mEq/L	35	32	36	15	8
Chloride, mEq/L	85	68	70	78	94
Net charge (Na + K – Cl)	45	39	44	9	–4

Question: What is this patient's acid base disorder on day three? What therapy should be initiated to correct it on the fifth hospital day?

Answer: Hyperkalemia of type IV renal tubular acidosis.

Discussion: The kidney is an important regulator of acid base status. To remain in balance, the kidney must excrete the approximately one mmol/kg body weight of acid generated by the average western diet daily. Net acid excretion by the kidney is determined by the reabsorption of filtered bicarbonate and by the excretion of ammonium and titratable acid primarily in the form of phosphate. Disorders in any of these processes can lead to a metabolic acidosis. **Impaired renal ammoniagenesis** is characteristic of acute and chronic renal failure, and is primarily responsible for the acidosis of type IV distal RTA.

Ammonium excretion in the urine is the result of an interplay of factors, including the generation and secretion of ammonium by cells in the proximal tubule, reabsorption in the medullary thick ascending limb of the loop of Henle, and secretion into the distal convoluted tubules and cortical and medullary collecting duct. Hyperkalemia can impair ammonium excretion by interfering at a number of these steps. The enzymes responsible for the generation of ammonium in the proximal tubule cell are glutaminase and phosphoenolpyruvate carboxykinase. Glutaminase is upregulated by metabolic and respiratory acidosis, and downregulated by hyperkalemia. In animals, hyperkalemia also has been shown to impair secretion of ammonium from the interstitium into the collecting duct. These two processes result in decreased ammonium excretion and hyperkalemic metabolic acidosis.

A variety of factors can contribute to hyperkalemia, including diet, drugs, and mineralocorticoid-deficient and -resistant states. In the present patient, hyperkalemia was the result of the **hyporeninemic hypoaldosterone state characteristic of many diabetics**. Hypoaldosteronism leads to impaired renal potassium excretion and hyperkalemia. Hyperkalemia in turn contributes to impaired ammoniagenesis and metabolic acidosis (see figure).

The modest hyperkalemia and metabolic acidosis of a type IV RTA often are well tolerated clinically. Over the long term, however, chronic metabolic acidosis leads to buffering of acid by bone hydroxyapatite, calcium loss, and osteopenia. Marked hyperkalemia may result when the kidney's potassium excretory capacity is further hampered by the addition of angiotensin-converting enzyme inhibitors or potassium-sparing diuretics. Additionally, the kidney's impaired ammoniagenesis will result in inability to compensate for superimposed metabolic acidosis, such as diarrhea, or respiratory acidosis. As seen in the present patient, when stressed to muster a metabolic response to a respiratory

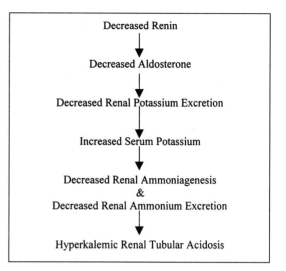

Pathogenesis of hyperkalemic renal tubular acidosis due to hyporenemic hypoaldosteronism.

acidosis, her inability to increase ammonium excretion resulted in a severe acidosis.

When confronted with a nonanion gap metabolic acidosis, the separation of renal from nonrenal causes often can be accomplished by history alone. Further assistance can be obtained from the examination of the urine net charge. As previously stated, the kidney is responsible for excreting approximately 1 mmol/kg body weight of acid/day, and at baseline the kidney will excrete >30 mEq of NH_4^+ daily. In response to a superimposed acidotic state, e.g., due to diarrhea or respiratory failure, this can increase several fold. The urinary net charge assumes that the sum of urinary cations (largely Na^+, K^+, and NH_4^+) equals the sum of urinary anions (largely Cl^-). As NH_4^+ ordinarily is not measured, the urinary net charge is normally negative:

Urine net charge = [Na] + [K] – [Cl]

In states of impaired ammoniagenesis, such as type IV RTA, the urine net charge may be zero or positive.

While the modest hyperkalemia and metabolic acidosis of a type IV RTA do not mandate intervention acutely, concerns for the long-term effect on bones suggest a benefit of treatment. Correction of the hyperkalemia with the use diuretics, and of the acidosis with $NaHCO_3$, may be beneficial. Alternatively, despite its low palatability, cation exchange resins such as sodium polystyrene (Kayexelate) effectively decrease potassium and result in improved ammonium excretion. Although mineralocorticoid deficiency underlies the disorder, the use of supraphysiologic doses of mineralocorticoid are undesirable due to the risk of volume overload and hypertension.

On the third day of her hospitalization, the present patient had a combined nonanion gap metabolic and respiratory acidosis. She was admitted with an underlying type IV distal renal tubular acidosis (RTA), also known as hyperkalemic renal tubular acidosis, due to hyporeninemic hypoaldosteronism, which is common in diabetics. The exacerbation of the COPD led to a superimposed respiratory acidosis. Initiation of sodium polystyrene therapy on the fifth hospital day to treat her hyperkalemia restored her kidney's ability to generate ammonium and thus compensate for her respiratory acidosis.

The hyperkalemia of the present patient's type IV RTA impaired her ability to metabolically compensate for her respiratory acidosis (respiratory failure). After sodium polystyrene was added on the fifth hospital day, her potassium decreased from 5.9 to 3.9 mEq/L over the ensuing 48 hours. As a result, her renal ammoniagenesis was restored, as demonstrated by a decrease in her urine net charge from 44 to 9 and then to −4, reflecting the appearance of ammonium in the urine. Her serum bicarbonate rose from 20 to 29 mEq/L by the ninth hospital day, allowing adequate compensation for her respiratory acidosis.

Clinical Pearls

1. Hyperkalemia impairs renal ammonium excretion by inhibiting proximal tubule ammoniagenesis and decreasing ammonium secretion into the distal nephron.

2. The correction of hyperkalemia can correct hyperkalemic metabolic acidosis (type IV RTA)

3. The inability of the kidney to increase ammoniagenesis in a type IV RTA leads to marked acidosis when coexisting respiratory or metabolic acidoses arise.

REFERENCES

1. Szylman P, Better O, Chaimowitz C, et al: Role of hyperkalemia in the metabolic acidosis of isolated hypoaldosteronism. N Engl J Med 1976;294:361–365.
2. DuBose T, Good D: Effects of chronic hyperkalemia on renal production and proximal tubule transport of ammonium in rats. Am J Phys 1991;260:F680–F 687.
3. DuBose T, Good D: Chronic hyperkalemia impairs ammonium transport and accumulation in the inner medulla of the rat. J Clin Invest 1992;90:1443–1449.
4. Battle D, Flores G: Underlying defects in distal renal tubular acidosis: New understandings. Am J Kidney Dis 1996;27:896–915.
5. DuBose T: Hyperkalemic hyperchloremic metabolic acidosis: Pathophysiologic insights. Kidney Int 1997;51:591–602.

C. Crawford Mechem, MD

PATIENT 18

A 29-year-old woman with dyspnea and chest pain

A 29-year-old woman with no significant past medical history comes to the emergency department with the acute onset of dyspnea and pleuritic chest pain. Her symptoms developed shortly prior to presentation while she was "partying" with friends. The patient denies recent cough, chest trauma, or prolonged immobilization. When further questioned, she admits that she was drinking alcohol and smoking crack cocaine when her symptoms developed. In the emergency department her room air pulse oximetry reading is 92%. Oxygen is administered by non-rebreather mask, with mild improvement of symptoms.

Physical Examination: Temperature 37.1°; pulse 112; respirations 28; blood pressure 102/60. General: thin and dyspneic; in obvious discomfort. HEENT: unremarkable. Cardiac: regular rate without murmurs. Neck: supple; no jugular venous distention. Chest: decreased breath sounds on right side. Abdomen: soft, nontender; bowel sounds present. Extremities: unremarkable.

Laboratory Findings: WBC and blood chemistries: normal. Electrocardiogram: sinus tachycardia with normal complexes and intervals. Chest radiograph: see below.

Question: What abnormality is present on the chest radiograph? What is the most likely etiology?

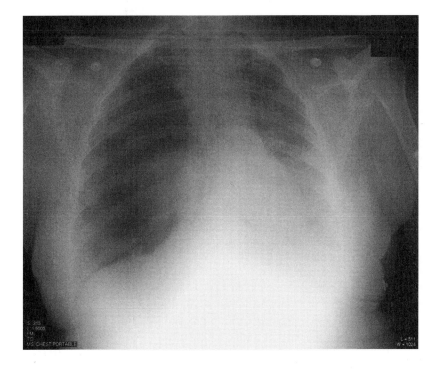

Diagnosis: Right-sided pneumothorax due to crack cocaine use.

Discussion: Pneumothorax is one of the many pulmonary complications associated with crack cocaine use. Pneumomediastinum or pneumopericardium also may be seen. These are manifestations of **barotrauma** resulting from increased airway pressures and alveolar rupture. Air subsequently dissects along fascial planes into the mediastinum, pericardium, neck, or pleural space. Barotrauma may result from the patient's coughing against a closed glottis or performing a Valsalva maneuver after inhaling in order to hasten absorption of the drug into the pulmonary circulation. Another cause of barotrauma is the practice of one person forcibly exhaling crack smoke into another person's mouth to enhance absorption. Finally, drug abusers with poor intravenous access may attempt to inject cocaine directly into a subclavian vein, a so-called "pocket shot," which can induce pneumothorax or pneumomediastinum.

Cocaine is an alkaloid extracted from the leaves of the shrub *Erythroxylon coca*. Cocaine hydrochloride is a heat-labile white powder that is snorted or injected intravenously. When it is boiled in water and baking soda and the resultant precipitate extracted with ether, the product is "crack": a heat-stable, free-base form that may be smoked. Its name comes from the characteristic crackling sound it makes when burned. Crack is rapidly absorbed into the pulmonary circulation and reaches the central nervous system in a matter for seconds.

While commonly associated with cardiac and behavioral effects, crack use can cause a variety of pulmonary complications in addition to barotrauma. Many crack users develop dyspnea, cough, pleuritic chest or back pain, and fever. Patients with underlying asthma can experience exacerbation of symptoms, while nonasthmatics can develop bronchospasm with wheezing. Hemoptysis or melanoptysis (black sputum production) may be noted. The local anesthetic properties of cocaine also predispose abusers to direct thermal injury to the airway from deep inhalation of hot smoke. "Crack lung" refers to a combination of fever, hypoxemia, hemoptysis, and eosinophilia that develops within 1–48 hours of crack use. Chest radiograph reveals diffuse alveolar, perihilar, or interstitial infiltrates. This may be a variation of Löffler's syndrome.

Chronic crack use can cause diffuse alveolar damage, alveolar hemorrhage, bronchiolitis obliterans with organizing pneumonia (BOOP), noncardiogenic pulmonary edema, pulmonary fibrosis, interstitial pneumonitis, pulmonary hypertension, and pulmonary infarction. Abnormalities of gas transfer and reduced carbon monoxide diffusion capacity also have been reported.

Barotrauma associated with techniques of smoking crack accounts for several of the pulmonary sequelae of cocaine abuse. The pathophysiology of cocaine's other pulmonary effects appears to involve a combination of tissue ischemia, direct cellular toxicity, effects on endothelial cells, and induction of an inflammatory response. Diagnosis of pulmonary complications of crack use is based on a careful history and physical examination, supplemented with determination of oxygenation and chest radiography. Laboratory studies are only valuable in excluding other potential etiologies for the patient's symptoms. Urine or serum toxicology screens may be helpful if the diagnosis is in doubt. Otherwise, they contribute little to the evaluation.

The management of pneumothorax will, in most cases, involve placement of a **thoracostomy tube** on the affected side. In clinically stable patients with small pneumothoraces, needle aspiration or expectant management may be considered. Treatment of other pulmonary complications of cocaine abuse is supportive. Oxygenation should be optimized. Bronchodilators are administered to patients with bronchospasm. Corticosteroids are appropriate for patients with crack-induced asthma exacerbation. The role of steroids in the management of "crack lung" is less clear. No large, prospective studies of the subject exist. However, steroid administration has been associated with improvement in some patients. In the presence of pulmonary infiltrates, administration of empiric antibiotics is prudent until infection is excluded by sputum cultures. Given the transient lifestyle of many cocaine abusers, the diagnoses of tuberculosis and HIV infection should be entertained in patients presenting with pulmonary infiltrates. Once stabilized, all patients should be referred for substance abuse counseling.

In the present patient, the diagnosis was made by physical examination and chest radiography. While initially reluctant to admit that she had been smoking crack, the patient ultimately revealed this information when pressed. This illustrates the value of a detailed history, including social history. A thoracostomy tube was placed on the right side with reexpansion of the lung, and the patient was admitted to a ward bed. She was discharged 2 days later with referral for out-patient substance abuse counseling.

Clinical Pearls

1. Because the pulmonary manifestations of crack toxicity may be nonspecific, a careful social history is helpful in making the diagnosis.

2. On initial presentation, "crack lung" may be indistinguishable from pneumonia.

3. Consider tuberculosis and HIV infection in patients presenting with pulmonary symptoms after cocaine abuse.

4. The role of corticosteroids in the management of non-asthma pulmonary complications of crack use is controversial.

REFERENCES

1. Forrester JM, Steele AW, Waldron JA, Parsons PE: Crack lung: An acute pulmonary syndrome with a spectrum of clinical and histopathologic findings. Am Rev Respir Dis 1990;142:462–467.
2. Tashkin DP, Gorelick D, Khalsa M, et al: Respiratory effects of cocaine freebasing among habitual cocaine users. J Addict Dis 1992;11:59–70.
3. Nadeem S, Nasir N, Israel RH: Löffler's syndrome secondary to crack cocaine. Chest 1994;105:1599–1600.
4. Albertson TE, Walby WF, Derlet RW: Stimulant-induced pulmonary toxicity. Chest 1995;108:1140–1149.
5. Haim DY, Lippmann ML, Goldberg SK, Walkenstein MD: The pulmonary complications of crack cocaine: A comprehensive review. Chest 1995;107:233–240.
6. Thadani PV: NIDA conference report on cardiopulmonary complications of "crack" cocaine use: Clinical manifestations and pathophysiology. Chest 1996;110:1072–1076.
7. Albertson TE, Walby WF: Respiratory toxicities from stimulant use. Clin Rev Allergy Immunol 1997;15:221–241.
8. Osborn HH, Tang M, Bradley K, Duncan BR: New-onset bronchospasm or recrudescence of asthma associated with cocaine abuse. Acad Emer Med 1997;4:689–692.

Thomas J. Kayani, MD
Thomas A. Golper, MD

PATIENT 19

A 49-year-old man with acute renal failure

A 49-year-old man with a long history of alcohol abuse and cirrhosis is admitted to the intensive care unit (ICU) with pancreatitis. Gram-negative sepsis with multisystem organ failure complicated by oliguric renal insufficiency subsequently develops. Obligatory fluid requirements result in massive volume overload. He becomes encephalopathic and increasingly obtunded, necessitating intubation. Anuria develops on hospital day number seven, along with systemic hypotension requiring vasopressor support. The ensuing metabolic and acid-base derangements led to nephrologic consultation.

Physical Examination: Temperature 38.3°; pulse 135; respirations 24; blood pressure 79/23 mmHg; weight 100 kg (increased 20 kg from admission). General: anasarca; jaundiced. HEENT: scleral icterus. Cardiac: 1/6 holosystolic murmur at apex. Chest: diffuse rhonchi and wheezes; decreased breath sounds at bases. Abdomen: distended; no bowel sounds. Extremities: pitting edema. Neurologic: asterixis; obtunded.

Laboratory Findings: WBC 24,000/μl with 10% bands. Sodium 127 mEq/L, potassium 5.7 mEq/L, chloride 93 mEq/L, bicarbonate 12 mEq/L, BUN 122 mg/dl, creatinine 5.3 mg/dl. Urine sodium < 10 mEq/L. Chest radiograph: pulmonary edema and bilateral pleural effusions.

Question: What mode of renal support would be appropriate for this patient?

Answer: Continuous renal replacement therapy (CRRT).

Discussion: The goal in acute renal failure is to provide renal support while awaiting recovery of native function. Patients do not have time to develop the adaptive responses that patients with end-stage renal disease achieve in regard to metabolic, acid-base, and extracellular water abnormalities. Therefore, renal replacement in patients with acute renal failure should be initiated before they develop progressive uremia.

CRRT was introduced in 1977 as a means to remove fluid in volume overloaded patients who were resistant to diuretics. Since that time, refinements have occurred in vascular access, volumetrically controlled pumps, membranes, anticoagulation in extracorporeal circuits, and replacement fluids. The veno-venous approach, requiring placement of a dual lumen catheter into a central vein in conjunction with a blood pump, has largely replaced arterio-venous techniques. Solute removal occurs either by convection or diffusion. **Hemofiltration** takes advantage of the frictional forces between water and solutes, known as *solvent drag*, as a pressure gradient is applied across a membrane to achieve convective clearance of molecules up to 5000 Daltons. Volume balance is maintained by replacing the amount of discarded ultrafiltrate with infusion of replacement fluid which resembles nonuremic plasma water. **Hemodialysis** removes smaller molecular weight molecules based on concentration gradients between dialysate and plasma. Combining the two methods in **hemodiafiltration** provides a broad spectrum of efficient solute removal.

ICU patients often have comorbid conditions—myocardial ischemia, gastrointestinal bleeding, sepsis, hepatic failure—that render them too hemodynamically unstable for rapid solute and fluid shifts associated with intermittent hemodialysis (IHD). The more gradual alterations provided by CRRT lead to less hypotension and cardiac arrhythmias. Ischemic tubular necrosis due to hypotension may delay recovery of renal function in patients with acute renal failure.

ICU patients with acute renal failure frequently become volume overloaded due to multiple intravenous medications, nutritional support, and volume trials. Fluid removal during IHD can only occur during the procedure, and the longer the procedure, the slower the rate of removal to protect hemodynamic stability. Instability generally precludes further ultrafiltration. CRRT allows complete control over fluid balance. The ultrafiltration rate can be altered based on hemodynamic status or obligatory fluid intake, or targeted to achieve a particular pulmonary capillary wedge pressure. As residual renal function declines, adjustment of the CRRT prescription is accomplished by increasing the dialysate inflow rate or the rate of ultrafiltration and replacement fluid administration. ICU patients often require total parenteral nutrition to provide nutritional support and prevent breakdown of endogenous body proteins. The large volume requirements associated with parenteral nutrition are easily accommodated by increasing the ultrafiltration rate in CRRT. Studies have shown a positive correlation between improved nutritional support and survival.

Likewise, replacement fluid and dialysate composition can be readily adjusted to achieve control of serum electrolytes or targeted to specific metabolic goals. Control over solute balance is dissociated from fluid balance. Lactate-buffered replacement solutions can worsen acidosis in patients with hepatic failure or prolonged hypotension who are unable to metabolize lactate. In these situations, bicarbonate-based fluids can be used.

In hypercatabolic patients with high urea generation rates, IHD will not maintain the BUN < 50–80 mg/dl. With continuous veno-venous hemodiafiltration (CVVHDF), urea clearances of 20–30 ml/min can be achieved and used to sustain milder levels of azotemia. Based on estimates of the urea generation rate and a desired BUN level, the required extracorporeal urea clearance rate can be calculated. In CVVHDF, the dialysate outflow rate—the sum of the inflow rate plus the ultrafiltration rate—equals this clearance rate.

Besides solute and fluid removal, CRRT has potential uses in several specialized situations. Body temperature regulation via heat loss in the extracorporeal circuit may be useful in hyperpyretic patients. Modulation of the body's inflammatory response by removal of certain cytokines or utilizing the absorptive capacity of the membrane for endotoxin elimination may play a role in the future treatment of sepsis. Patients with hepatic encephalopathy or neurologic trauma who undergo IHD may develop worsened neurologic dysfunction due to the dysequilibrium syndrome associated with rapid changes in serum osmolality. IHD has been shown to decrease cerebral perfusion pressure secondary to systemic hypotension, increase intracranial pressure due to intracellular fluid shifts, and induce seizures. CRRT causes slower changes in osmolality and is the therapy of choice in patients with cerebral edema.

CRRT may require constant **anticoagulation** to prevent clotting of the membrane and the extracoporeal circuit. Insufficient anticoagulation results in loss of solute removal capacity, while prolonged exposure increases the potential of bleeding. System clotting also interrupts the continuity of CRRT, further decreasing extracorporeal solute clearance rates. Patients with hepatic failure, coagulopathy, heparin-induced thrombocytopenia, or gastrointestinal bleeding can undergo therapy without anticoagulation, but will need replacement of clotted filters every 24–36 hours. Other drawbacks to CRRT include limited patient mobility due to vascular access and the continuous nature of the therapy; the potential for volume depletion if ultrafiltration is not closely monitored; air embolism or accidental disconnection of lines; and the increased expense compared with IHD.

In the present patient, CVVHDF was instituted for fluid management, permitting initiation of parenteral nutrition. A negative fluid balance despite persistent hypotension was achieved 24 hours after therapy was begun. His multisystem organ dysfunction and sepsis failed to improve, and the decision was made to withdraw all life-support therapy on hospital day sixteen.

Clinical Pearls

1. Solute balance can be manipulated independent of fluid balance.
2. Continuous therapies allow aggressive fluid management that can be targeted to specific hemodynamic parameters, and the slower rate of fluid removal protects hemodynamic stability.
3. Patients with cerebral edema and ARF are best served with CRRT.

REFERENCES

1. Kramer P, Wigger W, et al: Arteriovenous haemofiltration: A new and simple method for treatment of over-hydrated patients resistant to diuretics. Klin Wochenschr 1977;55:1121–1122.
2. Golper, TA: Continuous arteriovenous hemofiltration in acute renal failure. Am J Kidney Dis 1985;6:373–386.
3. Conger JD: Does hemodialysis delay recovery from ARF? Semin Dial 1990;3:146–148.
4. Golper TA: Indications, technical considerations, and strategies for renal replacement therapy in the intensive care unit. J Intensive Care Med 1992;7:310–317.
5. Bellomo R, Ronco C: Continuous versus intermittent renal replacement therapy in the intensive care unit. Kidney Int 1998;53S66:125–128.
6. Schetz M: Classical and alternative indications for continuous renal replacement therapy. Kidney Int 1998;53S66:129–132.
7. Davenport A: Is there a role for continuous renal replacement therapies in patients with liver and renal failure? Kidney International 1999;56S72:62–66.
8. Druml W: Metabolic aspects of continuous renal replacement therapies. Kidney Int 1999;56S72:56–61.

Bruce Y. Tung, MD
Kris V. Kowdley, MD

PATIENT 20

A 34 year-old man with ulcerative colitis, jaundice, pruritus, and low-grade fevers

A 34-year-old man with a history of ulcerative colitis presents with 1 week of jaundice, fatigue, and pruritus. He was diagnosed with ulcerative colitis at age 12, and underwent a subtotal colectomy at age 22 for subfulminant colitis. One week ago, he noted yellowness of the eyes, dark urine, and acholic stool. He has had low-grade fevers, fatigue, and generalized pruritus. He denies a history of known liver disease or intravenous drug use, but did require blood transfusions with his colectomy 12 years ago.

Physical Examination: Temperature 37.9°; pulse 68; respirations 22; blood pressure 108/72. General: thin; obvious jaundice. Skin: no spider angiomata or palmar erythema. HEENT: icteric sclerae, otherwise unremarkable. Cardiac: regular rhythm without murmur. Chest: clear. Abdomen: liver edge palpable 1 cm below costal margin, without tenderness; no splenomegaly or abdominal distension.

Laboratory Findings: WBC 6400/μl. Total bilirubin 12.9 mg/dl, direct bilirubin 10.3 mg/dl, albumin 3.3 g/dl, alkaline phosphatase 318 U/L, AST 125 U/L, ALT 108 U/L, prothrombin time 21.1 sec, INR 2.1. Abdominal ultrasound: dilation of common hepatic duct and intrahepatic ducts; gallbladder with sludge, but no stones. Endoscopic retrograde cholangiopancreatography (ECRP; see below): stricture of common bile duct (*white arrow*) with irregular, dilated common hepatic duct; abnormal intrahepatic ducts with areas of stricturing (*black arrow*) and dilation.

Question: What clinical condition explains this patient's symptoms and ERCP findings?

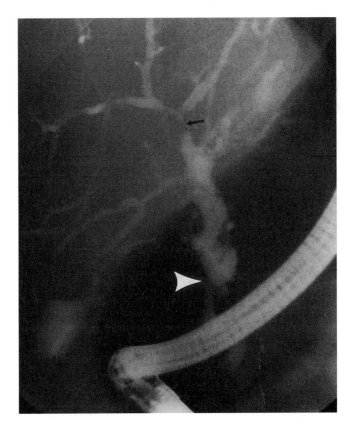

Answer: Primary sclerosing cholangitis.

Discussion: Primary sclerosing cholangitis (PSC) is a cholestatic liver disorder of unknown etiology that is characterized by inflammation, fibrosis, and destruction of the intra- and extrahepatic biliary tree. It is a chronic, progressive disorder that often leads to the development of biliary cirrhosis.

PSC is rare, with an estimated prevalence of 6 per 100,000. The mean age at diagnosis is 40 years, with a slight male predominance. One of the most interesting facets of PSC is its strong association with **inflammatory bowel disease:** 75–90% of PSC patients have underlying inflammatory bowel disease, and of these, 85–90% have **ulcerative colitis**. Overall, PSC affects 2–4% of all patients with ulcerative colitis.

The etiology of PSC is unknown, but because of its association with inflammatory bowel disease, chronic portal bacteremia has been postulated to play a role. However, there is no correlation between the severity of colitis and that of PSC. As illustrated in the present patient, PSC may develop years after colectomy. Alternatively, the diagnosis of PSC may precede the development of colitis. Other possible etiologic factors in the development of PSC include ischemic vascular injury, toxic bile acids, and disorders of immunoregulation.

Many patients are asymptomatic at the time of diagnosis. Elevations of serum alkaline phosphatase or bilirubin in a patient with inflammatory bowel disease should raise suspicion for the diagnosis of PSC. In some cases, features of low-grade bacterial cholangitis are present: fever, night sweats, right upper quadrant pain, and jaundice, often associated with pruritus.

Patients with PSC are at particularly high risk for the development of **cholangiocarcinoma**, which affects 10–15% of all PSC patients. This is a difficult diagnosis to make, as the sensitivities of endobiliary brush cytology and endobiliary biopsies are relatively poor. PSC patients with ulcerative colitis are also at an increased risk for **colorectal cancer**. The incidence of colonic dysplasia or cancer approaches 50% in PSC patients after 25 years of colitis. Other complications of PSC include steatorrhea due to inadequate concentration of bile salts for efficient fat emulsification, and osteoporosis, as seen in other cholestatic liver diseases.

The diagnosis of PSC is made cholangiographically, typically by endoscopic retrograde cholangiography. More recently, magnetic resonance cholangiography (MRC) has been developed to allow noninvasive evaluation of the biliary tract. MRC has largely supplanted the need to perform percutaneous transhepatic cholangiography. The typical cholangiographic appearance of PSC involves both intra- and extrahepatic biliary strictures. There often are alternating areas of stricturing and pre-stenotic dilation, leading to a chain-of-lakes appearance of the biliary tree. Dominant strictures should be brushed and/or biopsied to evaluate for cholangiocarcinoma. Liver biopsy is useful in staging the degree of hepatic fibrosis, and provides prognostic information. However, liver biopsy findings alone often are nonspecific for the diagnosis of PSC.

No specific treatment has been shown to conclusively alter the natural history of PSC. Dominant biliary strictures should be endoscopically or percutaneously dilated and/or stented. Although ursodiol therapy at a dose of 13–15 mg/kg/day improves serum biochemical markers of liver function, it does not delay the time to treatment failure or liver transplantation. Therefore, the routine use of ursodiol in patients with PSC is not currently supported by available data. Other medical therapies such as methotrexate, corticosteroids, azathioprine, D-penicillamine, colchicine, and cyclosporine have shown no clinical benefit in the treatment of PSC.

When hepatic decompensation develops, such as the onset of synthetic dysfunction (hypoalbuminemia or coagulopathy), ascites, or encephalopathy, consider liver transplantation. PSC patients with recurrent bouts of cholangitis that are difficult to medically manage also should be considered for liver transplantation. Overall, patients with PSC have an excellent prognosis after liver transplantation, with a 5-year patient survival rate exceeding 80%.

In the present patient, the diagnosis was made by characteristic cholangiographic findings at ERCP (see figure). The patient's common bile duct stricture was treated with successive endoscopic dilations and biliary stents. Although multiple endobiliary brushings were negative for malignancy, a mass was seen eroding into the duodenum at follow-up endoscopy. Biopsies of the duodenal mass showed poorly differentiated adenocarcinoma, most consistent with cholangiocarcinoma. Despite radiation therapy and chemotherapy, the patient died 5 months later.

Clinical Pearls

1. Patients with inflammatory bowel disease who have jaundice or asymptomatic elevations of serum alkaline phosphatase and/or serum bilirubin should undergo cholangiography to evaluate for primary sclerosing cholangitis.

2. Patients with primary sclerosing cholangitis are at significantly increased risk of developing cholangiocarcinoma, as well as colorectal carcinoma.

3. No medical therapy has been clearly proven to alter the natural history of primary sclerosing cholangitis.

4. Liver transplantation is an effective therapy for patients with advanced liver disease or recurrent cholangitis from primary sclerosing cholangitis.

REFERENCES

1. Lee YM, Kaplan MM: Primary sclerosing cholangitis. N Engl J Med 1995; 332;924–933.
2. Brentnall TA, Haggitt RC, Rabinovitch PS, et al: Risk and natural history of colonic neoplasia in patients with primary sclerosing cholangitis and ulcerative colitis. Gastro–enterology 1996; 110:331–338.
3. Lindor KD: Ursodiol for primary sclerosing cholangitis. N Engl J Med 1997; 336:691–695.
4. Graziadei IW, Wiesner RH, Marotta PJ, et al: Long-term results of patients undergoing liver transplantation for primary sclerosing cholangitis. Hepatology 1999; 30:1121–1127
5. Kim WR, Poterucha JJ, Wiesner RH, et al: The relative role of the Child-Pugh classification and the Mayo natural history model in the assessment of survival in patients with primary sclerosing cholangitis. Hepatology 1999; 29:1643–1648.

William D. Haire, MD

PATIENT 21

A 19-year-old man with pain and swelling in his left arm

A 19-year-old, previously healthy man presents with discomfort and "tightness" in his left arm for the last week, with more recent swelling in his left hand. He is a left-handed pitcher on a full athletic scholarship for his college baseball team. He hopes to base a professional athletic career on his ability as a "southpaw" pitcher.

Physical Examination:　Vital signs: normal. Extremities: slight asymmetry to arms and shoulder girdle, with left side slightly larger, compatible with either work hypertrophy of musculature or edema; ring on left-hand finger too tight to rotate, compressing soft tissues; ring on right hand fits normally.

Question:　Do the patient's complaints and clinical findings represent pathology, or a normal response to his protracted, vigorous use of his left arm and shoulder girdle?

Diagnosis: Axillary/subclavian vein thrombosis (Paget-Schroetter syndrome)

Discussion: Initially described in Europe in the 1880s independently by Drs. Paget and von Schroetter, Paget-Schroetter syndrome was first introduced to the American literature in 1934. Defined by spontaneous thrombosis of the veins of the upper arm, this syndrome has been considered to be a rare occurrence caused by unusually strenuous use of the arm. This relationship to exertion accounts for its alternative name of **effort thrombosis**.

Paget-Schroetter syndrome usually affects otherwise healthy, vigorous young people, as opposed to the more common type of axillo-subclavian vein thrombosis that occurs with the use of indwelling venous access devices. The latter syndrome affects older patients with severe underlying disease. The Paget-Schroetter syndrome usually results from an underlying anatomic abnormality that compresses the veins of the thoracic outlet, causing localized damage to the venous endothelium and distal "stasis" of venous blood flow that eventually results in thrombosis. The thrombus often propagates distally to involve the axillary and, less commonly, the cephlaic veins. The occluding lesion can be quite variable, but most often is due to compression against the first rib by hypertrophied scalene or subclavius tendons or between the clavicle and a cervical rib. Chronic compression of the vein and the resultant inflammatory reaction can lead to perivenous fibrosis, which may leave chronic venous obstruction even after surgical correction of the underlying anatomic lesion.

The anatomic abnormalities occasionally are bilateral, predisposing to contralateral thrombosis at a future date. Though not classically believed to be related to systemic "prothrombotic" states, such abnormalities can be found with some frequency—especially if there is no history suggestive of protracted vigorous use of the arm.

The diagnosis is relatively straightforward once the condition is considered. The main difficulties with diagnosis derive from its occurrence in outwardly healthy young people and the often subtle clinical findings. As in this patient, the subjective complaints often are out of proportion to the physical findings. Typically, patients have only subtle evidence of hand edema or, less commonly, enlarged subcutaneous collateral veins over the shoulder and chest. A number of imaging techniques, from ultrasound to MRI, can visualize the thrombus. Unfortunately, these non-invasive imaging techniques generally do not provide sufficient anatomic detail to guide therapy, which requires **venography**.

Clinical dilemmas are encountered when making therapeutic decisions. To make a logical therapeutic decision, clinicians need to accurately predict the natural history of the disease and the likely effects therapy will have on its course. Unfortunately, neither of these factors are predictable in patients with Paget-Schroetter syndrome. Classically, most patients with this condition are considered to have a poor prognosis, with symptoms of chronic venous insufficiency that cause protracted pain, swelling, and functional limitations. Recent prospective studies, however, suggest that severe symptoms occur in as little as 13% of patients. Because of the potential for a poor outcome and its frequent occurrence in patients who depend on vigorous use of their arms vocationally or for sports-related recreation, an aggressive approach to therapy usually is taken.

Considering these therapeutic uncertainties, the therapeutic approach must be tailored to match the patient's long-term lifestyle goals for the arm. More aggressive, risky, and costly treatments are reserved for patients who need to maintain full function of their arm, such as the present patient. In such patients, catheter-directed thrombolytic therapy followed by surgical correction of any remaining obstruction is a reasonable consideration. For other patients, anticoagulant therapy for 3 or more months, until the thrombus organizes, is an alternative approach. For those patients with persistent, debilitating symptoms of venous obstruction, surgical reconstruction of the venous drainage of the arm can be considered.

The present patient's severe symptoms, unilateral distribution of hand edema, and absence of lympadenopathy as a cause of lymphedema warranted further evaluation. An ultrasound examination demonstrated a noncompressible subclavian and axillary vein. Arm venography (see top figure, *arrow*) showed complete occlusion of the axillary vein. The patient was treated with catheter-directed fibrinolysis, which lysed the thrombus. A repeat venogram demonstrated a persistent obstruction in the middle portion of the subclavian vein (see bottom figure, *arrow*). This defect persisted after first rib resection and remained after balloon dilation. Stent placement was avoided because of reports of a high frequency of stent fractures when used in this location. Prolonged anticoagulant therapy was recommended, but declined by the patient because of his desire to maintain an active lifestyle. At a 5-year follow-up, the patient was asymptomatic (though not a professional pitcher). He declined follow-up imaging studies to determine patency of the subclavian vein.

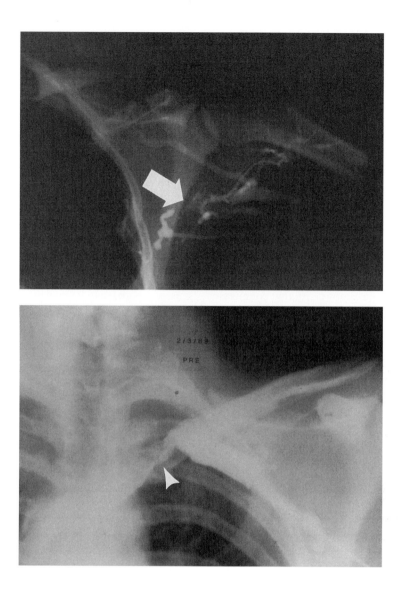

Clinical Pearls:

1. Subtle signs of hand and finger edema may be the only objective evidence of Paget-Schroetter syndrome.

2. As opposed to deep vein thrombosis of the legs, the cause of the Paget-Schroetter syndrome usually is mechanical venous damage and/or obstruction rather than a "hypercoagulable" state.

3. The natural course of the disease and response to therapy is not predictable for any specific patient, necessitating a highly individualized approach to treatment.

REFERENCES

1. Haire WD: Arm vein thrombosis. Clin Chest Med 1995;16:341–351.
2. Heron E, O Lozinguez O, Emmerich J, et al. Long term sequelae of spontaneous axillary-subclavian venous thrombosis. Ann Intern Med 1999:131;510-513.
3. Heron E, Lozinguez O, Alhenc-Gelas M, et al: Hypercoagulable states in primary upper-extremity deep vein thrombosis. Arch Intern Med 2000;160:382–386.

Steven M. Kawut, MD
Selim M. Arcasoy, MD

PATIENT 22

A 49-year-old man with left shoulder pain and arm weakness

A 49-year-old man presents with a 2-month history of left shoulder pain and left arm weakness. He denies cough, sputum production, hemoptysis, or weight loss. He has smoked three packs of cigarettes per day for 35 years.

Physical Examination: Vital signs: normal. General: no distress. HEENT: left ptosis. Cardiac: regular rate without murmurs. Chest: clear breath sounds. Abdomen: soft, nontender. Extremities: clubbing. Neurologic: decreased strength in left hand.

Laboratory Findings: Chest radiograph: see figure, *top*. Chest CT: see figure, *bottom*.

Question: What syndrome explains this patient's signs and symptoms?

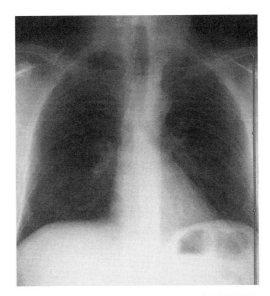

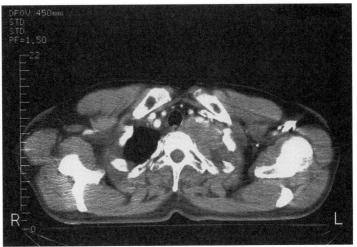

Diagnosis: Pancoast's syndrome.

Discussion: Pancoast's syndrome is defined by the presence of shoulder and arm pain, neurologic deficits in the distal upper extremity, or Horner's syndrome, usually caused by an apical lung tumor located at the thoracic inlet. These tumors also are called superior pulmonary sulcus tumors, apical chest tumors, or Pancoast's tumors. The vast majority are non-small cell bronchogenic carcinomas, usually squamous cell or adenocarcinoma. Other causes of Pancoast's syndrome include various primary and metastatic neoplasms, infection, and inflammatory and structural lesions.

The most common symptom upon presentation is **shoulder pain**, caused by involvement of the brachial plexus, parietal pleura, vertebral bodies, and ribs. The pain may radiate to the head, neck, scapula, axilla, anterior chest, or ipsilateral arm. Presumptive treatment for osteoarthritis or bursitis often leads to a delay in diagnosis. It is important to note that pulmonary symptoms are infrequent in the early stages of the disease.

Ipsilateral ptosis, miosis, and anhidrosis are the classic triad of **Horner's syndrome**, caused by invasion of the paravertebral sympathetic chain and the inferior cervical (stellate) ganglion. Irritation of the sympathetic chain prior to frank invasion may cause ipsilateral flushing and hyperhydrosis of the face before the development of Horner's syndrome.

Tumor extension to the C8 and T1 nerve roots results in pain or paresthesia along the distribution of the ulnar nerve, and weakness and atrophy of the intrinsic muscles of the hand. Tumor extension through the intervertebral foramina may cause spinal cord compression and paraplegia.

Chest radiographic findings of superior sulcus tumors include a unilateral apical cap, asymmetry of bilateral apical caps, an apical mass, and bony destruction. Computed tomography (CT) of the chest provides information about the extent of disease and may identify unsuspected pulmonary nodules, parenchymal disease, chest wall involvement, and mediastinal lymphadenopathy. Magnetic resonance imaging is especially useful to evaluate the brachial plexus, subclavian vessels, vertebral bodies, and spinal canal for tumor extension.

The diagnostic yield of sputum cytology is low in the work-up of superior sulcus tumors. Fiberoptic bronchoscopy with cytology and biopsy may provide a diagnosis in 30–40% of patients. The highest diagnostic yield is achieved with **percutaneous transthoracic needle biopsy**, which may be performed via a posterior or cervical approach, guided by fluoroscopy, ultrasonography, or CT. Video-assisted thoracoscopy or thoracotomy is performed if less invasive methods are nondiagnostic. A definitive diagnosis is required before embarking on therapy, because of the many etiologies of Pancoast's syndrome.

Superior sulcus tumors are staged in a fashion similar to other non-small cell bronchogenic carcinomas. Detailed history, physical examination, and blood tests are performed to evaluate the presence of distant metastases. CT of the chest and abdomen should be obtained to examine the mediastinum, liver, and adrenal glands. Bone scanning also may be indicated. Although not routinely recommended for asymptomatic patients with bronchogenic carcinoma, preoperative neuroimaging should be performed in all patients with superior sulcus tumors who are surgical candidates because of the high incidence of brain metastases. By definition, Pancoast's tumors are classified as T3 (chest wall involvement) or T4 lesions (invasion of the brachial plexus, mediastinal structures, or vertebral bodies). In the absence of distant metastases, these tumors are stage IIB or III (A or B).

Superior sulcus tumors are best treated with complete surgical resection. Preoperative radiotherapy frequently is used, despite a lack of conclusive evidence of benefit. In this approach, surgery usually is performed 2–4 weeks after completion of radiotherapy. As with other forms of non-small cell lung cancer, lobectomy is the procedure of choice for Pancoast's tumors. Surgical treatment usually involves en bloc resection of the tumor and chest wall and may require additional resection of subclavian vessels, lower trunks of the brachial plexus, paravertebral sympathetic chain, stellate ganglion, or portions of thoracic vertebrate. Surgical mortality is approximately 5–10%.

Radiotherapy is used as a primary treatment for patients with inoperable tumors or contraindications to surgery. This therapy appears to result in palliation of pain in most patients. Despite reported benefit of intraoperative or postoperative radiotherapy, the efficacy of this modality as an adjunct to complete resection is unproven, and it should be reserved for patients who are found to have unresectable tumors during surgery. The role of neoadjuvant chemotherapy for Pancoast's tumors is not clearly defined at this time.

The overall 5-year survival rate following combined preoperative radiotherapy and surgical resection is 20–35%, with a median survival of 7 to 31 months. With radiotherapy alone, the overall 5-year survival rate is 0–29%. Since patients with medical comorbidities and advanced-stage disease are more likely to receive primary radiotherapy, the pronounced differences in survival probably reflect this bias in patient selection, as well as efficacy. Good performance status and lack of significant weight loss are associated with improved survival. The presence of Horner's syndrome, tumor extension to the base of the neck, vertebral bodies or great vessels, or mediastinal lymph node involvement is associated with a worse prognosis.

In the present patient, the chest radiograph demonstrated a left apical cap, which was confirmed to be an apical mass by the chest CT scan. A diagnosis of squamous cell carcinoma was made by CT-guided transthoracic needle biopsy. Further work-up revealed Stage IIB disease. The patient underwent preoperative radiotherapy and surgical resection, and has done well postoperatively.

Clinical Pearls

1. Pancoast's syndrome usually is caused by non-small cell bronchogenic carcinoma.
2. Diagnosis of Pancoast's tumors is typically delayed for several months due to lack of pulmonary complaints. A high index of suspicion and careful review of radiographic studies are required for early diagnosis in patients with compatible signs and symptoms.
3. Histologic diagnosis should be established prior to treatment.

REFERENCES:
1. Pancoast HK: Superior pulmonary sulcus tumor: Tumor characterized by pain, Horner's syndrome, destruction of bone, and atrophy of hand muscles. JAMA 1932;99:1391–1396.
2. Arcasoy SM, Jett JR: Superior pulmonary sulcus tumors and Pancoast's syndrome. N Engl J Med 1997;337:1370–1376.
3. Detterbeck FC: Pancoast (superior sulcus) tumors. Ann Thorac Surg 1997;63:1810–1818.

John R. Bach, MD

PATIENT 23

A 15-year-old boy with a spinal cord injury and respiratory compromise

A 15-year-old boy was admitted to a trauma center after a diving accident in a local lake. While swimming with friends, he dove into a shallow area and struck his head on the lake bottom. His friends pulled him to shore and called an ambulance because he could not move his arms or legs.

Physical Examination: Vital signs: normal. General: awake and alert, but anxious; no respiratory complaints. Chest: clear. Cardiac: normal heart sounds. Neurologic: complete, flaccid paralysis of all extremities; motor level defect C2 tetraplegia.

Laboratory Findings: Chest radiograph: normal. Spine films: odontoid fracture.

Hospital Course: The patient was managed with neck stabilization bracing. On the day after admission, he complained of anxiety, difficulty falling asleep, and a sensation of not being able to take a deep breath. His vital capacity was 750 ml, and an ABG (room air) demonstrated a $PaCO_2$ of 55 mmHg.

Question: What complication of the patient's spinal cord injury is likely to occur? How should the patient be managed?

Answer: Respiratory failure related to spinal cord injury. Available management includes noninvasive ventilation.

Discussion: Spinal cord injuries present a considerable risk for respiratory complications, with up to 40% of patients developing ventilatory failure 1 to 6 days after the initial spinal injury. Respiratory muscle paralysis decreases the ability of patients to cough, which results in retained secretions and respiratory compromise. Muscle weakness further impairs ventilatory capacity, resulting in decreased vital capacity and progressive hypoventilation. When ambulatory patients with neuromuscular disorders develop ventilatory failure, dyspnea typically is the initial clinical manifestation. Dyspnea usually does not occur, however, in nonambulatory patients with spinal cord injuries who experience respiratory compromise. These patients often report anxiety and difficulty falling asleep as the initial portends of respiratory failure.

Conventional management of ventilatory failure due to spinal cord injury entails intubation and mechanical ventilation. Intubation, however, presents considerable risks for colonization of the airway with bacterial pathogens that promote increased airway secretions and risks for nosocomial pneumonia. Nosocomial pneumonia increases mortality and delays transfer to acute rehabilitation hospitals. Some trauma centers, therefore, manage some patients with spinal cord injuries and tetraplegia with alternative noninvasive ventilatory approaches.

Noninvasive methods for improving coughing and the mobilization of airway secretions is one alternative approach for ventilatory assistance. **Cough flows** can be increased by manually and mechanically assisted coughing. Because a normal cough expels approximately 2.3 L of air at flows of 6 to 20 L/sec, patients with vital capacities below approximately 1.5 L have a compromised cough. These patients need assistance to inhale a large volume of air or to "air stack" smaller volumes of air before coughing. The In-exsufflator (J. H. Emerson Co., Cambridge, MA) provides this assistance by delivering a deep insufflation, usually at a pressure of 40 to 60 cm H_2O, followed immediately by a deep exsufflation, usually at –40 to –60 cm H_2O. A manual abdominal thrust delivered by a bedside caregiver timed to the opening of the patient's glottis can also promote forceful expiration and an effective cough. With an abdominal thrust provided in conjunction with the In-exsufflator, coughing is maximally assisted.

Noninvasive positive-pressure ventilation is an alternative ventilatory approach that does not require airway intubation. Patient breathing is assisted by an **intermittent positive-pressure ventilation** (IPPV) device interfaced with the patient by a mouthpiece with or without a lipseal or a nasal or oro-nasal mask. Mouthpiece IPPV is most useful for long-term support during daytime hours. Some patients also may interface with IPPV through a mouthpiece without a lipseal during sleep, if they have an intact chemotaxic drive. They develop reflex efforts to periodically seal their lips during sleep to limit an airleak and promote full inspiration.

Most reports of the effectiveness of noninvasive ventilation have studied patients with chronic lung diseases, such as chronic obstructive pulmonary disease or asthma, during acute exacerbations of their airway disease. Reports of patients with neuromuscular disease usually have focused on the nocturnal use of noninvasive IPPV during sleep. Noninvasive ventilation also has been used continuously, 24 hours a day, for hundreds of patients in a few medical centers. Long-term, intermittent use of noninvasive IPPV can be used for patients with chronic neuromuscular conditions during potential episodes of respiratory failure—which would be precipitated by a weakened ability to cough during upper respiratory tract infections. These episodes can be prevented by the use of expiratory muscle aids.

Although only a limited number of centers regularly use noninvasive IPPV during the acute phase of spinal cord injury, this mode of ventilation combined with assisted coughing has been reported to be an effective substitute for intubation and tracheostomy in over 800 patients with neuromuscular disease or spinal cord injury. Unfortunately, only 20% of patients with traumatic quadraplegia and respiratory muscle failure admitted to level 1 trauma centers are candidates for noninvasive ventilation.

The present patient initially was managed with a chest shell ventilator, which improved his tidal volume and $PaCO_2$. He became dependent on the shell ventilator, which had to be removed 4 days later when he underwent placement of a halo brace with an anterior chest apron. He was switched to a portable volume ventilator for continuous IPPV, which can be used with a mouth piece (see figure, *left*); a mouth piece with lipseal retention (Malincrodt, Pickering, Ontario) for sleep (see figure, *right*); or a nasal continuous positive airway pressure mask. He chose to use a simple mouth piece during the day and a mouth piece with lipseal at night. During the next 2 weeks, he was progressively weaned from noninvasive IPPV support as his vital capacity improved.

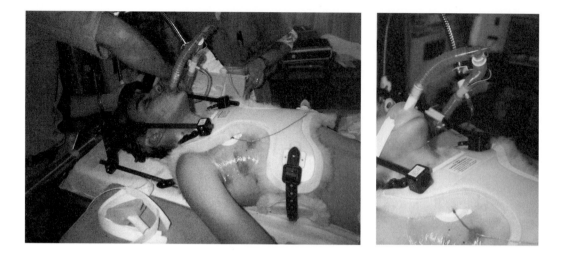

Clinical Pearls

1. Dyspnea portents respiratory failure for ambulatory patients with lung disease or ventilatory pump weakness. Anxiety and inability to fall asleep more commonly herald respiratory failure for nonambulatory patients with neuromuscular weakness.

2. Noninvasive IPPV with assisted coughing provide an effective approach in approximately 10% of patients with acute spinal cord injury to manage respiratory failure and avoid airway intubation.

3. Measure vital capacity (VC) every 6 hours during the first several days after admission of a patient with acute spinal cord injury. Symptoms or signs of respiratory failure or a VC less than 1.5 L signifies a need for continuous pulse oximetry and training of the patient for noninvasive IPPV with assisted coughing. Avoid using supplemental oxygen, unless the patient has coexisting lung disease or requires intubation.

4. Noninvasive ventilation for patients with ventilatory pump failure (VC < 1.5 L) is best provided by portable volume-cycled ventilators. Portable pressure-cycled and ICU volume-cycled ventilators are impractical: the patient cannot air stack with the former, and the volume alarm systems on the latter sound inappropriately when patients use noninvasive IPPV intermittently or exhale through their mouths, so that air does not flow back into the ventilator system.

REFERENCES

1. Raphael J-C, Chevret S, Chastang C, Bouvet F: Randomised trial of preventive nasal ventilation in Duchenne muscular dystrophy. Lancet 1994;343:1600–1604.
2. Bach JR, Robert D, Leger P, Langevin B: Sleep fragmentation in kyphoscoliotic individuals with alveolar hypoventilation treated by nasal IPPV. Chest 1995;107:1552–1558.
3. Bach JR (ed): Pulmonary Rehabilitation: The Obstructive and Paralytic Conditions. Philadelphia, Hanley & Belfus, Inc., 1996.
4. Bach JR, Saporito LR: Criteria for extubation and tracheostomy tube removal for patients with ventilatory failure: A different approach to weaning. Chest 1996;110:1566–1571.
5. Bach JR, Ishikawa Y, Kim H: Prevention of pulmonary morbidity for patients with Duchenne muscular dystrophy. Chest 1997;112:1024–1028.
6. Bach JR, Rajaraman R, Ballanger F, et al: Neuromuscular ventilatory insufficiency: The effect of home mechanical ventilator use vs. oxygen therapy on pneumonia and hospitalization rates. Am J Phys Med Rehabil 1998;77:8–19.

Andrew P. Keaveny MB, MRCPI
Nezam H. Afdhal MD, FRCPI

PATIENT 24

A 44-year-old woman with sonographic evidence of gallstones

A 44-year-old woman presents with increased belching and nausea. She had been adhering strictly to an 800-kilocalorie/day weight-reducing diet for the management of obesity for the previous 4 months. During that time, she reduced her weight from 290 pounds to 234 pounds. While following the diet, the patient experienced no gastrointestinal symptoms. She now notes the onset of belching and nausea after resuming a regular diet. The patient has a history of diabetes mellitus and mild hypertension.

Physical Examination: Vital signs: normal: General: morbidly obese. Abdomen: normal bowel sounds, no organomegaly.

Laboratory Findings: CBC, electrolytes, renal indices, liver function tests: normal. Abdominal ultrasound: multiple defects within the gallbladder with echogenic shadows, diagnostic of gallstones (see figure). Radiological Murphy's sign: negative.

Question: Are the patient's symptoms related to the finding of gallstones? How should the patient be advised regarding her gallstones?

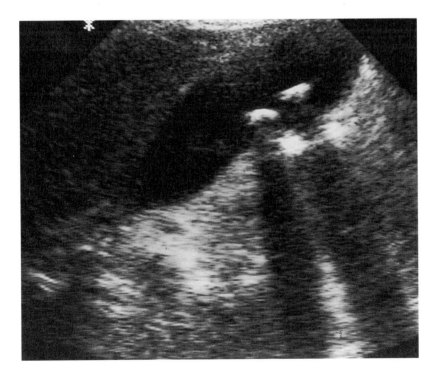

Answer: Her symptoms are not related to the finding of gallstones. Watchful waiting is advisable.

Discussion: Multiple risk factors exist for the development of gallstones. Female gender, older age, obesity, parity, rapid weight loss, and hypertryglyceridemia are commonly associated with the disease. Other risk factors include genetic background (higher risk in Pima Indians and Chileans), use of certain medications (e.g., estrogen, clofibrate, ceftriaxone, sandostatin), terminal ileal resection, gallbladder hypomotility (pregnancy, diabetes mellitus, post-vagotomy), somatostatinomas, total parenteral nutrition, and spinal cord injury

The prevalence of gallstones, as determined by screening ultrasonography, is 15% and 7% in adult women and men, respectively. Approximately 80% of affected individuals are asymptomatic, with so-called **incidental gallstones**. Twenty to 25% of persons with incidental gallstones become symptomatic with biliary pain within 20 years. The 1–2% chance per year of having an episode of biliary pain may actually decrease over time. Pain precedes the development of gallstone-related complications in over 90% of patients.

Although no prospective studies have evaluated the relative benefits of different therapeutic approaches to patients with asymptomatic gallstones, decision analysis models in the pre-laparoscopic era showed no benefit with prophylactic cholecystectomy. Survival was not increased, and there was no appreciable increase in discounted life-years gained.

Laparoscopic cholecystectomy has revolutionized the management of cholelithiasis in terms of length of hospital stay and patient morbidity. It has been estimated that the maximum increase in discounted life-years gained by the laparoscopic approach amounts to approximately 2 weeks more than gains from prophylactic open surgery. Furthermore, a sensitivity analysis assuming operative mortality to be zero for prophylactic cholecystectomy, by any technique, resulted in a gain in life expectancy of only 7 and 6 days for a 30-year-old man and woman, respectively. Higher rates of gallstone-related complications would likely result in additional small increases in survival advantage for intervention over expectant management. However, since most people with incidental gallstones remain asymptomatic, and symptoms in the vast majority of cases precede complications, *prophylactic* cholecystectomy usually is not indicated.

It is important to determine, therefore, if patients have symptoms related to their gallstones. Characteristic manifestations of symptomatic cholelithiasis or complications related to the disease include biliary colic, acute cholecystitis, acute pancreatitis, biliary obstruction, ascending cholangitis, gallbladder cancer, and gallstone ileus. Pain located in the epigastrium or right upper quadrant, especially if it radiates to the right shoulder and develops soon after meals in the absence of heartburn, has been significantly associated with gallstones. Once biliary pain occurs, cholecystectomy should be considered, especially in younger persons, as the likelihood of recurrent attacks may be as high as 30–50% per year.

The presence of gallstones has been associated with an increased risk for the development of **gallbladder cancer**. While the absolute incidence of gallbladder cancer is very low, this form of cancer has a high fatality rate. Therefore, younger subjects with asymptomatic gallstones have been considered by some as candidates for prophylactic cholecystectomy. However, because of the low incidence rate of gallbladder cancer, prophylactic intervention in asymptomatic individuals does not appear to be justified, except in certain situations.

One special circumstance derives from the observation that an increased risk of gallbladder carcinoma has been associated with the presence of a porcelain gallbladder or adenomas within the gallbladder. The risk of malignant change in an adenoma appears to be size dependent. Cholecystectomy has been recommended in asymptomatic patients with polyps when gallstones are present, or when an adenoma is greater than 10 mm in diameter in the absence of gallstones. A high association with gallbladder cancer also is seen in patients with anomalous drainage of the pancreatic duct into the common bile duct. These patients should undergo prophylactic cholecystectomy.

Also consider a cholecystectomy in patients with sickle cell disease if abdominal surgery is being performed for another reason. However, prophylactic cholecystectomy *per se* is not recommended, despite the high prevalence of pigment gallstones in these patients. In a recent study, patients with sickle cell anemia undergoing cholecystectomy were found to have a perioperative morbidity of 39%.

Patients who undergo gastric bypass surgery have a greater than 30% chance of developing postoperative gallbladder disease. Therefore, prophylactic cholecystectomy is recommended at the time of the initial surgery.

During **weight-reducing diets**, gallbladder disease (sludge and stones) can develop rapidly. In one study, 26% of subjects developed sonographic abnormalities within 8 weeks of dieting. In another study, gallstones developed in 28% of patients enrolled in a 16-week, 520-kcal/day liquid protein diet program. Prophylaxis with ursodeoxycholic acid (UDCA) is effective in reducing the risk of gallstone development during rapid weight loss by dieting, or after gastric by-pass surgery.

Consider prophylactic cholecystectomy at the time of other intra-abdominal surgery in patients with benign underlying disorders in whom long-term survival is anticipated.

In asymptomatic patients with other underlying conditions, the role of prophylactic cholecystectomy is less certain, and definitive recommendations cannot be made. For instance, gallstones are more common in patients with diabetes mellitus. Predominately anecdotal evidence suggests that patients with diabetes have an increased risk of developing severe, gangrenous cholecystitis. However, the benefits of prophylactic cholecystectomy are unclear. In a study of 47 patients with non-insulin-dependent diabetes who were evaluated 5 years after incidental gallstones had been diagnosed, 15% of initially asymptomatic patients had become symptomatic, a figure similar to non-diabetics. While only two patients presented with complications of gallstones, one patient died post-operatively after surgery for obstructive jaundice.

Asymptomatic subjects who have gallstones with diameters greater than 3 cm are considered by some as candidates for prophylactic cholecystectomy.

The present patient's rapid weight loss from a very low calorie diet was likely an important factor – in addition to her female gender and obesity – in the development of gallstones. Somewhat unusual was her lack of symptoms, which are common in patients with weight-loss related cholelithiasis. She should have been treated with UDCA 600 mg/day, started *before* she began her weight-loss diet. Because her symptoms (nonspecific dyspnea) were not suggestive of a gallbladder origin, prophylactic cholecystectomy was not recommended. Surgery will be recommended if she develops biliary colic or other complications of gallstones.

Clinical Pearls

1. In the vast majority of patients who are found to have incidental gallstones, no intervention is required.

2. Prophylactic cholecystectomy should be considered in asymptomatic patients with a porcelain gallbladder, gallbladder adenoma(s), or anomalous pancreatic ductal drainage, and at the time of bariatric surgery.

3. Obese patients who commence a rapid weight loss dieting program should take UDCA 600 mg daily while dieting.

REFERENCES

1. Gracie WA, Ransohoff DF: The natural history of silent gallstones: The innocent gallstone is not a myth. N Engl J Med 1982;307(13):798–800.
2. Ranosohoff DF, Gracie WA, et al: Prophylactic cholecystectomy or expectant management for silent gallstones. A decision analysis to assess survival. Ann Intern Med 1983;99(2):199–204.
3. Barbara L, Sama C, et al: A population study on the prevalence of gallstone disease: The Sirmione Study. Hepatology 1987;7(5):913–917.
4. Broomfield PH, Chopra R, et al: Effects of ursodeoxycholic acid and aspirin on the formation of lithogenic bile and gallstones during loss of weight. N Engl J Med 1988;319(24):1567–1572.
5. Liddle RA, Goldstein RB, et al: Gallstone formation during weight-reduction dieting. Arch Intern Med 1989;149(8):1750–1753.
6. Attili AF, Carulli N, et al: Epidemiology of gallstone disease in Italy: Prevalence data of the Multicenter Italian Study on Cholelithiasis. Am J Epidemiol 1995;141(2):158–165.
7. Attili AF, De Santis A, et al: The natural history of gallstones: The GREPCO experience. The GREPCO Group. Hepatology 1995; 21(3):655–660.
8. Shiffman ML, Kaplan GD, et al: Prophylaxis against gallstone formation with ursodeoxycholic acid in patients participating in a very-low-calorie diet program. Ann Intern Med 1995;122(12):899–905.
9. Festi D, Sottili S, et al: Clinical manifestations of gallstone disease: Evidence from the multicenter Italian study on cholelithiasis (MICOL). Hepatology 1999; 30(4):839–846.

Helen E. Bateman, MD
Robert S. Pinals, MD

PATIENT 25

A 70-year-old woman with pain and swelling in multiple joints

A 70-year-old woman presents with a 4-day history of pain and swelling in her hands and wrists, left ankle, and right knee. The symptoms began suddenly and worsened over the last 24 hours. She had one previous episode of painful swelling in her feet and knees, but denies other articular problems. She also notes "lumps" on her elbows. Her past medical history is significant for hypertension, mild congestive heart failure, and diabetes. Her medications include furosemide 40 mg daily, aspirin 325 mg daily, glipizide 5 mg daily, calcium, and multivitamins. She denies any allergies and other recent problems, other than a tooth extraction 10 days ago. The patient drinks three cocktails every evening, but denies smoking and recent sexual activity.

Physical Examination: Temperature 38°. General: rather hirsute. Extremities: erythema, swelling, decreased range of motion and tenderness in the metacarpalphalangeal (MCP) joints, bilaterally, left ankle and right knee; moderate effusion right knee; nontender, nodular swellings over the olecranon bilaterally (see figure, *left*).

Laboratory Findings: WBC 12,000/μl, Hct 35%. Rheumatoid factor: positive 1:80. BUN 30 mg/dl, creatinine 1.7 mg/dl, serum uric acid 9.0 mg/dl. Hand radiographs obtained after a fall 3 months ago: see figure, *right*.

Questions: What is the most likely diagnosis for this patient? What further investigation would you perform?

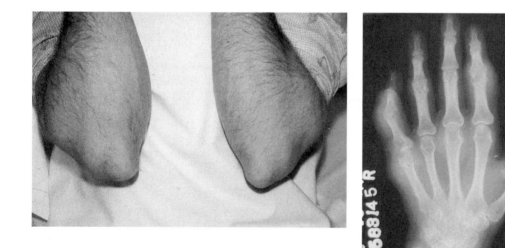

Diagnosis: Acute polyarticular gout.

Discussion: The differential diagnosis of a patient presenting with inflammatory polyarthritis includes bacterial infection, rheumatoid arthritis, systemic lupus erythematosus (SLE), and crystal–induced arthropathy. Septic arthritis is suggested by the presence of fever and leukocytosis, but is typically monarticular except in patients with Neisserial infection. A history of recurrent synovitis suggests the possibility of rheumatoid arthritis, but this diagnosis is unlikely in patients with asymmetric polyarthritis. SLE is an additional consideration, but it rarely presents with synovitis in the absence of other manifestations of the disease. Pseudogout, a crystal-induced arthropathy due to calcium pyrophosphate deposition, most often affects older patients and may mimic rheumatoid arthritis; an acute, polyarticular onset of pseudogout, however, does not usually occur. Among the remaining considerations, acute polyarticular gout is the most likely explanation for this patient's symptoms.

Gout presents with polyarticular symptoms in up to 39% of patients. Although gouty attacks are more common in elderly men than women, the diagnosis should be considered in post-menopausal women presenting with acute arthritis. Women are more likely to present with polyarticular symptoms. Acute podagra—the sudden onset of a painful, inflamed great toe—occurs less commonly in women, and therefore is misdiagnosed frequently. In elderly women, polyarticular gout may be superimposed on osteoarthritis with tophaceous deposits occurring in Heberden's nodes.

The diagnosis of gout is supported by the presence of **tophi over articular surfaces**, which may develop even before the onset of articular symptoms. Tophi are subcutaneous nodules that may simulate rheumatoid nodules. Most tophi, however, have a yellowish hue in contrast to rheumatoid nodules. Note that this discoloration can be difficult to appreciate when tophi are over the elbow, as compared with over the fingers or toes.

The presence of radiographic evidence of cystic-erosive changes in the interphalangial and MCP joints suggests the diagnosis of gout or rheumatoid arthritis. Erosions can occur in both diseases and often are radiographically indistinguishable. The serum uric acid level may be normal during an acute gouty attack.

The appropriate approach for establishing the diagnosis of acute gout is examination of synovial fluid aspirated from an inflamed joint or aspirates from tophi for **urate crystals**. The synovial fluid cell count is less discriminative because it is elevated in patients with acute gout and rheumatoid arthritis. The detection of urate crystals, however, is diagnostic of gout. Aspirated fluid should be cultured even if urate crystals are detected, because crystal-induced and septic arthritis can coexist. It is not unusual for a low-titer, positive rheumatoid factor to be a nonspecific finding when evaluating older patients, as in the present patient. A synovial fluid aspiration from this patient's right knee showed a white count of 50,000/μl with 97% neutrophils, negative gram stain, and intracellular, negatively birefringent crystals, consistent with sodium urate.

Therapeutic options for acute gouty polyarthritis include nonsteroidal anti-inflammatory drugs (NSAIDs), colchicine, and oral or intra-articular corticosteroids. The use of NSAIDs for elderly patients requires caution, however, because these drugs may worsen renal insufficiency, heart failure, and hypertension. Also, colchicine toxicity is greatly enhanced in the setting of renal insufficiency. For patients with these underlying conditions and polyarticular gout, a short course of oral steroids may be appropriate, but requires close monitoring of blood sugars in patients with diabetes. If gouty arthritis affects only one or two joints, intra-articular corticosteroids may be the safest therapeutic option. Prophylaxis with allopurinol is indicated for patients with tophaceous gout, but only after recovery from the acute attack. Earlier initiation of allopurinol may cause a recurrent exacerbation of gout.

The nodules over the present patient's elbows were compatible with tophi. Her hand radiograph demonstrated cystic-erosive changes at the 2nd proximal interphalangeal joint and 5th MCP joint, with surrounding tophi. She was found to have urate crystals on microscopic examination of synovial fluid obtained from her right knee. Her serum uric acid level was elevated, probably due to the combined effects of her renal insufficiency and treatment with furosemide and aspirin. She was treated with a short course of oral prednisone, with rapid resolution of her symptoms.

Clinical Pearls

1. Post-menopausal women, as compared to elderly men, are more likely to present with polyarticular manifestations of gout and to have normal serum uric acid levels.

2. Polyarticular gout may mimic not only rheumatoid arthritis with its manifestations of subcutaneous nodules and joint erosions, but also septic arthritis with its presentation with fever and leukocytosis.

3. Up to 39% of patients with polyarticular gout present with polyarticular involvement with their first gouty attack.

4. Synovial fluid analysis or tophus aspiration for identification of intracellular, negatively birefringent urate crystals remains the gold standard for diagnosis of gout.

5. Do not start allopurinol for prophylaxis against further gouty attacks during an acute episode, as it may worsen the attack.

REFERENCES

1. Hadler NM, Franck WA, Bress NM, Robinson DR: Acute polyarticular gout Am J Med 1974;56:715–719.
2. LawryGV, Fan TP, Bluestone R: Polyarticular versus monoarticular gout: A prospective, comparative analysis of clinical features. Medicine 1988;67:335–343.
3. Groff GD, Franck WA, Raddatz DA: Systemic steroid therapy for acute gout: A clinical trial and review of the literature. Semin Arthritis Rheum 1990;19:329–336.
4. Puig JG, Michan AD, Jimenez ML, Perez de Ayala C, et al: Female gout—Clinical spectrum and uric acid metabolism. Arch Int Med 1991;151:726–732.
5. Alloway JA, Moriaty MJ, Hoogland YT, Nashel DJ: Comparison of triamcinolone acetonide with indomethacin in the treatment of acute gouty arthritis. J Rheumatol 1993;20:111–113.
6. Pinals RS: Polyarthritis and fever. New Engl J Med 1994;330:769–774.
7. Pinals RS: Polyarticular joint disease. In Klippel JH (ed): Primer on the Rheumatic Diseases, 11th ed. 1997, pp 119–122.
8. Eliseo P, Batlle-Gualda E, Martinez A, Rosas J, et al: Diagnosis of inter-critical gout. Ann Intern Med 1999;131:756–759.
9. Schlessinger N, Bater D, Schumacher JR: How well have diagnostic tests and therapies for gout been evaluated. Curr Opin Rheumatol 1999;11:441–445.

Peter S. Guido, MD
Lee K. Brown, MD

PATIENT 26

A 45-year-old man with sleepiness, snoring, and disturbed nocturnal sleep

A 45-year-old man with a history of hypothyroidism and allergic rhinitis complains of a 3-month history of progressive fatigue and nocturnal awakenings associated with acid brash and nocturia. He denies any changes in sleep hours, but notes increased stress at work. He has gained 20 pounds over the last year, and his wife says that he is irritable and "lays around the house all day." She describes his sleep as restless, with heavy snoring and frequent changes in sleep position. He has been experiencing difficulty concentrating at work, and often catches himself feeling drowsy when seated at his office computer and during staff meetings. His current medications include levothyroxine 0.75 mcg daily for hypothyroidism and nonprescription antacids for heartburn. Review of systems was notable for profuse nocturnal perspiration and depressed mood.

Physical Examination: Pulse 72; respirations 14; blood pressure 146/88. General: obese (height 70 inches; weight 217 pounds). HEENT: enlarged, elongated uvula; palatine tonsils markedly enlarged but not acutely inflamed; large tongue; mild retrognathia, dentition in poor repair (see figure); nasal septum moderately deviated to left; scanty clear nasal secretions. Cardiac: normal. Chest: clear. Abdomen: obese. Extremities: normal. Neurologic: normal reflexes.

Laboratory Findings: Hemogram and blood chemistries: normal. TSH: 1.57 (normal).

Question: What laboratory test should be performed next?

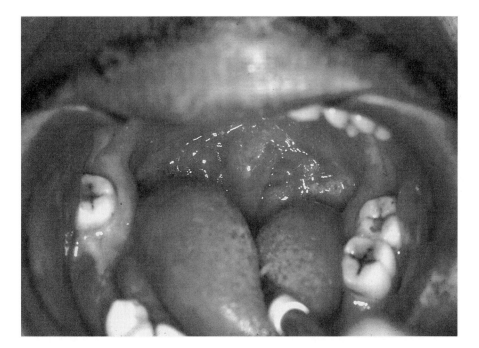

Answer: Nocturnal polysomnography.

Discussion: Obstructive sleep apnea syndrome (OSAS) is a disorder of respiration that is characterized by recurrent episodes of apnea or hypopnea during sleep despite continued inspiratory effort. Loud snoring during hypopneas, or between respiratory events, and repetitive arousals from sleep are the hallmarks of this condition. The disorder is quite common; prevalence is estimated at 4% of middle-aged men, and 2% of middle-aged women. This is comparable to other well-recognized disorders such as chronic obstructive pulmonary disease or asthma, but sleep apnea tends to be overlooked or minimized by medical professionals.

The upper airway involved in the pathogenesis of OSAS consists of the anatomic regions between the nares and the glottis, and includes the nasopharynx, oropharynx, and hypopharynx. Patency of the upper airway depends on the balance between pharyngeal dilator muscles and negative intraluminal pharyngeal pressures which are produced by inspiration. There are interactive factors that predispose to upper airway collapse and development of OSAS. Obesity, palatine tonsillar hypertrophy, nasal obstruction, and retrognathia may cause narrowing of the upper airway even during wakefulness. During sleep, physiologic changes occur which further promote airway collapse. Some of these mechanisms include reduced upper airway dilator muscle tone; changes in CO_2 chemoreceptor set point, causing respiratory instability during transitions between wakefulness and sleep; and reduction of airway reflexes that normally promote patency of the upper airway. Partial upper airway collapse is associated with snoring and obstructive hypopneas (reduction in airflow), while complete occlusion results in apnea (cessation of airflow). Most such events result in an arousal from sleep that leads to increased upper airway dilator tone and thereby terminates the apnea or hypopnea. The repetitive arousals lead to sleep fragmentation and daytime sleepiness.

Chronic loud snoring and **excessive sleepiness**, as was found in this individual, are the two major markers of OSAS. The snoring may be described as intermittent or resuscitative. Snoring is absent during the apneas, resulting in the intermittent nature; snoring increases in volume during the hyperpneic periods between respiratory events and is thus characterized as resuscitative. Symptoms of sleepiness can be difficult to elicit reliably, since patients may minimize symptoms or be so accustomed to sleepiness that they view it as normal. Validated questionnaires such as the Epworth Sleepiness Scale or Sleep-Wake Activity Inventory are easy to use in the office to quantify sleepiness.

Frequent arousals and brief awakenings from sleep may be noted, but complaints of difficulty initiating sleep or prolonged nocturnal awakenings are uncommon. Other common complaints include night sweats, restless sleep, nocturnal gastroesophageal reflux, nocturia, enuresis, dry mouth and sore throat upon awakening, impaired memory and cognition, and automatic behavior (due to lapses in attention and impaired vigilance).

Physical examination typically reveals an obese individual with a thick neck and crowded oropharyngeal airspace. Measure neck circumference, as neck sizes ≥ 17 inches in males and ≥ 16 inches in females are associated with significant risk for obstructive sleep apnea. Systemic hypertension is frequently detected. Patients may present with profound cardiopulmonary dysfunction, with evidence of daytime hypoxemia and hypercapnia, pulmonary hypertension, and cor pulmonale (the obesity-hypoventilation or "Pickwickian" syndrome).

Patients suspected of having OSAS should be evaluated by nocturnal polysomnography to confirm the diagnosis, as was performed in this case (see figure, page 78). A polysomnogram includes **electroencephalography**, **electro-oculography**, and **electromyography** (these allow the determination of sleep stage); as well as **electrocardiography**, respiratory effort, nasal and oral airflow, and oxyhemoglobin saturation (these determine the severity of sleep-disordered respiration based upon the number of respiratory events, disturbance of sleep architecture, and effects on cardiac rate and rhythm). The presence of other sleep disorders also can be determined with polysomnography; anterior tibialis electromyography, for instance, is typically included to diagnose periodic leg movements of sleep.

Treatment options for obstructive sleep apnea include nasal continuous positive airway pressure (CPAP) therapy, upper airway surgery, oral appliances, and behavioral therapies (see table, next page). Pharmacotherapies generally have not been effective, and oxygen alone may prolong respiratory events and is not recommended. The goals of treatment not only include reducing symptoms such as sleepiness, snoring, sleep disruption, and cognitive disturbances, but also minimizing long-term cardiovascular morbidity and mortality.

The present patient's oral examination demonstrated severe crowding due to palatine tonsillar enlargement; enlarged, elongated uvula; and macroglossia. His nocturnal polysomnogram revealed 72 episodes of obstructive apnea or hypopnea for every hour of sleep (respiratory disturbance index or RDI of 72). Nadir oxyhemoglobin saturation was 68%. A second night of polysomnography was performed with nasal CPAP, and RDI declined to 4.8 with the application of CPAP at 10 cm H_2O. He began CPAP treatment at home, and at follow-up 2 months later reported increased energy and improved mood; his wife reported resolution of his snoring when using CPAP.

Common Treatment Options For Obstructive Sleep Apnea

Treatment	Advantages	Disadvantages
Nasal continuous positive airway pressure (CPAP)	Most effective overall, including in severe disease Noninvasive; quickest means to symptomatic improvement No contraindications for majority of patients Increasing number of mask types and sizes has resulted in improved likelihood of finding proper mask fit Nasal/oral side effects can be treated with humidification, chinstrap or full face mask to prevent mouth leaks, nasal corticosteroids or disodium cromoglycate, or oral antihistamines/decongestants	Long-term compliance may be as low as 50% Mask fit can be problematic Some patients complain of claustrophobia Social stigma Local nasal/oral side effects may occur: rhinorrhea, sneezing, nasal congestion, epistaxis, nasal/oral dryness
Mandibular advancement device (oral appliance)	Effective in about 50% of patients overall Usually well-tolerated Easy to take along on trips; can be used away from electrical power (e.g., camping)	Less effective in severe OSAS Temporomandibular joint symptoms may occur Excess salivation, choking may occur
Uvulopalatopharyngoplasty (UPPP)	Effective in about 50% of patients overall Can result in a permanent cure	Less effective in severe OSAS Does not address "base-of-tongue" (hypopharyngeal) obstruction Carries usual operative risks: bleeding; airway edema; infection Small incidence of long-term adverse effects: nasal regurgitation of liquids; change in voice (rhinolalia aperta) OSAS can return with weight gain
Base-of-tongue procedures: genioglossal advancement, hyoid myotomy, inferior sagittal osteotomy, etc.	Can improve efficacy of UPPP slightly by treating hypopharyngeal obstruction	Additional operative/postoperative risk
Maxillary and mandibular osteotomies with advancement	High likelihood of success Done as a staged procedure if uvulopalatopharyngoplasty and base-of-tongue procedures fail	Additional operative/postoperative risk Radical procedure, requiring expert head and neck surgeon
Behavioral therapies: weight loss, sleep position training, avoidance of alcohol and sedative medications	Can be effective in mild OSAS and an adjunct to treatment in more severe disease	Weight loss may be difficult to achieve and maintain

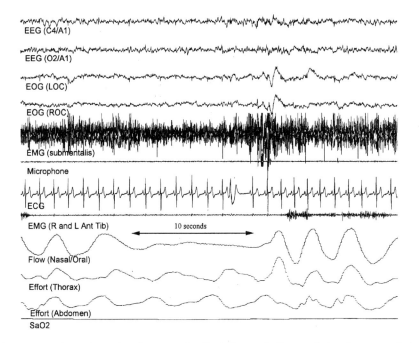

EEG (C4/A1)

EEG (O2/A1)

EOG (LOC)

EOG (ROC)

EMG (submentalis)

Microphone

ECG

EMG (R and L Ant Tib) ←——— 10 seconds ———→

Flow (Nasal/Oral)

Effort (Thorax)

Effort (Abdomen)

SaO2

Diagnostic polysomnography performed on the present patient, demonstrating an obstructive apnea during stage 1 and non-REM sleep lasting just over 10 seconds (*arrow*). The electroencephalograms (EEG), electro-oculograms (EOG), and submentalis electromyogram (EMG) show low-voltage, mixed-frequency activity, lack of eye movements, and moderate muscle tone (respectively) consistent with stage 1. Nasal/oral air flow is absent, while thoracic and abdominal effort signals demonstrate continued respiratory attempts that are out-of-phase (paradoxic), consistent with an obstructive apnea. The electrocardiogram (ECG) records a ventricular premature contraction as the apnea terminates. The microphone, placed on the neck, demonstrates snoring as normal breathing resumes.

Clinical Pearls

1. OSAS often has an insidious onset, and the patient may minimize symptoms. Interviewing a spouse or roommate often is useful in determining the diagnosis.

2. Symptoms of OSAS, such as depressed and irritable mood, cognitive difficulties, lack of motivation, and disturbed sleep, may be attributed to psychiatric disorders and inappropriately treated unless a high index of suspicion for sleep disorders is maintained.

3. Neck circumference and the upper airway physical examination can provide important clues to the presence of OSAS.

4. The mainstay of treatment remains nasal CPAP; a variety of techniques are available to the skillful clinician to minimize side effects from this device and improve compliance.

REFERENCES

1. Johns MW: A new method for measuring daytime sleepiness: The Epworth Sleepiness Scale. Sleep 1991;14:540–545.
2. Davies RJ, Ali NJ, Stradling JR: Neck circumference and other clinical features in the diagnosis of the obstructive sleep apnoea syndrome. Thorax 1992;47:101–105.
3. Rosenthal L, Roehrs TA, Roth T: The Sleep-Wake Activity Inventory: A self-report measure of daytime sleepiness. Biol Psychiatry 1993;34:810–820.
4. Young T, Palta M, Dempsey J, et al: The occurrence of sleep-disordered breathing among middle-aged adults. N Engl J Med 1993;328:1230–1235.
5. Sher AE, Schectman KB, Piccirillo JF: The efficacy of surgical modifications of the upper airway in adults with obstructive sleep apnea syndrome. Sleep 1996;19:156–177.
6. American College of Chest Physicians and American Association of Cardiovascular and Pulmonary Rehabilitation Pulmonary Rehabilitation Guidelines Panel: Pulmonary Rehabilitation: Joint ACCP/AACVPR Evidence-Based Guidelines. Chest 1997;112:1363–1396.
7. Quan SF, Howard BV, Iber C, et al:. The Sleep Heart Health Study: Design, rationale, and methods. Sleep 1997;20:1077–1085.
8. Young T, Evans L, Finn L, et al: Estimation of the clinically diagnosed proportion of sleep apnea syndrome in middle-aged men and women. Sleep 1997;20:705–706.

John E. Pandolfino, MD
Peter J. Kahrilas, MD

PATIENT 27

A 25-year-old man with progressive dysphagia

A 25-year-old man presents with progressive dysphagia of 6-month duration. He states that food has been "hanging up" behind his sternum. His symptoms initially occurred only with steak and bread, but now have progressed to also occur with liquids. He denies weight loss, abdominal pain, and visible blood in his stool. Last year he sustained an anterior cruciate ligament tear and has been taking ibuprofen for pain relief. His only other medication is occasional Maalox for intermittent heartburn. The patient is a never-smoker, and he consumes about three alcoholic beverages a month.

Physical Examination: Vital signs: normal. HEENT: unremarkable. Lymph nodes: none palpable. Chest: normal. Cardiac: normal heart sounds. Abdomen: soft, not distended, nontender. Rectal exam: brown stool.

Laboratory Findings: Barium upper gastrointestinal: see below.

Question: What is the most appropriate next diagnostic study? What is the likely cause of his dysphagia?

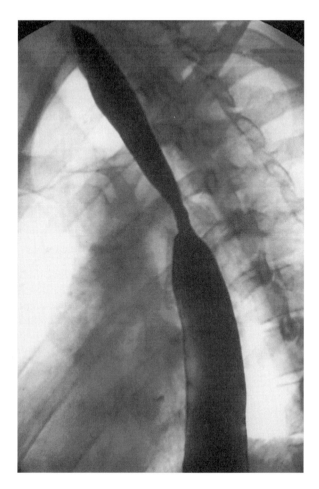

Answer: Endoscopy and, if necessary, ambulatory pH monitoring. The likely diagnosis is peptic stricture secondary to reflux.

Discussion: The differential diagnosis for a mid-esophageal stricture—as for a distal esophageal stricture—includes neoplasia, caustic injury (including pill esophagitis), and gastroesophageal reflux. Esophageal cancer presenting in the mid-esophagus most likely is squamous cell carcinoma, as opposed to adenocarcinoma, which most frequently occurs distally. Squamous cell cancers typically occur in older patients with a long history of smoking and drinking alcohol. Caustic injury secondary to medications is a well-documented cause of stricturing and is attributable to a wide array of medications, including nonsteroidal anti-inflammatory drugs, antibiotics, and potassium chloride. Pill esophagitis most commonly presents with segmental esophagitis that is not contiguous with the squamocolumnar junction; this is distinct from peptic esophagitis, which always involves the most distal mucosa. Pill esophagitis also can present with stricture in the mid-esophagus.

However, the most common etiology of esophageal stricture is reflux esophagitis. Reflux strictures typically occur in the distal esophagus at the squamocolumnar junction, because this is the region with the greatest exposure to the caustic gastric refluxate. However, if columnar metaplasia is present (Barrett's epithelium), the metaplastic epithelium is resistant to acid-induced injury. Thus, in the presence of Barrett's metaplasia, strictures occur at the superior margin of the metaplastic epithelium that can be in the mid- or even proximal esophagus.

Gastroesophageal reflux disease (GERD) is a clinical condition that results from the reflux of noxious gastric contents into the esophagus. It is a common malady and is estimated to affect 40% of the adult American population. Seven percent of U.S. adults experience severe symptoms of heartburn that may occur daily. Reflux disease is a chronic and recurrent condition that usually requires repeated or sustained therapy.

The pathophysiology of GERD is multifactorial, with the disease ultimately related to the balance between factors tending to erode the esophageal epithelium and those tending to preserve it. Esophagitis occurs when the balance between the caustic factors (acid reflux, causticity of refluxate) and defensive mechanisms (esophageal acid clearance, mucosal resistance) tilts in the favor of the aggressive forces. Under normal conditions, reflux episodes are prevented by the anti-reflux barrier located at the esophagogastric junction (EGJ). The integrity of the anti-reflux barrier is compromised via three dominant mechanisms: (**1**) transient lower esophageal sphincter relaxations, (**2**) lower esophageal sphincter hypotension, or (**3**) anatomic disruption of the EGJ usually associated with hiatal hernia. Transient lower esophageal sphincter relaxations are the predominant mechanism in mild to moderate reflux, while a hypotensive lower esophageal sphincter is found in more severe cases, including essentially every instance with a long segment of Barrett's metaplasia.

The most common clinical symptoms of GERD are **heartburn** and **acid regurgitation**. These two symptoms are considered to be quite specific, but not sensitive. Patients also may present with dysphagia, epigastric pain, nausea, and belching. Atypical symptoms such as asthma, laryngitis, chronic cough, and recurrent pneumonitis also are associated with GERD. However, it is difficult to prove causality in the case of these extraesophageal manifestations given the poor specificity of GERD as the inciting cause.

GERD typically is diagnosed by a careful history, and usually is treated empirically with antisecretory medications. Patients who do not respond to therapy, or are found to have clinical warning signs (anemia, weight loss, dysphagia / odynophagia, occult blood in the stool, and advanced age) should be referred for upper endoscopy. Barium studies are not very useful in the diagnostic evaluation of GERD, but may be helpful in identifying strictures and hiatus hernia. Endoscopy has the greatest sensitivity to document mucosal injury. Unfortunately, approximately 50% of patients will not have esophagitis on endoscopy. These patients have *nonerosive* GERD, and may require alternative diagnostic tests if they do not respond to treatment. Ambulatory pH monitoring may provide useful quantitative data; this currently is the most sensitive test for diagnosing reflux.

The natural history of reflux disease is variable, but is estimated to be chronic in 80% of cases. Patients may have minimal symptoms requiring only symptomatic treatment, or they may develop esophagitis and its complications. There is an imperfect correlation between symptom severity and either the amount of reflux or the presence of esophagitis. Patients with Barrett's esophagus also may present with minimal symptoms because of reduced esophageal sensitivity. Regardless of this ambiguity, patients with GERD typically have an excellent prognosis. Although chronic antisecretory therapy often is required, disease progression is very slow, and relatively few patients develop severe complications of the disease.

Some degree of **dysphagia** is reported by more than 30% of individuals with GERD. Dysphagia can be caused by peptic stricture, peristaltic dysfunction, or simply by mucosal inflammation. The prevalence of peptic stricture is from 8–20% in patients with esophagitis. Strictures initially are treated by dilation. Dilation to a diameter of 14 mm generally provides good relief. With the advent of proton pump inhibitor therapy, strictures are no longer an indication for surgery.

Another important complication of GERD is the development of **Barrett's metaplasia**. Barrett's metaplasia is metaplastic columnar epithelium that has replaced the normal squamous epithelium of the esophagus. It is found in 10–15% of GERD patients undergoing endoscopy, and its pathogenesis is unclear. Barrett's esophagus is a premalignant condition associated with an estimated 40-fold increased risk of developing adenocarcinoma of the esophagus relative to the general population. Neither antisecretory therapy nor antireflux surgery causes Barrett's to regress. Screening programs have been devised to identify patients at greatest risk for malignancy. Surveillance endoscopy should be done every 2–5 years with a standardized biopsy protocol. Patients found to have high-grade dysplasia should be referred for esophagectomy, mucosal ablation, or intensive surveillance. Patients with low-grade dysplasia should be surveyed at a more frequent interval.

The present patient presented with dysphagia and evidence of a mid-esophageal stricture on a barium esophogram. His endoscopy revealed severe erosive esophagitis with a peptic stricture and Barrett's metaplasia without dysplasia. He underwent successful dilation with a Savary-Guilliard dilator to 14 mm. He requires lifelong acid suppression, or he may opt for antireflux surgery. He also requires lifelong surveillance endoscopy for his Barrett's metaplasia.

Clinical Pearls

1. Peptic stictures may present in the mid-esophagus in patients with Barrett's metaplasia.
2. Esophagitis is not evident on upper endoscopy in approximately 50% of GERD patients.
3. Peptic strictures require lifelong therapy with proton pump inhibitors to prevent recurrence.
4. Barrett's esophagus is a premalignant condition with a 40-fold increased risk for adenocarcinoma of the esophagus compared to the general population.

REFERENCES
1. Kahrilas PJ, Dodds WJ, Hogan WJ, et al: Esophageal peristaltic dysfunction in peptic esophagitis. Gastroenterology 1986;91:897.
2. Mittal RK, Balaban D: Mechanism of diseases: The esophagogastric junction. N Engl J Med 1997;336:924–933.
3. Richter JE: Long-term management of gastroesophageal reflux disease and its complications. Am J Gastroenterol 1997;92(4 suppl):30S–34S.
4. Sampliner RE: Practice guidelines on the diagnosis, surveillance, and therapy of Barrett's esophagus. The Practice Parameters Committee of the American College of Gastroenterology. Am J Gastroenterol 1998;93(7):1028–1032.
5. Spechler SJ: AGA technical review on treatment of patients with dysphagia caused by benign disorders of the distal esophagus. Gastroenterology 1999;117:233–254.

Lee K. Brown, MD

PATIENT 28

A 69-year-old woman with frequent nocturnal awakenings and daytime sleepiness

A 69-year-old woman presents with frequent nocturnal awakenings and daytime sleepiness. She has had difficulty falling asleep since childhood largely because of an "achy" feeling in her legs. Once asleep, she thinks that she drifts in and out of sleep throughout the night, with frequent tossing and turning. She maintains a regular sleep schedule, with lights out at 10:00 PM and lights on at 7:00 AM every day. Her bedroom environment is conducive to sleep, and she does not "clockwatch." Her sleep quality is the same when she is away from home, and she usually awakens unrefreshed. She does not consume alcoholic or caffeine-containing beverages before bedtime, takes no hypnotics, and denies having experienced cataplexy, hypnagogic or hypnopompic hallucinations, or sleep paralysis.

She has never been told that she snores, does not wake up with dyspnea, and denies morning headaches or nausea. Her legs feel "achy" most days in the late afternoon, especially when sitting or lying still; the ache is relieved by vigorously rubbing her legs or walking. Her father was a chronic insomniac who also complained of pain in his legs that kept him awake at night.

Physical Examination: Vital signs: normal. General: moderately overweight (height 67 inches, weight 191 pounds). HEENT: no retrognathia or micrognathia; widely patent oropharynx; no gross nasal obstruction. Chest: clear. Cardiac: regular rhythm, no murmurs or gallops. Abdomen: nontender, without organomegaly. Extremities: no cyanosis or edema.

Laboratory Findings: CBC, blood chemistries, TSH: normal. Nocturnal polysomnography (see figure, next page): clusters of leg movements during non-rapid eye movement sleep; average of 61 movements in each cluster, with movements separated by an average interval of 23 seconds; last leg movement frequently followed by an arousal or brief awakening; 136 leg movements each hour of sleep; 34 leg movements per hour of sleep associated with arousals.

Question: What class of medications is best used to treat this disorder?

A 2-minute segment of the present patient's nocturnal polysomnogram. A series of five periodic leg movements is demonstrated on the combined right and left anterior tibialis electromyogram (LEGS EMG). The movements are separated by approximately 20-second intervals. Electroencephalogram (EEG) recordings do not show evidence of arousal, but respiratory effort irregularity (EFRT THOR and EFRT ABD) suggests subcortical arousal following each leg movement. The other channels depict left and right eye movements (EOG LOC and EOG ROC), chin electromyogram (CHIN EMG), audio recording from the anterior neck (MIC SNOR), electrocardiogram (EKG), airflow at the nose and mouth (FLOW THRM), and oxyhemoglobin saturation (SAO2). The vertical lines are at 30-second intervals.

Answer: Dopaminergic medications are most effective for restless legs syndrome/periodic limb movement disorder.

Discussion: Restless legs syndrome (RLS) and periodic limb movement disorder (PLMD; also called nocturnal myoclonus) usually are considered to be different manifestations of one neurological disorder. RLS is defined as an irresistible need to move the limbs (usually the legs) in order to relieve a **dysesthesia**. The dysesthesia often is poorly characterized by the patient, but may be described as itching, burning, crawling, tingling, pricking, tension, or aching. Patients most often resort to walking, rubbing the legs, or constantly moving the legs to relieve the sensation. The severity of the symptoms usually follows a circadian rhythm, with worsening in the evening and at night. Consequently, one of the most bothersome effects of the disorder is interference with sleep onset, as well as delaying the return to sleep if the patient awakens during the night. Patients may express difficulties with sitting still, e.g., in airplanes, automobiles, and movie theatres.

The diagnosis of RLS almost always is established on clinical grounds, with the minimal criteria defined as: (**1**) desire to move the limbs, usually associated with a dysesthesia; (**2**) motor restlessness; (**3**) symptoms worse or only present at rest, and at least partially (but transiently) relieved by activity; (**4**) symptoms worse in the evening or nighttime. RLS often is familial—63% of first-degree relatives of patients complained of RLS symptoms in one study. In addition, approximately 40% of adult idiopathic or familial RLS patients report the onset of their symptoms during childhood, when it was often ascribed to "growing pains."

PLMD is characterized by stereotypical limb movements occurring during sleep. Most commonly, patients dorsiflex the ankle and extend the big toe; sometimes they may flex the knee and/or hip, and overall the movement often resembles the **Babinski reflex**. The movements must occur as part of a sequence of four or more, each lasting 0.5–5 seconds and separated by an interval of 10–90 seconds, to be considered as evidence of PLMD. Some movements are accompanied or followed by electroencephalographic evidence of arousal, and are thereby felt to result in symptoms of insomnia or daytime sleepiness. However, PLMD frequently may be an incidental, asymptomatic finding on polysomnography (the recording of multiple physiological signals during sleep) performed for other indications. The polysomnographic criterion for establishing the diagnosis of PLMD consists of a **periodic limb movement index** (the number of periodic limb movements per hour of sleep) of five or greater. Electromyographic or other types of limb movement recordings are included in the polysomnogram for this purpose.

The existence of a variety of **mutual attributes** suggests that RLS and PLMD share a common pathogenesis. The prevalence of both disorders increases with age, with an overall prevalence in adults of about 10%. Approximately 80% of individuals with symptoms of RLS are found to meet criteria for PLMD if subjected to polysomnography. Both disorders are more common in patients with a list of illnesses and conditions that includes renal failure, diabetes, neuropathies, spinal cord disorders, pregnancy, and iron-deficiency anemia, and both seem to worsen with the use of antidepressant medications. Finally, RLS and PLMD respond to the same types of medications, particularly dopaminergic substances, opioids, and the anticonvulsant neurontin (see table, next page).

The fact that periodic leg movements closely resemble the Babinski reflex has led to the theory that PLMD (and by extension, RLS) represents the loss of the descending inhibitory drive that tonically suppresses that polysynaptic spinal cord reflex. The high prevalence of RLS and PLMD in spinal cord disorders (e.g., intervertebral disk disease, tumors, multiple sclerosis) tends to support this pathogenetic theory. However, this theory fails to account for the high prevalence of RLS/PLMD in other disorders (e.g., neuropathies, renal failure) that should not affect descending inhibitory tone. Other pathogenetic theories involve subcortical or reticular alerting mechanisms or imbalance of CNS dopaminergic, opiate, or adrenergic systems. The association of RLS/PLMD with iron-deficiency anemia is intriguing in that regard, since iron is known to be involved in dopamine synthesis. Serum ferritin levels less than 45-50 mcg/L have been correlated with worsening symptoms in some studies.

Treatment consists of screening for the disorders mentioned above, with appropriate treatment if they are detected, as well as appropriate medication (see table, next page). Levodopa/carbidopa, followed by pergolide, have been the most common choices in the recent past, but rapidly are being superceded by the synthetic dopaminergic agonists in the view of many experienced clinicians. Benzodiazepines frequently are used by physicians not acquainted with recent advances in the therapy of these disorders; these should be reserved as second-line agents.

The present patient was begun on levodopa/carbidopa (controlled-release formulation), 50/200 mg at bedtime. She reported being able to fall asleep consistently in 15 minutes, and was able to achieve 4–6 hours of consolidated sleep per night without perceived awakenings. She awakened feeling refreshed in the morning, and denied daytime sleepiness.

Drugs Commonly Used to Treat RLS and PLMD

Class	Drug Examples	Comments Applicable to Class
Dopamine precursor	Levodopa/carbidopa	Inexpensive Effective in many cases No evidence that RLS/PLMD patients develop dyskinesia May cause rebound or augmentation
Ergot-derived dopaminergic agonist	Pergolide Cabergoline Bromocriptine	Pergolide most commonly used Can cause nausea, orthostatic hypotension Potential for retroperitoneal, mediastinal, or pulmonary fibrosis with long-term use
Synthetic dopaminergic agonist	Ropinirole Pramipexole	May be the most effective agents, but costly Side effects include nausea, edema
Anticonvulsant	Neurontin	Degree of efficacy yet to be demonstrated
Benzodiazepine	Clonazepam Lorazepam Temazepam	Does not suppress PLMD, but blunts arousal response Sedating Potential for abuse/addiction Previously was first-line choice; now second-line
Opioid agonist	Codeine Oxycodone Methadone	Effective Potential for abuse/addiction, making these second-line agents Sedating
Mineral supplement	Iron Magnesium	May be useful if ferritin $\leq$ 45-50 mcg/L Anecdotal reports of efficacy

Clinical Pearls

1. Restless legs syndrome is diagnosed using *clinical* criteria: inexorable need to move legs due to a dysesthesia at least partially relieved by the movement, motor restlessness, symptoms worse or exclusively at rest, and peak in symptoms during the evening and nighttime.

2. Periodic limb movement disorder is a *clinical and laboratory* diagnosis: nocturnal polysomnography demonstrating a PLMS index of 5 or greater, with symptoms of nocturnal awakenings or daytime sleepiness attributable to PLMD.

3. Approximately 80% of patients with RLS have polysomnographic evidence of PLMD.

4. Most RLS/PLMD is familial, but also may be related to other diseases and conditions such as renal failure, diabetes, iron-deficiency anemia, and pregnancy.

5. Both RLS and PLMD respond best to dopaminergic medications. The most common choices are levodopa/carbidopa, pergolide, and, more recently, ropinirole and pramipexole.

REFERENCES.
1. Smith RC: Relationship of periodic movements in sleep (nocturnal myoclonus) and the Babinski sign. Sleep 1985; 8:239–243.
2. Walters AS: Toward a better definition of the restless legs syndrome. Movement Disorders 1995; 10:634–642.
3. Trenkwalder C, Walters AS, Hening W: Periodic limb movements and restless legs syndrome. Neurol Clin 1996; 14:629–651.
4. Montplaisir J, Boucher S, Poirier G, et al: Clinical, polysomnographic, and genetic characteristics of restless legs syndrome: A study of 133 patients diagnosed with new standard criteria. Movement Disorders 1997; 12:61–65.
5. Earley CJ, Yaffee JB, Allen RP: Randomized, double-blind, placebo-controlled trial of pergolide in restless legs syndrome. Neurology 1998; 51:1599–1602.
6. Picchietti DL, England SJ, Walters AS, et al: Periodic limb movement disorder and restless legs syndrome in children with attention-deficit hyperactivity disorder. J Child Neurol 1998; 13:588-594.
7. Sun ER, Chen CA, Ho G, et al: Iron and the restless legs syndrome. Sleep 1998; 21:371–377.
8. Bene H, Kurella B, Kummer J, et al: Rapid onset of action of levodopa in restless legs syndrome: A double-blind, randomized, multicenter, crossover trial. Sleep 1999; 22:1073–1081.
9. Montplaisir J, Nicolas A, Denesle R, Gomez-Mancilla B: Restless legs syndrome improved by pramipexole. A double-blind randomized trial. Neurology 1999; 52:938–943.

Richard W. Light, MD

PATIENT 29

A 62-year-old male with shortness of breath and a pleural effusion following coronary artery bypass surgery

A 62-year-old man returns to his primary care physician complaining of shortness of breath. Six weeks ago, he was hospitalized with an acute myocardial infarction and underwent coronary artery bypass graft (CABG) surgery. He received two internal mammary artery grafts and two saphenous vein graphs during that hospitalization. His immediate postoperative course was uncomplicated, except for one brief episode of atrial fibrillation. After discharge, he did well for the first 3 weeks. He then gradually experienced increasing shortness of breath and fatigue. The patient can presently walk only 50 feet before becoming dyspneic. He denies chest pain, fever, peripheral edema, orthopnea, and paroxysmal nocturnal dyspnea.

Physical Examination: Temperature 37.0°, pulse 96, respirations 24, blood pressure 130/80. General: mild dyspnea while talking. Chest: dullness to percussion; absent tactile fremitus and decreased breath sounds over the lower one half of the left hemithorax. Cardiac: no jugular venous distention, murmurs, gallops, or rubs. Abdomen: no organomegaly. Extremities: no edema or calf tenderness.

Laboratory Findings: WBC 9600/μl with a normal differential. Chest radiograph: pleural effusion occupying 50% of left hemithorax (see figures, below and next page); no infiltrates or cardiomegaly. Thoracentesis: clear yellow fluid; WBC 1600/μl, with 61% small lymphocytes, 27 % mesothelial cells, and 2% neutrophils. Glucose 96 mg/dl, protein 4.4 gm/dl (simultaneous serum 7.3 gm/dl), and lactic acid dehydrogenase (LDH) 280 IU/L (simultaneous serum 220 IU/L; upper limits of normal 300 IU/L). Pleural fluid adenosine deaminase: 20.5 U/L.

Question: What is the most likely explanation for this patient's pleural effusion?

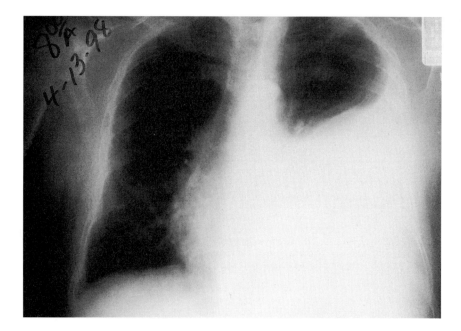

Diagnosis: Lymphocytic pleural effusion post-CABG surgery—pathogenesis unknown.

Diagnosis: More than 50% of patients undergoing CABG surgery have a pleural effusion in the first few days after the operation. Most of these effusions are left-sided, small, and asymptomatic. However, about 10% of patients have a larger, symptomatic pleural effusion within the first 3 months after surgery. More than 90% of the symptomatic pleural effusions are left-sided or, if bilateral, are larger on the left. In general, these effusions can be divided into those that present early (within 30 days of surgery) and those that present later (more than 30 days postsurgery). With both types of effusions, patients present with shortness of breath; fever and chest pain are unusual.

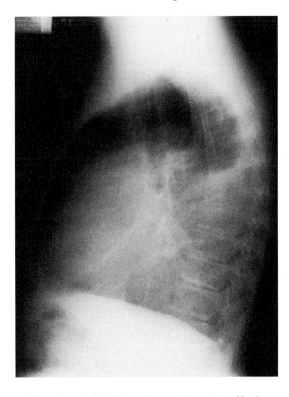

The pleural fluid in patients with **early effusions** is a bloody (mean hematocrit ~20%) exudate with a high percentage of **eosinophils** (median >40%). The eosinophilia is probably due to the blood in the pleural space. The pleural fluid LDH averages about twice the upper limit of normal for serum. These early pleural effusions probably are due to postoperative bleeding into the pleural space. Most patients with these early bloody post-CABG effusions are cured with one or two therapeutic thoracenteses.

The pleural fluid in patients with **late effusions** post CABG is usually a clear yellow exudate with an LDH approximately equal to the upper limit of normal for serum. The pleural fluid differential cell count reveals predominantly small **lymphocytes**. The pathogenesis of these late effusions is unknown, but probably has an immunologic basis. These effusions tend to recur more after therapeutic thoracentesis than do the early bloody effusions, but most are cured with a few therapeutic thoracenteses. Although NSAIDs and corticosteroids are frequently given to these patients, there is no good evidence that these medications are effective. An occasional patient will require tube thoracostomy with the instillation of a sclerosing agent such as doxycycline, or thoracoscopy to remove a pleural peel for the management of the effusion.

The differential diagnosis of pleural effusions in the patient post-CABG surgery includes congestive heart failure, chylothorax, pulmonary embolus, constrictive pericarditis, tuberculosis, and empyema. Patients with congestive heart failure or constrictive pericarditis usually have distended neck veins and peripheral edema. In addition, the pleural fluid is a transudate, rather than the exudate seen in patients with post-CABG effusion. The pleural fluid in chylothorax is distinctive in that it looks like milk. Patients with pulmonary embolism usually have a sudden onset of dyspnea, while patients with effusions post CABG have gradually increasing dyspnea. Always consider tuberculous (TB) pleuritis in patients with lymphocytic pleural effusions. Note that the adenosine deaminase level is elevated (>40 U/L) in TB pleuritis, but not in patients with effusions post CABG. Pleural fluids can be sent to Dr. Kent Miller (7380 Southwest 123 Terrace, Miami, Fl 33156, Telephone 305-243-6617) for ADA analysis. Patients with empyema usually are febrile and have purulent pleural fluid with a high percentage of neutrophils and positive bacterial cultures.

In the present patient, the diagnosis was made by the patient's history and the exclusion of the other main causes of pleural effusion in the patient post CABG. After the initial therapeutic thoracentesis, the patient required one additional therapeutic thoracentesis 3 weeks later. At followup 6 months post-CABG surgery, there was no evidence of pleural effusion on the chest radiograph.

Clinical Pearls

1. Large exudative pleural effusions frequently complicate coronary artery bypass surgery.

2. Effusions occurring within the first 30 days usually are bloody with a high percentage of eosinophils, while those occurring after 30 days usually are clear with a high percentage of lymphocytes.

3. The pleural fluid adenosine deaminase levels are not elevated in patients with post-CABG pleural effusions as they are in pleural tuberculosis.

4. Most pleural effusions post CABG can be managed with one to three therapeutic thoracenteses.

REFERENCES:

1. Light RW, Rogers JT, Cheng D-S, Rodriguez RM: Large pleural effusions occurring after coronary artery bypass grafting. Ann Intern Med 1999; 130:891–896.
2. Sadikot RT, Rogers JT, Cheng DS, et al: Pleural fluid characteristics of patients with symptomatic pleural effusion post-coronary artery bypass surgery. Arch Intern Med 2000 (in press).

John W. Doggett, MD
Lee K. Brown, MD

PATIENT 30

A 19-year-old woman with profound fatigue

A 19-year-old woman complains of an 8-year history of severe daytime fatigue. She first noted a strong tendency to fall asleep in class at age 11 and routinely came home after school to nap. She now sleeps 9 hours every night, but struggles to stay awake at work and frequently naps during her lunch break. She dreams during these short naps and awakens feeling refreshed and able to function with normal alertness for several hours. The patient notes drowsiness while driving, and once fell asleep at the wheel, awakening when she drove onto the roadway shoulder. Her family has described her sleep as quiet, without snoring or leg jerks. She dreams soon after falling asleep at night, and occasionally feels that her dreams start before she is fully asleep. Since age 15, she has experienced monthly episodes of being unable to move for a short time after awakening. For the last 3 years, she often has stumbled and almost fallen when startled or angry.

Physical Examination: Vital signs: normal. General: mildly overweight (height 64 inches, weight 160 pounds), depressed affect. Chest: clear. Cardiac: regular rhythm, no murmurs. Extremities: no cyanosis or edema. Neurologic: normal.

Laboratory Findings: Hemogram, blood chemistries: normal. Nocturnal polysomnogram (see figure): 41 obstructive hypopneas, 1 obstructive apnea, with a borderline elevated respiratory disturbance index of 6.0; most respiratory events occurred during rapid eye movement (REM) sleep; no periodic limb movements, normal sleep efficiency (96%); reduced sleep-onset latency (1 min); first REM sleep period began 3 minutes after sleep onset; numerous brief awakenings, most lasting < 1 minute. Multiple sleep latency test (MSLT): mean latency to sleep onset 2.4 min; episodes of REM sleep documented on all four naps.

Question: How are the MSLT findings related to her different symptoms?

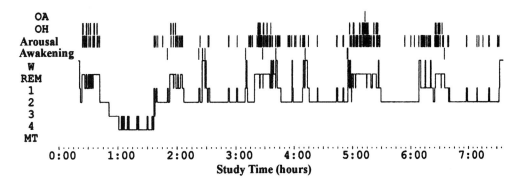

Hypnogram derived from the patient's nocturnal polysomnogram. The stages of sleep are plotted against study time (W = wakefulness; 1–4 = stages of nonREM sleep; MT = movement time.) Vertical bars depict the occurrence of obstructive apnea (OA), obstructive hypopnea (OH), arousals, and awakenings. Note the very brief time spent awake at the beginning of the study, with rapid transition into stage 1 sleep consistent with the short initial sleep latency. REM sleep occurs very shortly after sleep onset, a pathological finding. OH is seen occurring during REM sleep, and there are numerous brief arousals, but few are long enough to constitute awakenings.

Answer: The very short sleep-onset latency confirms the complaint of severe daytime sleepiness. The presence of REM sleep on each nap indicates a very disorganized REM-control mechanism, which supports the interpretation of her other complaints as hypnagogic hallucinations, sleep paralysis, and cataplexy.

Discussion: Narcolepsy is a genetically based, neurological disorder that is characterized by **excessive daytime sleepiness**. The sleepiness is virtually unremitting, although there may be a short period of improved functioning after a brief nap (known as a refractory period for sleepiness). The diagnostic tetrad classically includes excessive sleepiness, cataplexy, hypnagogic hallucinations, and sleep paralysis. Symptoms and severity of impairment can vary. Virtually all patients eventually complain of daytime sleepiness, but as many as one third never manifest the other symptoms of the tetrad. Persons with narcolepsy typically are symptomatic for years before they are diagnosed. They often are labeled as lazy, and have considerable difficulty with school and employment due to their overwhelming sleepiness. They also suffer from a substantially increased risk of motor vehicle accidents. Often the primary complaint is fatigue, rather than sleepiness, as many people have difficulty distinguishing the two symptoms. Narcolepsy most frequently presents at puberty or young adulthood, and is generally an uncommon cause of daytime sleepiness, with an estimated prevalence on the order of 0.05%.

The sleepiness is ascribed to a defective sleep/wake control mechanism in the sleep-generating centers of the brain, although an actual anatomic lesion has never been demonstrated. Narcolepsy has been associated with specific human HLA antigens, and certain families of dog have been identified with inherited narcolepsy. It is thought that the development of human narcolepsy requires both genetic predisposition and an unknown environmental factor. Genetic research in the canine model is focusing on a possible defect in lateral hypothalamic receptors for the neurotransmitter hypocretin-1. Recent human research suggests that a deficiency of hypocretin-1 may be causative in some patients.

Paradoxically, patients with narcolepsy also may complain of disturbed nocturnal sleep, thought to be another indication of a disruption in the sleep/wake control mechanism. In addition, there is disorganization in the normal temporal cycling of REM sleep. The predilection to exhibit REM sleep is tightly linked to the circadian rhythm that governs body temperature and sleepiness, and follows a regular pattern of cycles through the night. The first episode of REM begins 60–120 minutes after sleep onset, and returns roughly every 90 minutes during the sleep period, with increasing length of the REM episode each time. REM sleep generally does not occur during daytime naps in normal individuals, except occasionally in the early morning. On the other hand, persons with narcolepsy may have their first REM episode very early in the night, and are likely to have REM during brief daytime naps.

Cataplexy, sleep paralysis, and hypnagogic hallucinations are considered dissociated REM phenomena occurring during wakefulness. Characteristics of normal REM sleep include visual imagery (dreams), rapid eye movements, and skeletal muscle atonia. The muscle atonia is mediated by specific pontine nuclei acting on spinal interneurons, and teleologically is thought to prevent the acting out of dreams. **Cataplexy** is sudden muscle weakness triggered by a strong emotional stimulus, such as laughter, anger, or fear. **Sleep paralysis** is the inability to move either immediately upon awakening or just prior to sleep onset, usually associated with considerable anxiety (at least during the first few episodes.) Both represent the dissociated REM phenomenon of muscle atonia intruding upon wakefulness. **Hypnagogic hallucinations** are dream images (another dissociated REM phenomenon) intruding onto wakefulness, and may occur just before sleep onset or after awakening.

The diagnosis of narcolepsy is established by performing nocturnal polysomnography followed by a **multiple sleep latency test** (MSLT). Polysomnography consists of recording multiple physiological signals during sleep, including electroencephalograms (EEG), electrooculograms (EOG), and submental electromyogram (EMG) to define the presence and stage of sleep; respiratory signals to determine whether sleep-disordered breathing is present; and anterior tibialis EMG, to screen for periodic limb movement disorder. The nocturnal polysomnogram may demonstrate recurrent arousals without any precipitating events, consistent with the disturbed nocturnal sleep that narcoleptics often report; approximately 20% of individuals with narcolepsy demonstrate some degree of sleep apnea (as in this patient) or periodic limb movement disorder, adding to their sleep complaint. As was demonstrated in this individual, the time required to fall asleep (initial sleep latency) is usually short, and the first REM episode may occur much earlier than usual.

The MSLT is performed on the day after nocturnal polysomnography, and consists of a series of four or five nap opportunities separated by 2-hour intervals. The average time required to fall asleep during the MSLT is called the *mean sleep latency*, and is a measure of sleepiness; the presence of REM sleep during two or more naps indicates an abnormal tendency to exhibit REM sleep. If the nocturnal polysomnogram is relatively normal, mean sleep latency is reduced, and there are two or more naps containing REM sleep, the diagnosis of narcolepsy is established. The diagnosis is somewhat ambiguous if the nocturnal polysomnogram demonstrates significant degrees of sleep apnea or periodic limb movement disorder.

The present patient had only borderline obstructive sleep apnea and a markedly abnormal MSLT, confirming the diagnosis of narcolepsy. If a more severe degree of sleep apnea is demonstrated, treatment of the nocturnal sleep disorder followed by repeat MSLT usually is required to establish the additional diagnosis of narcolepsy.

Treatment of narcolepsy consists of stimulant medications to relieve daytime sleepiness and REM-suppressant medications to minimize dissociated REM symptoms. Conventional stimulants such as methylphenidate and dextroamphetamine are used most commonly. Modafinil, a wakefulness-promoting agent without CNS and cardiovascular stimulant effects, has been released recently and may be preferable in some patients. Significant dissociated REM symptoms (particularly cataplexy) can be treated with selective serotonin reuptake inhibitors (such as fluoxetine) initially. More severe symptoms may require tricyclic antidepressants or even monoamine oxidase inhibitors. Periodic brief naps are recommended, and psychiatric or social service counseling may be necessary due to the psychosocial effects of the disease.

The present patient presented with the characteristic clinical features of narcolepsy. The reduced mean sleep latency correlated with the patient's complaint of sleepiness, while the presence of REM sleep in her naps explained her hypnagogic hallucinations, hypnopompic sleep paralysis, and cataplexy. She was treated with modafinil and fluoxetine, as well as brief naps three times daily. She reported improved daytime functioning, substantial reduction in cataplexy episodes, and remission of hypnagogic hallucinations and hypnopompic sleep paralysis.

Clinical Pearls

1. Excessive fatigue or sleepiness in a young person with good sleep habits may be due to narcolepsy.

2. In the absence of dissociated REM symptoms, other common disorders causing excessive daytime sleepiness should be considered first. These include obstructive sleep apnea and insufficient sleep syndrome.

3. Persons with narcolepsy typically suffer symptoms for many years before diagnosis.

4. In addition to pharmacological therapy, narcolepsy treatment should include periodic brief naps and appropriate psychosocial intervention.

REFERENCES.
1. Wittig R, Zorick F, Piccione P, et al: Narcolepsy and disturbed nocturnal sleep. Clin Neurophysiol 1983; 14:130–134.
2. Aldrich MS: Narcolepsy. Neurology 1992; 42(suppl 6):34–43.
3. Mullington J, Broughton R: Scheduled naps in the management of daytime sleepiness in narcolepsy-cataplexy. Sleep 1993; 16:444-456.
4. Mitler MM, Aldrich MS, Koob GF, Zarcone VP: American Sleep Disorders Association Standards of Practice. Narcolepsy and its treatment with stimulants. Sleep 1994; 17:352–371.
5. U.S. Modafinil in Narcolepsy Multicenter Study Group: Randomized trial of modafinil for the treatment of pathological somnolence in narcolepsy. Ann Neurol 1998; 43:88–97.
6. Nishino S, Ripley B, Overeem S, et al: Hypocretin (orexin) deficiency in human narcolepsy. Lancet 2000; 355:39–40.

Richard J. Martin, MD

PATIENT 31

A 48-year-old woman with worsening bronchospasm

A 48-year-old woman presents with worsening asthma. She has a lifelong history of asthma that has required oral prednisone therapy for the last 4 years. She has recently used her inhaled β-agonist, albuterol, more frequently during the day because it does not seem to be as effective as in previous years. Her medications include fluticasone (110 μg/puff) by meter dose inhaler (MDI) at 2 puffs bid; albuterol MDI 2 puffs 5 to 8 times a day and 3 times during the night; ipratropium bromide 2 puffs qid; and prednisone 10–20 mg each morning between 7 and 8 AM.

Physical Examination: Temperature 36.9°; pulse 110; respiration 24; blood pressure 138/88. General: cushingoid appearance, slight respiratory distress. HEENT: small oropharynx; boggy nasal mucosa with clear secretions. Cardiac: normal. Chest: decreased breath sounds, no wheezes. Abdomen: striae. Extremities: trace edema. Neurologic: difficulty getting up from a chair; depressed about her illness.

Laboratory Findings: Chest radiograph: hyperinflated lung fields; bronchial wall thickening. Screening sinus CT: pansinusitis. Esophageal pH probe: no evidence of gastrointestinal reflux. Polysomnogram: 20 obstructive apneas per hour. Laryngoscopy: vocal cord function normal. Spirometry: severe airflow limiation with 18% improvement after bronchodilator; no inspiratory flow abnormality. Peak expiratory flow rates over 24 hours: see below. Bone densitometry: decreased density in the femor trochanter and lumbar spine. MDI technique: patient was observed to double-actuate her inhalers and have a rapid inspiratory phase.

Question: How should this patient's treatment regimen be changed to improve her severe asthma symptoms?

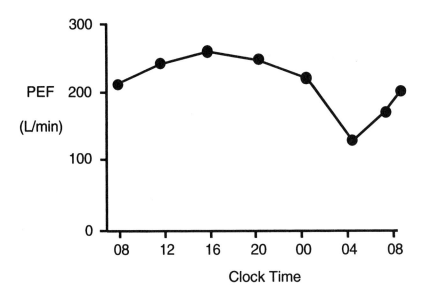

Diagnosis: Severe persistent asthma with pansinusitis.

Discussion: Asthma is classified as mild intermittent, mild persistent, moderate persistent, and severe persistent. This classification allows a stepwise approach to treatment based on the recommendations of the Expert Panel II report from the National Heart, Lung, and Blood Institute.

In managing patients with severe persistent asthma, the first step is to instruct them on the **proper technique for using an MDI**. Although this recommendation seems simplistic, studies demonstrate that 50% of patients and a large number of healthcare providers do not know how to use inhaled medications properly. This step alone frequently improves asthma control by promoting better delivery of drug to patients' lungs.

An additional step in managing severe persistent asthma is to **maximize the dose of inhaled corticosteroids**. Many patients benefit from a starting dose of fluticasone of 3 puffs of a 220 µg/ml formulation bid. Other inhaled steroids can be used at an equivalent dose, recognizing that each steroid preparation has a different potency. Recent studies also indicate that combining an inhaled steroid with a long-acting β-2 agonist such as salmeterol, a long-acting theophylline product, or a leukotriene modifer will produces better symptom control than relying on progressively higher doses of inhaled corticosteroids.

Clinicians should remember that the nocturnal worsening of asthma is a major risk factor for asthma morbidity and mortality. Additionally, when nocturnal asthma is controlled, daytime symptoms are more easily managed. There are two important points regarding nocturnal asthma. First, consider whether the patient has sleep apnea. Studies demonstrate that improving sleep-related apneas not only improves nocturnal asthma, but also improves daytime asthma symptoms. Second, airway inflammation from asthma is greatest during the night, and oral steroids given at 3 PM improve asthma control and do not increase systemic toxicity.

The control of naso-sinus disease is important to overall control of asthma. A screening sinus CT is more than adequate for determining the degree of chronic sinusitis. Saline naso-sinus irrigation followed by nasal steroids improves both the upper and lower airway disease.

Frequent doses of inhaled short-acting β-2 agonists down-regulate the β-2 receptors in the airway and make this class of medications less effective. Therefore, short-acting β-2 agonists should be reserved for "rescue" therapy.

For patients with steroid-induced osteoporosis and myopathy, the main intervention is to decrease the oral steroid dose to as low as possible, or discontinue these agents whenever possible. Patients who require long-term oral steroids and patients with established osteoporosis require careful management with calcium, vitamin D, hormonal agents, and newer drugs that restore calcium to bone to prevent progressive steroid-induced osteoporosis. The steroid-induced myopathy most commonly affects proximal muscle groups. Physical therapy and strengthening exercises are adjuncts to lowering or discontinuing oral corticosteroids.

Aggressive management of gastrointestinal reflux and immunotherapy for allergy-related symptoms are additional interventions for patients with severe persistent asthma.

The present patient had severe persistent asthma with steroid toxicity, and evidence of nocturnal bronchospasm as demonstrated by her 24-hour peak flow data (see figure). After improving her MDI technique and adding a spacer to her MDI, her symptoms improved. She increased her inhaled fluticasone dose to 660 µg bid and received a bid dose of inhaled salmeterol, 2 puffs. She also received therapy with a nocturnal continuous positive airway pressure device, which improved her sleep apnea and daytime asthma symptoms. Her oral prednisone dosing was changed to 3 PM daily. With these interventions, the patient's asthma dramatically improved over the following 4 weeks, allowing her prednisone to be tapered to 7.5 mg/day. The prednisone was not tapered below 7.5 mg/day until improvement in her adrenal gland supresion could occur. Her sinus disease was treated with saline naso-sinus irrigation, followed by sprays of nasal steroids.

Clinical Pearls

1. Proper technique for use of MDIs is mandatory for best therapeutic efficacy.
2. The inflammatory response in asthma increases during the night.
3. Efficient dose timing of certain medications improves asthma outcome.
4. Sleep apnea can worsen both nocturnal and daytime asthma.
5. Improving upper airway disease (rhinosinusitis) has a beneficial effect on asthma.
6. Chronic oral steroids can produce Cushing's syndrome, with adrenal suppression, osteoporosis, and myopathy.

REFERENCES

1. Chan CS, Woolcock AJ, Sullivan CE: Nocturnal asthma: Role of snoring and obstructive sleep apnea. Am Rev Respir Dise 1988;137:1503–1504.
2. Beam WR, Weiner DE, Martin RJ: Timing of prednisone and alterations of airways inflammation in nocturnal asthma. Am Rev Respir Dis 1992;146:1524–1530.
3. Corren J, Adinoff AD, Buchmeier AD, Irvin CG: Nasal beclomethasone prevents the seasonal increase in bronchial responsiveness in patients with allergic rhinitis and asthma. J Allergy Clin Immunol 1992;90:250–256.
4. Greening AP, Ind PW, Northfield M, Shaw G: Added salmeterol versus higher-corticosteroid. Lancet 1994;344:219–242.
5. National Asthma Education and Prevention Program. Expert Panel Report 2: Guidelines for the Diagnosis and Management of Asthma. Pub. no. 97-4051. Bethesda, MD, National Institutes of Health, 1997.
6. Laviolette M, Malmstrom K, Lu S, et al: Montelukast added to inhaled beclomethasone in treatment of asthma. Am J Respir Crit Care Med 1999; 160:1862–1868.

Glenn D. Braunstein, MD

PATIENT 32

A 35-year-old man with breast enlargement and a testicular mass

A 35-year-old man presents with a 3-month history of bilateral enlargement of both breasts associated with nipple tenderness without discharge. He denies chest trauma, presence of a cough, abdominal pain, and testicular masses. There is no history of cryptorchidism or use of medications known to be associated with gynecomastia. He does note a 1-month history of diminished libido.

Physical Examination: Blood pressure 130/80, pulse 68 and regular. Visual fields: full to confrontation. Thyroid: normal size and texture. Chest: clear to percussion and auscultation. Breasts: bilateral 4 cm gynecomastia tender to palpation. Cardiac: regular rate without murmur. Abdomen: liver, spleen, and kidneys not felt; bowel sounds present. GU: both testes in a scrotal position; right measures 15 ml, left 20 ml by Prader orchiodometer; no masses or tenderness.

Laboratory Findings: CBC, liver functions tests, creatinine, BUN, free thyroxine, TSH: normal. Serum human chorionic gonadotropin (hCG) and alpha-fetoprotein: undetectable. Serum testosterone 270 ng/dl (300–1000), estradiol 80 pg/ml (< 40), LH 1.5 mIU/ml (1–8), FSH 0.5 mIU/ml (1–7), serum dehydroepiandrosterone-sulfate (DHEA-sulfate) 300 ug/dl (100–450). Chest radiograph: normal. Testicular ultrasound: 2-cm hypoechogenic mass in left testis.

Question: What is the cause of this patient's gynecomastia?

Diagnosis: Leydig cell tumor.

Discussion: Gynecomastia is due to an imbalance between the estrogen and androgen concentrations or effects at the level of the breast glandular tissue. Such an imbalance may result from an increase in free estrogen levels, an absolute increase in estrogen levels, a decrease in endogenous free androgen concentrations, androgen receptor defects, or medications that interact with the estrogen receptor. This patient exhibited an elevated estradiol and slightly suppressed testosterone concentration in his serum. Such a combination can be found in an individual who is ingesting exogenous estrogens, has an estrogen-secreting neoplasm of the testes or adrenal, has primary hypogonadism with excessive gonadotropin stimulation of the Leydig cells, or has a condition associated with excessive aromatization of androgens to estrogens, such as obesity, hyperthyroidism, or liver disease. The elevated estradiol, suppressed testosterone, and normal concentrations of the adrenal androgen DHEA-sulfate, in association with hypoechogenic mass in the left testicle, indicates that this patient has an estradiol-secreting neoplasm of the testes.

Approximately 95% of testicular tumors are **germ cell tumors** of testes, and those that contain trophoblastic elements that secrete hCG may be associated with gynecomastia. The hCG, which biochemically resembles luteinizing hormone (LH), stimulates the normal Leydig cells to secrete testosterone and estradiol. The concentrations of the latter are increased out of proportion to the former in the presence of high levels of hCG. In addition, trophoblastic tumors have increased placental-type aromatase activity, which results in an increased production of estrogens from androgens. Therefore, testosterone is excessively converted to estradiol, and androstenedione is excessively converted to estrone. The resulting imbalance of estrogens to androgens then leads to gynecomastia. This patient does not have a germ cell tumor as a cause of his gynecomastia, since his hCG concentration is undetectable in the serum. In addition, many germ cell tumors also secrete alpha-fetoprotein, which also is undetectable in this patient.

Leydig cell tumors of the testes account for < 2% of all tumors. Approximately 90% of these tumors are benign, and the 10% that are malignant are associated with a median survival of about 4 years. Between 20 and 30% of patients with Leydig cell tumors experience gynecomastia, decreased libido, and possibly erectile dysfunction. The Leydig cells contain aromatase activity which converts testosterone to estradiol. The high intra-testicular estradiol concentration inhibits testosterone biosynthesis through a direct effect on the steroid biosynthetic enzymes as well as indirectly through inhibition of pituitary LH secretion, which results in decrease trophic hormone stimulation of the testes. Thus, the testicle contralateral to the one containing the tumor may exhibit some degree of atrophy. Although Leydig cell tumors may be small and nonpalpable, all men with an elevated estradiol and suppressed LH (a finding which rules out primary hypogonadism as a cause of the elevated estradiol) should undergo a **testicular ultrasound evaluation**. This is a sensitive technique for picking up such small tumors.

A rare neoplasm of the testes that also may be associated with gynecomastia and may present in a similar fashion to Leydig cell tumors, is the large cell calcifying **Sertoli cell tumor**. This is associated with increased aromatase activity. Although these tumors can occur sporadically, they often are seen in association with several complex syndromes including the Peutz-Jeghers syndrome (gastrointestinal polyposis and lip macules) and the Carney complex (atrial myxomas, skin pigmentation, and adrenal nodules).

The treatment of choice for Leydig cell tumors is **orchidectomy**. This results in a normalization of the serum estradiol and testosterone concentrations, resumption of appropriate spermatogenesis, and resolution of the decreased libido and erectile dysfunction. The gynecomastia may or may not regress, depending upon the length of time that it has been present. Gynecomastia that is present for 3 months or less demonstrates a florid pattern histologically, with marked proliferation of the breast glandular epithelial cells, stromal edema, and infiltration of the stroma with round cells. Correction of the estrogen-androgen imbalance during this stage generally leads to full resolution of the gynecomastia. However, gynecomastia that has been present for 12 months or more usually has entered a fibrotic stage, with hylinization of the stromal tissue, dilation of the ducts, and a decrease in the epithelial proliferation. Restoration of the normal estrogen-androgen balance at this stage is *unlikely* to lead to significant reduction in the size of the breasts. Although medical therapies such as anti-androgens (e.g., tamoxifen) or aromatase inhibitors (e.g., anastrozole) may resolve the gynecomastia during the florid stage of the disease, they also are unlikely to be of help once the patient is in the fibrotic stage. In that situation, reduction mammoplasty is the therapy of choice.

The present patient underwent a radical orchidectomy. The bisected left testes demonstrated a well-circumscribed, tan lesion; histological exam revealed a Leydig cell tumor containing numerous crystals of Reinke. Although occasional mitoses were seen, there was no evidence of vascular invasion, and a CT examination of the pelvis did not demonstrate any retroperitoneal adenopathy. Six weeks postoperatively, his testosterone had risen to 850 ng/dl, estradiol had decreased to 26 pg/ml, LH had risen to 5 mIU/ml, and FSH had risen to 4.5 mIU/ml. His breast and nipple pain had completely remitted, and the size of his gynecomastia had decreased to 1.5 cm bilaterally. He no longer complained of erectile dysfunction.

Clinical Pearls

1. In a patient with gynecomastia, an elevated serum estradiol and decreased testosterone with normal LH warrants an evaluation for testicular or adrenal neoplasms, as well as liver or kidney disease or hyperthyroidism.

2. Even if a testicular mass is not palpated, a testicular ultrasound should be carried out in a patient with an elevated estradiol and low testosterone with normal gonadotropins.

3. If gynecomastia has been present for a year or more, it is unlikely to respond to removal or correction of the cause of the estrogen-androgen imbalance, nor to administration of antiestrogens or aromatase-inhibiting drugs, because of underlying fibrosis.

4. Gynecomastia associated with germ cell tumors of the testes is associated with elevations of human chorionic gonadotropin concentrations.

REFERENCES

1. Fox H, Reeve NL: Endocrine effects of testicular neoplasms. Invest Cell Pathol 1979;2:63–73.
2. Bercovici J-P, Nahoul K, Ducasse M, et al: Leydig cell tumor with gynecomastia: Further studies—The recovery after unilateral orchidectomy. J Clin Endocrinology Metab 1985;61:957–962.
3. Mathur R, Braunstein GD: Gynecomastia: Pathomechanisms and treatment strategies. Horm Res 1997;48:95–102.
4. Junnila J, Lassen P: Testicular masses. Am Family Phys 1998;57:685–692.
5. Braunstein GD: Aromatase and gynecomastia. Endocrine-Related Cancer 1999;6:315–324.

Catherine J. Markin, MD
Alan Barker, MD

PATIENT 33

A 36-year-old man with worsening of a chronic cough

A 36-year-old man presents for evaluation of a recently worsening cough that has been present for several years. He also notes low-grade fevers, occasional chills, and night sweats. The patient denies a history of sinusitis or hemoptysis, but has noted occasional wheezing and dyspnea with exertion in the past. His PPD was positive 10 years ago when he immigrated to the United States from Mexico; he completed 12 months of isoniazid for treatment of latent tuberculosis. He denies frequent respiratory illnesses in childhood and does not drink alcohol, smoke, or use illicit drugs. He and his wife have been unable to conceive children. One of his six brothers is infertile.

Physical Examination: Temperature 37.5; pulse 60; respiration 14; blood pressure 90/60. General: weight 140 lbs; height 5'8". Lymph nodes: bilateral axillary adenopathy. Chest: scattered crackles and rhonchi throughout both lungs. Cardiac: normal. Extremities: no edema or clubbing.

Laboratory Findings: CBC: normal. Sputum culture: 3+ *Staphylococcus aureus*, 3+ *Pseudomonas aeruginosa*, 2+ aspergillus species. Three sputums for AFB stain and culture: negative. High-resolution chest CT: see below. Spirometry: FVC 2.57 L (58% of predicted), FEV_1 1.7 L (47% of predicted), FEV_1/FVC 0.66.

Question: What additional studies would define the underlying etiology of this patient's clinical problem?

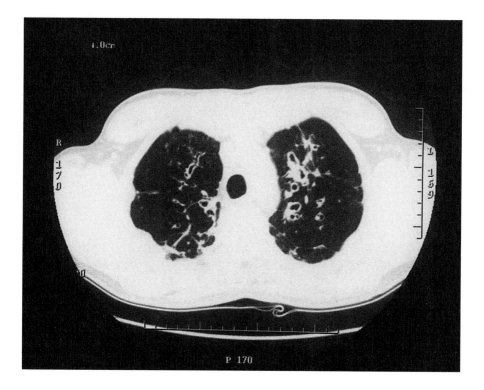

Answer: Serum immunoglobulin levels, serum aspergillus precipitins, nasal mucosal biopsy, sweat chloride test.

Discussion: Bronchiectasis is defined pathologically as irreversible, abnormal dilation of the bronchi. It is characterized clinically by chronic cough productive of purulent sputum, recurrent pulmonary infections, and progressive decline in lung function. Recurrent hemoptysis is common and sometimes life-threatening. Inflammation of the lower airways is critical in development of bronchiectasis, with proinflammatory cytokines, inflammatory cells, and proteolytic enzymes in the airways leading to permanent damage and dilation. The dilated airways have impaired ciliary action and mucus clearance. Colonization of micro-organisms occurs, with perpetuation of inflammation by host reaction to these organisms. The result is a vicious cycle of bronchial wall damage with ever increasing bronchiectasis.

Bronchiectasis is historically classified as cylindrical, varicose, or cystic based on the pattern of bronchial dilation. A clinically more important distinction considers the extent of lung involvement: localized versus diffuse. Although most patients with bronchiectasis have an abnormal chest radiograph (85–95%), the distribution and extent of disease is better visualized with CT. **High-resolution CT scanning** (HRCT) has become the imaging procedure of choice. The use of thin or medium (1- to 4-mm) sections at close intervals has improved the sensitivity and specificity of HRCT over conventional imaging techniques. HRCT findings include bronchial wall thickening, signet ring sign (bronchi on end with internal diameter greater than the adjacent pulmonary artery), bronchi extending to the costal margin and/or abutting mediastinal structures, and loss of bronchial wall tapering.

Focal bronchial obstruction is the most common cause of **localized bronchiectasis**, such as from a foreign body, broncholith, stricture, or endobronchial mass. Localized bronchiectasis may result from necrotizing pneumonia, although this is uncommon in the era of antibiotics. Surgical resection remains the mainstay of treatment for localized bronchiectasis.

The etiologies of **diffuse bronchiectasis** are more numerous than localized disease. Diffuse bronchiectasis is associated with chronic pulmonary infections, such as tuberculosis and non-tuberculosis mycobacterial infections. Childhood immunizations have resulted in a significant decrease in post-infectious bronchiectasis from severe pneumonia (i.e., adenovirus, pertussis, or measles). Immunologically mediated airway inflammation is the mechanism of bronchiectasis in allergic bronchopulmonary aspergillosis (ABPA) and lung allograft

rejection, with similar immune-mediated mechanisms occurring in bronchiectasis associated with rheumatoid arthritis, Sjögren's disease, and ulcerative colitis.

The most common causes of diffuse bronchiectasis are related to impaired local or systemic host defenses. **Local impaired host defenses** include dyskinetic cilia syndrome, cystic fibrosis, and Young's syndrome (obstructive azoospermia). Syndromes with **systemic impaired host defenses** include X-linked agammaglobulinemia, common variable immunodeficiency, chronic granulomatous disease of childhood, and selective immunoglobulin deficiency. Bronchiectasis also occurs in the setting of HIV disease, resulting from recurrent bacterial, *Pneumocystis carinii*, or mycobacterial infections.

Cystic fibrosis is the most common congenital cause of diffuse bronchiectasis. There is considerable heterogeneity in disease severity among patients with cystic fibrosis. Adult presentation of cystic fibrosis is relatively uncommon; most patients present in early childhood with pulmonary involvement and/or pancreatic insufficiency, or with meconium ileus in severely affected newborns. The respiratory syndromes in patients with cystic fibrosis consist of recurrent lung infections associated with diffuse bronchiectasis, asthma, and chronic obstructive pulmonary disease. The presence of *Pseudomonas aeruginosa* and/or *Staphylococcus aureus* in a patient's sputum should raise suspicion of cystic fibrosis.

The gene responsible for cystic fibrosis was identified in 1989 and encodes for cystic fibrosis transmembrane conductance regulator (CFTR), a protein that controls chloride and water transport from cells into the lumen of the airway. Patients can be homozygote or heterozygote for the abnormal allele. Cystic fibrosis appears to be a monogenic disease, although hundreds of mutations within the CFTR gene have been identified. Phenotypic variability is a result of the variety of mutations within the CFTR gene, as well as homozygote versus heterozygote genotype. In addition, it is well documented that patients with the same CFTR mutation(s) have variable disease severity, suggesting that there probably are modifier genes and/or environmental factors that also affect phenotypic expression.

In the present patient, diffuse bronchiectasis was evident on his HRCT. The presence of aspergillus in the sputum raised the possibility of ABPA. The family's difficulty having children suggested the possibilities of cystic fibrosis or a dyskinetic cilia syndrome. The patient underwent further laboratory evaluation with the following results—serum immunoglobulin levels: mildly elevated IgA, normal IgG, IgE and IgM; serum aspergillus precipitins: negative; nasal mucosal biopsy: ciliary structure normal on electron microscopy, cilia motility normal; sweat chloride test: 85 mmol/L (normal 4–56 mmol/L). The normal serum immunoglobulin levels did not entirely eliminate the possibility of an IgG subclass deficiency, in which the total IgG level can be normal. The elevated sweat chloride with a normal ultrastructural respiratory mucosal biopsy, however, confirmed the diagnosis of cystic fibrosis.

Clinical Pearls

1. Recurrent respiratory infections, chronic productive cough, obstructive impairment on spirometry, and shadowing of airway dilation or thickening on chest radiograph should raise suspicion of bronchiectasis.

2. HRCT scanning is a noninvasive, sensitive test for detection of the airway abnormalities in bronchiectasis and has become the imaging procedure of choice.

3. Diffuse bronchiectasis is a common manifestation of a wide variety of diseases that are characterized by local or systemic host defense dysfunction.

4. Substantial variability in phenotypic expression of cystic fibrosis occurs with less severely affected patients, who sometimes present in adulthood.

REFERENCES

1. Kang EY, Miller RR, Müller NL: Bronchiectasis: Comparison of preoperative thin-section CT and pathologic findings in resected specimens. Radiology 1995;195:649–654.
2. Van der Bruggen-Bogaarts BA, van der Bruggen HM, van Waes PF, Lammers JW: Screening for bronchiectasis: A comparative study between chest radiography and high resolution CT. Chest 1996;109:608–611.
3. Stern RC: The diagnosis of cystic fibrosis. New Engl J Med 1997;336:487–491.
4. Delen FM, AF Barker: New concepts in diagnosis and management of bronchiectasis. Resp Crit Care Med 1999;20:311–320.

PATIENT 34

A 52-year-old man with hepatocellular carcinoma and a wife who requests aggressive life-supportive care

A 52-year-old man with a long history of alcoholism, a 2-year history of Child's Class C cirrhosis, and a recent diagnosis of hepatocellular carcinoma is brought to the emergency department after two episodes of hematemesis at home. He is confused and disoriented, but his wife reports that he was felling well until the morning of admission, when he developed hematemesis. She reports that he has a good quality of life at home. He does not leave the house, but at baseline is not confused and enjoys communicating with her, watching television, and visiting with his adult children. His past medical history is significant for three episodes of esophageal variceal bleeding in the past year.

Physical Examination: Blood pressure 82/50; pulse 145; temperature 37.5. General: thin, jaundiced, confused, lethargic. HEENT: scleral icterus. Cardiac: tachycardic, without murmur. Abdomen: protruberant with caput medusa, but nontender. Extremities: no edema.

Laboratory Findings: Hematocrit 22%, WBC 8800/μl with normal differential, electrolytes normal. BUN 52 mg/dl, creatinine 1.4 mg/dl, INR 3.2.

Hospital course: The patient was admitted to the intensive care unit (ICU), where he received blood product support including 12 units of packed red blood cells and 4 units of fresh frozen plasma. He also received volume resuscitation with intravenous saline and was treated for hepatic encephalopathy with lactulose per rectum. He underwent endoscopy, which showed bleeding varices that were banded. Throughout his early ICU stay, the patient's wife seemed worried that intensive care might be withheld against her wishes. On the second hospital day, the patient aspirated and developed acute respiratory distress syndrome (ARDS) and septic shock. He required endotracheal intubation and mechanical ventilation for adequate oxygenation and airway protection. He also required dopamine infusion to maintain his systolic blood pressure over 90 mmHg. The patient's wife requests that the medical team "do everything" to keep him alive.

Question: Should life-sustaining therapy be continued?

Diagnosis: Terminal liver disease with a very low chance of survival.

Discussion: Death is common in the ICU, due to patients' severity of illness. Of patients who die in the hospital, approximately half are cared for in an ICU within 3 days of their death. Currently, almost 90% of deaths in the ICU involve withholding or withdrawing at least one life-supporting intervention—a dramatic increase compared to 10–15 years ago. Thus, the ICU has become a setting where decisions about managing the death of patients are made on a frequent basis.

In the presented case, the patient is admitted to the hospital with two terminal diseases, hepatocellular carcinoma and Child's class C cirrhosis. His upper gastrointestinal bleeding is a potentially reversible problem, and there is a reasonable chance he could return home with his current quality of life. His wife, the surrogate decision-maker, tells the doctors that the patient would want to receive intensive care for his upper gastrointestinal bleeding. At this point in his care, intensive life-support therapy is reasonable and was provided, even though some of the physicians caring for this patient felt that they would not want such care if they were in the patient's position.

Communication with families about end-of-life care in the ICU is an important skill for physicians and nurses. Family members with loved ones in the ICU rate communication with healthcare providers as extremely important—yet there is some evidence that such interactions are lacking. Early in the ICU stay, communication with this patient's wife should focus on building rapport, understanding her concerns about her husband's medical care, and educating her about the disease prognosis, treatment options, and possible outcomes. In addition, since she expresses some concern that life-sustaining therapy might be withheld against her wishes, explore why she feels that way and what experiences she has had to cause such feelings. These concerns often are best pursued in a family meeting with the physicians and nurses providing the major part of the patient's care. If there are other physicians involved in this patient's outpatient care, it can be useful to involve them as well. Additional family members and other support people for the wife also should be invited to attend. These meetings should occur in a private and quiet setting, without interruptions. Take the time to elicit the family's understanding of what is happening and their perspective on the patient's life, goals, and values and what his wishes would be in this situation. **Listening** is an important part of the physician's role in these conferences—yet there is evidence that physicians spend only 25% of the time in such conversations listening.

During the second hospital day, the clinical picture changed dramatically after the patient developed ARDS and septic shock. At this point, another family conference should be arranged to discuss these changes with the wife. Educate the family about the change in condition and the effect this has on the treatment options and the prognosis. It is important to be supportive of the wife and sensitive to the burden and stress on her. Given the clinical picture, discuss the option of withdrawing life-sustaining therapy, and focus the wife on what her husband would want in this situation. Focusing on what the patient would want, rather than what the family wants, can make it much easier for families to face these difficult situations. Make recommendations, but without trying to coerce the family into a decision. Note that offering a series of options without making any recommendations leaves the family feeling unsupported.

Allow families some time in facing these difficult decisions. Often, the medical team comes to the decision before the family does that withdrawing life-sustaining therapy is in the patient's best interest. Sometimes, **giving the family some time to adjust** to withdrawing life support can be a good use of intensive care resources. In this case, the wife initially was adamantly opposed to withdrawing life support. The medical team listened to her perspective and let her know that life-sustaining therapy would be continued if that is what she thought her husband would want. This approach reduced the pressure on her, and she felt that the medical team was "on her side." Within 24 hours after the second meeting, she decided that her husband would not want life support, given an extremely poor prognosis for short-term survival and dismal prognosis for long-term survival.

Conduct withdrawal of life support with the same care and attention that you perform other procedures. Develop a protocol that allows this to be done in a way that assures patient comfort and makes this as good an experience for the family as possible . In this case, once the patient's wife made the decision to withdraw life support, the team allowed the family to visit the patient and say their good-byes. Another family conference was held to educate the family about the withdrawal process and how long the team expected the patient to survive. The patient was on moderate levels of vasopressor medication and high levels of ventilator support, so the team expected the patient to die within an hour.

After the family has said good-bye, all life-sustaining therapies should be stopped. The only rationale for weaning any therapy is when its abrupt removal will cause discomfort. The ventilator is the only therapy that can cause discomfort when it is abruptly removed; therefore rapid terminal weaning should be performed to allow titration of medication for control of dyspnea and discomfort.

The present patient's dopamine was turned off; all laboratory and radiologic tests were stopped; and all medications were discontinued except for those medications that provided for comfort, including a continuous infusion of a narcotic and a benzodiazepine. Sometimes patients require very high doses due to tolerance developed over a long ICU stay: *no dose is too high if lower doses fail to achieve comfort*. The patient appeared comfortable, so the PEEP was removed, and the FiO2 was turned to room air. This caused an increase in respiratory rate and grimacing, so the morphine drip was increased until the grimacing resolved. Then the respiratory rate set on the ventilator was turned down while the physician observed for evidence of discomfort. The morphine rate was again increased for evidence of dyspnea, but then the patient appeared comfortable and the ventilator was removed from the room. At this point, the EKG leads were removed, and the patient was extubated. Sometimes physicians and families may decide to leave the endotracheal tube in place to allow suctioning and avoid any upper airway obstruction. Both approaches are acceptable. This patient's family wanted the endotracheal tube out so they could feel closer to him. They stayed in his room, and he died within 15 minutes.

Clinical Pearls

1. Sensitive but honest communication with patients and families about end-of-life care in the ICU is an important skill for providing high-quality ICU care.

2. Once the decision is made to withdraw or withhold life-sustaining treatments, all treatments and tests that do not provide for comfort should be stopped, including nutritional support. The only rationale for weaning any therapy is when its abrupt removal will cause discomfort.

3. In the setting of withdrawal of the ventilator, abrupt removal can cause discomfort in some patients. In this situation, the ventilator should be rapidly weaned, using the weaning process to assess for and treat evidence of patient discomfort.

4. High doses of narcotics and benzodiazapines sometimes are required to assure patient comfort during the withdrawal of life support. No dose is too high if lower doses have failed to achieve comfort.

REFERENCES

1. Tulsky JA, Chesney MA, Lo B: How do medical residents discuss resuscitation with patients? J Gen Intern Med 1995;10(8): 436–442.
2. The SUPPORT Principal Investigators: A controlled trial to improve care for seriously ill hospitalized patients: The study to understand prognoses and preferences for outcomes and risks of treatments (SUPPORT). JAMA 1996;274:1591–1598.
3. Brody H, Campbell ML, Faber-Langendoen K, Ogle KS: Withdrawing intensive life-sustaining treatment: Recommendations for compassionate clinical management. New Engl J Med 1997; 336(9):652–657.
4. Pendergast TJ, Luce JM: Increasing incidence of withholding and withdrawal of life support from the critically ill. Am J Respir Crit Care Med 1997;155:15–20.
5. Johnson D, Wilson M, Cavanaugh B, et al: Measuring the ability to meet family needs in an intensive care unit. Critical Care Medicine 1998;26:266–271.
6. Curtis JR, Patrick DL: How to discuss dying and death in the ICU. In Curtis JR, Rubenfeld GD (eds): Managing Death in the Intensive Care Unit: The Transition from Cure to Comfort. New York, NY, Oxford University Press, 2000.
7. Rubenfeld GD, Crawford S: Principles and practice of withdrawing life-sustaining treatments in the ICU. In Curtis JR, Rubenfeld GD (eds): Managing Death in the Intensive Care Unit: The Transition from Cure to Comfort. New York, NY, Oxford University Press, 2000.

Colleen L. Bailey, MD
Lewis J. Rubin, MD

PATIENT 35

A 32-year-old, HIV-positive man with syncope and dyspnea

A 32-year-old, HIV-positive man with a CD4 count of 385 cells/μl presents to his primary care physician after an episode of syncope. He was well until 1 month previously, when he noted mild dyspnea while performing household chores. Yesterday while jogging he experienced dyspnea, substernal chest pain, and loss of consciousness for several seconds. He denies any recent fevers, chills, sweats, weight loss, headaches, seizures, cough, orthopnea, abdominal pain, edema, or neurological deficits.

Physical Examination: Temperature 38.0°, pulse 80, blood pressure 116/80, respirations 12, oxygen saturation 99% on room air. General: well appearing, in no apparent distress. HEENT: unremarkable. Cardiac: right ventricular lift, accentuated pulmonic component of the second heart sound, II/VI systolic murmur at left lower sternal border without radiation; right-sided S4 gallop; jugular venous pressure 8 cm above the sternal angle with a prominent *a* wave. Chest: normal breath sounds. Abdomen: soft, nontender, liver span 10 cm, no ascites. Extremities: no cyanosis, clubbing, or edema. Neurologic: unremarkable. Skin: unremarkable.

Laboratory Findings: WBC and platelets normal, Hct 35.7%. Chemistry and liver panels: normal. EKG: right ventricular hypertrophy with strain pattern, right bundle branch block, left posterior fasicular block (see figure, *top*). Chest radiograph: cardiomegaly, enlarged pulmonary arteries bilaterally (see figure, *bottom*). Lung ventilation/perfusion scan: normal. Echocardiography: enlarged right heart chambers with depressed right ventricular function, severe tricuspid regurgitation, normal left ventricular function.

Question: What condition has caused this patient's dyspnea and syncope?

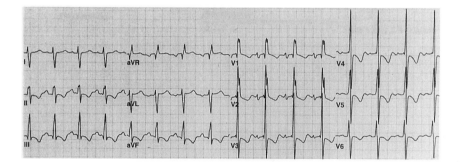

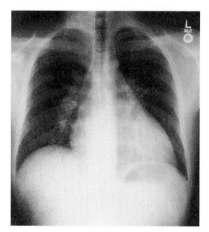

Diagnosis: HIV-associated pulmonary hypertension

Discussion: Pulmonary hypertension (PH) is an uncommon, but well-recognized complication of human immunodeficiency virus infection. The incidence of PH in HIV-infected patients has been estimated to be as high as 0.57%, compared with an incidence of 0.02% for primary pulmonary hypertension (PPH) in the general population.

HIV-associated PH (HIV-PH) does not have a universally accepted definition. Many investigators have applied the criteria of the National Institute of Health Patient Registry for the Characterization of PPH to patients with concomitant HIV: a mean pulmonary artery pressure (mPAP) > 25 mmHg at rest or > 30 mmHg with exercise, a pulmonary capillary wedge pressure (PCWP) < 15 mmHg, and the absence of other secondary causes of PH including parenchymal lung or valvular disease, chronic thromboembolic disease, collagen vascular disease, portal hypertension, or exposure to certain drugs or toxins.

The pathogenesis of HIV-PH remains unclear, but does not appear to be directly due to the virus. One hypothesis suggests an indirect role of HIV in the production of mediators leading to abnormal endothelial and smooth muscle proliferation.

As in other forms of PH, patients with HIV-PH often delay seeking medical attention because their symptoms initially are subtle and are attributed to other disease processes. In most cases, HIV is recognized before the first manifestation of PH. The interval between the diagnosis of HIV infection and PH has been reported to range from 1 to 9 years. PH can occur in any stage of HIV infection with over one-third of patients having CD4 counts > 200 cells/μl.

Consider the diagnosis of PH when an HIV+ patient seeks evaluation for dyspnea on exertion, syncope, chest pain, or fatigue. Initial assessment should consist of a thorough history and physical exam, as well as chest radiograph and EKG. If PH is suspected, the patient should undergo echocardiography to evaluate for evidence of PH and to rule out other secondary cardiac causes. Further work-up includes a ventilation/perfusion scan, pulmonary function tests, and connective tissue serologic studies. Right heart catheterization is necessary to confirm the diagnosis of PH and determine disease severity. Short-acting pulmonary vasodilators may be given during catheterization to assess for pulmonary vascular reactivity and guide treatment.

Given the low prevalence of PH in HIV-infected patients, screening for PH with a transthoracic echocardiogram is recommended only for those patients with symptoms consistent with this diagnosis.

Many of the treatment options for HIV-PH have been extrapolated from studies performed in PPH patients. In PH, venous stasis, slowed pulmonary blood flow, and right heart enlargement combine to increase the risk of developing in situ pulmonary thrombosis and thromboembolism. Several studies have suggested that anticoagulation might improve survival in patients with PPH; however, it is unknown if anticoagulation affects the survival of patients with HIV-PH.

The role of oral vasodilators in the long-term therapy of HIV-PH is unknown. As in primary PH, patients with HIV-PH should first undergo acute vasoreactivity testing with vasodilators (intravenous prostacyclin or adenosine, or inhaled nitric oxide) during right heart catheterization. Those who are responsive to acute vasodilator testing may derive benefit from treatment with oral calcium channel blockers, while those who are unresponsive acutely are unlikely to experience clinical benefit from oral vasodilators.

Prostacyclin, a potent vasodilator with antiplatelet aggregating properties, improves hemodynamics and survival in PPH. One report has described beneficial results with the long-term use of aerosolized prostacyclin in patients with HIV-PH. Long-term results from the use of continuous intravenous prostacyclin have not been reported.

Some case reports have described an improvement in pulmonary hypertension after the institution of combination antiretroviral therapy in patients with HIV-PH, while others have indicated no significant beneficial effect.

The survival of patients with HIV-PH is poor, and is not substantially different from that of primary PH. One study reported a 2-year survival of 46% in 20 patients with HIV-PH, compared to 53% in 71 patients with primary PH. Patients with HIV-PH have a much shorter survival (1.3 versus 2.6 years, respectively), compared to HIV-infected patients without PH. Death in patients with HIV-PH is attributable to pulmonary hypertension in 81% of cases.

This patient reported classic symptoms consistent with the diagnosis of PH, including the subacute onset of dyspnea on exertion, chest pain, and syncope. Physical examination findings of an increased pulmonic component of the second heart sound, a prominent *a* wave in the jugular venous pulse, a right-sided gallop, and a right ventricular lift indicate the presence of pulmonary hypertension and right ventricular pressure overload. Right ventricular hypertrophy and right bundle branch block, as noted on this patient's EKG, are commonly seen in PH. His chest radiograph shows enlargement of the main pulmonary arteries, a finding seen in 90% of patients with PPH.

The diagnosis of PH was confirmed with a right-heart catheterization, which showed a mPAP of 43 mmHg, PCWP of 7 mmHg, right atrial pressure of 14 mmHg, cardiac output 4.8 L/min, and pulmonary vascular resistance 600 dynes·sec/cm^5. He underwent an acute vasodilator trial without any significant change in hemodynamic parameters. He was started on an oral anticoagulant and antiretroviral therapy, and is being closely followed for any evidence of deterioration.

Clinical Pearls

1. The diagnosis of pulmonary hypertension should be considered in an HIV+ patient with dyspnea, exercise intolerance, chest pain, and syncope.

2. HIV-PH occurs in all stages of stages of HIV infection and is not related to the degree of immunodeficiency.

3. Combination antiretroviral therapy may have beneficial effects on pulmonary hypertension and should be considered in all patients, regardless of CD4 count or viral load.

4. The survival of patients with HIV-PH is similar to patients with primary PH, and is significantly worse than HIV-infected patients without PH.

REFERENCES

1. Mette SA, Palevsky HI, Pietra GG, Williams TM, et al: Primary pulmonary hypertension in association with human immunodeficiency virus infection. A possible viral etiology for some forms of hypertensive pulmonary arteriopathy. Am Rev Respir Dis 1992; 145(5):1196–1200.

2. Petitpretz P, Brenot F, Azarian R, et al: Pulmonary hypertension in patients with human immunodeficiency virus infection: Comparison with primary pulmonary hypertension. Circulation 1994; 89:2722–2727.

3. Opravil M, Pechere M, Speich R, et al: HIV-associated primary pulmonary hypertension: a case control study. Am J Respir Crit Care Med 1997; 155:990–995.

4. Rubin LJ: Primary pulmonary hypertension. New Engl J Med 1997; 336(2):111–117.

5. Stricker H, Domenighetti G, Mombelli G: Prostacyclin for HIV-associated pulmonary hypertension. 1997; 127(11):1043.

6. Golpe R, Fernandez-Infante B, Fennandez-Rozas S: Primary pulmonary hypertension associated with human immunodeficiency virus infection. Postgrad Med J 1998; 74(873):400–404.

7. Pellicelli AM, Palmieri F, D'Ambrosio C, et al: Role of human immunodeficiency virus in primary pulmonary hypertension: Care reports. Angiology 1998; 49(12):1005–1011.

8. Rich S: Primary pulmonary hypertension: Executive summary. World Symposium on Primary Pulmonary Hypertension 1998: 1–27.

Winston Sequeira, MD

PATIENT 36

A 63-year-old man with a painful wrist

A 63-year-old man presents with pain and swelling in his right hand that started the previous day. He has had similar episodes in the past and has responded to nonsteroidal anti-inflammatory drugs. Between episodes he is asymptomatic, aside from occasional aches and pains in both hands, which are readily relieved by analgesics. He also notes increasing dyspnea on exertion. In 1975, he was diagnosed with sarcoidosis by transbronchial biopsy and was treated briefly with steroids. He also has a history of renal stones, hypertension, and coronary artery disease. His medications include low-dose aspirin and hydrochlorothiazide.

Physical Examination: Vital signs: normal. General: no respiratory distress. Lymph nodes: none palpable. Chest: crackles. Extremities: dorsum of right hand diffusely swollen with marked tenderness over both wrists; digits of right index and middle finger diffusely swollen and tender; no subcutaneous nodules or clubbing.

Laboratory Findings: Radiograph of right hand: see below. Right wrist aspiration: joint fluid cultures negative; negatively birefringent crystals of sodium urate present. Serum angiotensin-converting enzyme 156 U (normal 8–52), uric acid 9.1 mg/dl, serum and urinary calcium normal; rheumatoid factor positive.

Question: Consider the etiology of the patient's joint complaints.

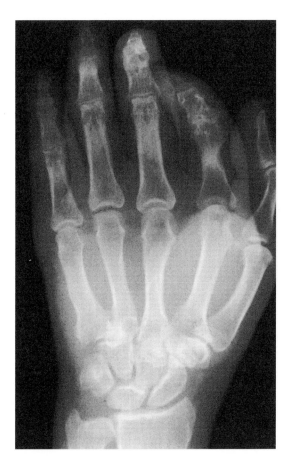

Diagnosis: Sarcoid dactylitis with gout.

Discussion: Patients with sarcoidosis may have joint pains with articular or periarticular swelling. Joint symptoms may be acute or chronic, with the acute arthritis tending to occur in the spring. A triad of acute polyarthritis with hilar lymph nodes and erythema nodosum is referred to as **Lofgren's syndrome**. The ankles are involved in 90% of cases; obtain a chest radiograph to exclude sarcoidosis in any patient presenting with bilateral ankle pain and swelling. Acute onset of joint pains is usually associated with a periarthritis involving the wrists and ankles, though other joints may be involved. The periarthritis has been demonstrated on the ankles using ultrasound. Effusions, when present, tend to be small and noninflammatory. This is a self-limiting condition, and more than two thirds of patients improve within 2 years. ACE levels may or may not be elevated. Patients with normal ACE levels tend to recover completely over time without recurrence of symptoms. However, some individuals—particularly those with elevated ACE levels—may have a more prolonged course.

In children, sarcoid arthritis may be misdiagnosed as juvenile rheumatoid arthritis. Liver disease is present in 30–50% of these patients, as an enlarged liver and/or abnormal enzymes.

Chronic sarcoid arthritis may be of three types: a nondeforming granulomatous synovitis, Jaccoud's arthritis, and a joint swelling adjacent to a sarcoid bone lesion. ACE levels are generally elevated. The diagnosis is made in an individual with sarcoidosis when other causes are excluded.

A diffuse, sausage-shaped digit or **dactylitis** is noted most commonly with seronegative spondyloarthropathy and sarcoid. Some patients have symptoms in a joint adjacent to sarcoid bone involvement. Sarcoid dactylitis is one such example, as demonstrated in our patient. Bone involvement in sarcoid is rare, estimated to occur in 1–7% of patients. In more than two-thirds of patients it is associated with skin lesions. Skin lesions over the face and nose, referred to as **lupus pernio**, are associated with lytic lesions of the flat bones of the scalp and nose. In the latter, Wegener's granulomatosis may need to be excluded. In sarcoidosis there is no necrosis, an important feature in Wegener's. Dactylitis may be mildly symptomatic. On x-ray, a **lacy pattern** (see figure, previous page) is very characteristic of sarcoid dactylitis. Patients complain of an ache or may present more acutely with

a pathological fracture as the granuloma expands and finally erodes the cortex. Rare bone lesions observed in sarcoid, either lytic or blastic lesions of the vertebrae, may occur as isolated disease, and a diagnosis can be confirmed only on biopsy.

Gout has been reported with sarcoidosis. It presents as an acute joint swelling that requires confirmation by identifying urate crystals using a polarized microscope.

The diagnosis of sarcoidosis usually requires tissue from a transbronchial biopsy, with a lymph node or skin demonstrating a noncaseating granuloma. However, note that the triad of symmetrical hilar lymph node enlargement, erythema nodosum, and acute polyarthritis seldom requires tissue to make a diagnosis of sarcoidosis. Fever is an unusual manifestation, though it can occur, but other conditions should be excluded. These include histoplasmosis, lymphoma, and tuberculosis. It is extremely rare for sarcoid to involve the bone marrow, and if observed, consider an alternate diagnosis.

There are two **characteristic patterns of Gallium scans** used to evaluate activity and extent of disease: a λ pattern, reflecting uptake in the hilar and right paratracheal lymph nodes, and a panda pattern, reflecting uptake in the lacrimals and parotids. *An elevated angiotensin-converting enzyme and characteristic patterns of gallium uptake have diagnostic specificity greater than 99%.*

Autoantibodies in low titers may occur in some patients with sarcoidosis, and an autoimmune disease like lupus or rheumatoid arthritis may coexist. These diseases have many features in common, so it often is difficult to decide if more than one disease is present.

Most patients with sarcoid arthritis respond to nonsteroidal anti-inflammatories alone. Some, however, may require low doses of steroids and even methotrexate before the joint symptoms are brought under control. Methotrexate is well tolerated even when used over a prolonged period. Osteoporosis observed in many patients may be exacerbated by the use of steroids. Calcium and vitamin D supplements require monitoring of the urinary and serum calcium, as hypercalciuria and renal stones are common in sarcoidosis.

The present patient had gout with sarcoidosis and dactylitis; the latter is not found in rheumatoid arthritis. He improved with nonsteroidal anti-inflammatory drugs.

Clinical Pearls

1. Sarcoidosis is associated with dactylitis.
2. The treatment includes steroids and methotrexate.
3. Calcium and vitamin D therapy should be carefully monitored with urinary calcium.
4. Gout may occur with sarcoidosis. Interestingly, the first description of sarcoid arthritis was not intended as such; Hutchinson thought it was gout.

REFERENCES

1. Glenas A, Kvein TK, Melby K, et al: Acute sarcoid arthritis: Occurrence onset, clinical features, and outcome. Br J Rheum 1995;34(1):45–50.
2. Kaye O, Palazzo, Grossin M, et al: Low-dose methotrexate: An effective corticosteroid sparing agent in the musculoskeletal manifestations of sarcoidosis. Br J Rheum 1995;34(7):642–644.
3. Lower EE, Baughman: Prolonged use of methotrexate for sarcoidosis. Arch Int Med 1995;155(8):846–851.
4. Gran JT, Bohmer E: Acute sarcoid arthritis: A favorable outcome? A retrospective survey of 49 patients with review of the literature. Scand J Rheumatol 1996;25(2):70–73.
5. Harvey JA, Pak CY: Gouty diathesis and sarcoidosis in patients with recurrent calcium nephrocalcinosis. J Urol 1998;139(6):287–289.
6. Rothschild BM, Pingitore C, Eaton M: Dactylitis: Implications for clinical practice. Semin Arthritis Rheum 1998;28(1):41–47.
7. Mana J, Gomez-Vaquera C, Montero A, et al: Lofgren's syndrome revisited. Am J Med 1999;107(3):240–245.
8. Gulati M, Sanjay S, Tierney L: Impatient inpatient care. N Engl J Med 2000;342:37–40.

Bruce A. Runyon, MD

PATIENT 37

A 42-year-old man with cirrhosis and sudden bizarre behavior

A 42-year-old man was found by his wife "on all fours" on the top of the kitchen table "barking like a dog." She had never seen him behave like this before and called 911. The paramedics could not obtain his cooperation. Finally, the police brought the patient to the hospital for evaluation. During transport to the emergency department, he became somnolent. He has a past history of alcoholic cirrhosis complicated by ascites.

Physical Examination: Temperature 38.4°; pulse 112; respirations 24; blood pressure 94/70. General: lethargic, emaciated. HEENT: scleral icterus. Chest: clear. Cardiac: tachycardia without murmur. Abdomen: moderate ascites, nontender, no palpable organs, active bowel sounds. Extremities: pitting edema of legs.

Laboratory Findings: WBC 8200/μl, with 61% neutrophils and 30% bands; platelets 141,000/μl. Hct 26%. Albumin 2.8 g/dl, total bilirubin 7.2 mg/dl, INR 2.0.

Question: What diagnostic procedure should be performed in the evaluation of this patient?

Diagnosis: Spontaneous bacterial peritonitis.

Discussion: Spontaneous bacterial peritonitis (SBP) is a common complication of ascites in the setting of cirrhosis. The bacteria that cause this life-threatening infection reside in the gut and can "translocate" across the leaky gut mucosa of the patient with cirrhosis. Once extra-intestinal, the bacteria can traverse mesenteric lymphatics and reach the systemic circulation, entering the peritoneal cavity in lymph that weeps across Glisson's capsule. If the peritoneal macrophages fail to kill the bacteria, neutrophils are attracted into the ascitic fluid. If they fail to kill the bacteria and an antibiotic is not given rapidly, the patient dies. The risk of SBP is inversely proportional to the protein concentration of the ascitic fluid. The protein concentration does not increase with development of infection. Low-protein fluid is opsonin-deficient and prone to infection.

The keys to survival of a patient with cirrhosis, ascites, and SBP are: (1) a high index of suspicion of this infection, (2) a low threshold for performing a diagnostic paracentesis, and (3) prompt initiation of a broad-spectrum non-nephrotoxic antibiotic.

Fever is the most common (69%) symptom of SBP, followed by abdominal pain (59%), hepatic encephalopathy (54%), and abdominal tenderness (49%). Some patients have mental status change as the only clinical evidence of infection. Young patients can have a hyperactive, delirious phase of their encephalopathy before they become lethargic, as in this patient.

The astute clinician performs an **abdominal paracentesis** when evaluating (1) patients with new onset ascites, (2) patients hospitalized with ascites, and (3) patients who deteriorate as inpatients or outpatients. This deterioration can be manifested by fever, abdominal pain, confusion, leukocytosis, or azotemia. Most patients with liver disease severe enough to be complicated by SBP have coagulopathy, including prolonged INR and thrombocytopenia. Many physicians are reluctant to perform the required procedure in this setting. However, studies have demonstrated the safety and utility of this simple procedure in this very context. Prophylactic transfusions are not required nor advised. Use sterile gloves and sterile technique. Inoculate blood culture bottles at the bedside with ascitic fluid. Submit the cell count in a purple-top EDTA tube and "chemistries" in a red-top tube. If there is high suspicion of infection, blood also should be cultured, as well as urine. Urinary tract infections in the setting of cirrhosis may progress to urosepsis without localizing signs. Because of multiple defects in cellular and humoral immunity, patients with cirrhosis can develop septic arthritis, meningitis, or spontaneous empyema. Obtain a fluid sample for testing from any body cavity with local evidence of infection.

SBP can be fatal in a period of minutes to hours. Therefore, initiate empiric antibiotic therapy when there is convincing evidence of infection, after appropriate cultures and samples are obtained. An ascitic fluid absolute neutrophil count ≥ 250/µl warrants antibiotic treatment. A temperature > 37.8° and/or diffuse recent-onset abdominal pain also warrants treatment, even if the neutrophil count is not elevated. The infection can be detected before there is a neutrophil response. If the cultures are sterile, and an alternative explanation for a fever (e.g., alcoholic hepatitis) is evident, treatment can be stopped after 24 hours. If there is a dramatic response to treatment, even if cultures are sterile, a full course is warranted.

Cefotaxime is the drug with the largest data base for empiric and definitive treatment of SBP. If bacterial antibiotic susceptibility testing indicates that a narrower-spectrum antibiotic is enough, it should be substituted for cefotaxime. A 5-day course of 2 g of cefotaxime intravenously every 8 hours is adequate treatment, based on a large randomized trial. Prolonged treatment is not needed. The dose can be reduced for azotemia, but there is no toxicity associated with standard dosing in the setting of renal failure. Avoid aminoglycosides because of nephrotoxicity and poor efficacy compared to cefotaxime.

Patients who survive one episode of SBP are at high risk of another infection. Randomized trials have shown that selective intestinal decontamination with norfloxacin decreases this risk and is cost-effective. SBP is a marker of advanced liver disease. Patients who survive this infection should be considered for liver transplantation.

The present patient underwent abdominal paracentesis. The ascitic fluid was turbid, and WBC was 17,750/µl with 91% neutrophils and an absolute neutrophil count of 16,153/µl. Total protein was 0.8 g/dl with albumin of 0.2 g/dl and serum-ascites albumin gradient of 2.6 g/dl. Glucose was 59 mg/dl (serum 83 mg/dl), amylase 35 IU/L (serum 30 IU/L), and lactate dehydrogenase 71 IU/L (serum 150 IU/L). Ascitic fluid was inoculated into blood culture bottles at the bedside; the next morning both bottles were growing *Escherichia coli.* Cultures of blood were sterile. He received 5 days of cefotaxime IV. Norfloxacin 400 mg orally per day was then initiated to decrease gut levels of gram-negative bacteria and prevent a future infection.

Clinical Pearls

1. Spontaneous bacterial peritonitis (SBP) is a common complication of ascites in patients with advanced cirrhosis.

2. SBP is rapidly fatal if not detected and treated early.

3. This infection can be prevented in high-risk patients by use of selective intestinal decontamination.

REFERENCES

1. Runyon BA, McHutchison JG, Antillon MR, et al: Short-course vs long-course antibiotic treatment of spontaneous bacterial peritonitis: A randomized controlled study of 100 patients. Gastroenterology 1991;100:1737–1742.

2. Runyon BA, Squier SU, Borzio M: Translocation of gut bacteria in rats with cirrhosis to mesenteric lymph nodes partially explains the pathogenesis of spontaneous bacterial peritonitis. J Hepatol 1994;21:792–796.

3. Guarner C, Runyon BA, Young S, et al: Intestinal bacterial overgrowth and bacterial translocation in an experimental model of cirrhosis in rats. J Hepatol 1997;26:1372–1378.

4. Runyon BA: Management of adult patients with ascites due to cirrhosis: AASLD Practice Guideline. Hepatology 1998;27:264–272.

5. Such J, Runyon BA: Spontaneous bacterial peritonitis. Clin Infect Dis 1998;27:669–676.

6. Rimola A, Garcia-Tsao G, Navasa M, et al: Diagnosis, treatment and prophylaxis of spontaneous bacterial peritonitis: A consensus document. J Hepatol 2000;32:142–153.

Mark Cohen, MD

PATIENT 38

A 42-year-old man with asthma and a spontaneous pneumothorax

A 42-year-old man with a life-long history of asthma presents with sharp, right-sided chest pain associated with severe dyspnea of 1-hour duration. He denies recent coughing or trauma. He had a "lung biopsy" 5 years earlier and was told that he had a "fungus," but never received any specific treatment for this problem.

Physical Examination: Temperature 36.4°; respirations 36; pulse 110; blood pressure 105/60; O_2 saturation (room air) 84%. General: thin, moderate respiratory distress. HEENT: normal. Chest: absent breath sounds on right, wheezing on left. Cardiac: tachycardic. Abdomen: nontender, without organomegaly. Extremities: no clubbing or cyanosis.

Laboratory Findings: WBC 10,700/μl, neutrophils 80%, lymphocytes 7%, monocytes 6%, eosinophils 7%, Hct 41%, platelet count 245,000/μl. Chemistry and coagulation tests: normal. Chest radiograph: see below.

Questions: What diagnosis should be considered? How would you explain the pneumothorax?

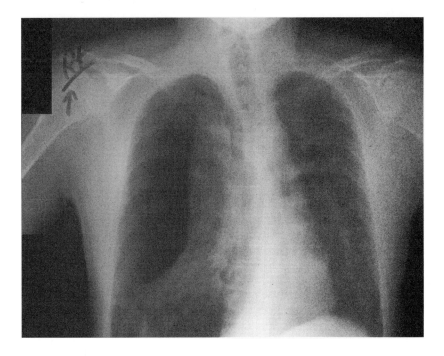

Diagnosis: Allergic bronchopulmonary aspergillosis (ABPA).

Discussion: ABPA is a hypersensitivity disease of the lungs usually caused by *Aspergillus fumigatus*, but it may be caused by any fungus. It is a potentially crippling complication of asthma and cystic fibrosis. Of patients with corticosteroid-dependent asthma, 7–37% meet the generally accepted definitions for ABPA. Although Aspergillus colonizes 40–57% of cystic fibrosis patients, only 6–10% manifest the typical features of ABPA.

The immune response to Aspergillus antigens in ABPA appears to be quantitatively greater than in allergic asthma or cystic fibrosis patients. In ABPA, inhaled *A. fumigatus* spores are trapped by the luminal mucus and form a mycelium. *A fumigatus* mycelium releases antigens that are processed by antigen-presenting cells and presented to T cells. The T-cell response to *A. fumigatus* antigens is skewed towards a Th$_2$ response, manifested by production of IL-4, IL-5, IL-10, and IL-13. Consistent with a predominant Th$_2$ response, IgG- and IgA-specific antibodies are also produced in addition to anti-*A. fumigatus* IgE antibodies.

The disease progresses through **five clinical stages:** (1) *Acute*—patients present with cough and wheezing, identical to any asthmatic, but also complain of malaise, fever, and cough productive of brown mucus plugs; peripheral eosinophilia and elevated serum precipitans and IgE levels (> 2500 ng/ml) are characteristic. (2) *Remission*—following therapy, patients enter a stage characterized by a prolonged or even permanent freedom from asthma symptoms and a decrease or normalization of IgE. (3) *Exacerbation*—symptoms are similar to those of the acute stage, or patients may be asymptomatic with only a rise in IgE levels or new chest x-ray infiltrates to mark disease activity. (4) *Steroid-dependent*—gradually, the exacerbations progress to a more permanent corticosteroid-dependent type of wheezing, cough, or dyspnea, associated with elevated IgE, serum precipitans, and eosinophilia. (5) *Fibrotic end stage*—patients manifest with severe cough productive of profuse amounts of sputum, dyspnea on exertion, and increasing bronchiectasis. Honeycombing is seen on standard chest x-rays, and the response to high-dose corticosteroids is poor. Fatalities due to respiratory failure, septicemia from opportunistic infections, severe bronchospasm, and terminal fibrotic lung disease often occur in the fourth decade. Long-term corticosteroid therapy in the early stages of ABPA may prevent the development of the fibrotic changes.

The most common radiographic finding is fleeting infiltrates, which can appear in any part of the lung, but predominate in the upper lobes and usually are bilateral. Permanent radiographic findings include interstitial fibrosis and, more commonly, central bronchiectasis with normal distal bronchi— a feature only seen in cystic fibrosis and ABPA. The latter findings are better assessed with high-resolution computed tomography.

Spontaneous pneumothorax is an extremely rare complication of ABPA, with only three reported cases in the literature. The presumed mechanisms for the development of the pneumothorax include an impacted mucus plug that acts as a "ball valve," causing post-mucus plug air trapping until a bronchus ruptures; pleural perforation of a pseudo-cavity containing aspergillomas; and, as in this case, a ruptured apical bleb.

Since no single test is specific for ABPA, diagnostic criteria have been proposed, incorporating the clinical, immunologic, and radiographic features of the disease. A step-wise approach for diagnosing or excluding ABPA has been proposed by Patterson and coworkers. When a patient with asthmatic symptoms and peripheral eosinophilia is encountered, a skin test with *Aspergillus* mixed extract is performed; if the skin test is negative, ABPA is excluded. If positive, serum IgE levels and precipitins for *Aspergillus* antigens are performed. If IgE levels are greater than 500 U/ml, and the precipitin tests are positive, IgE and IgG antibodies against *A. fumigatus* are obtained and compared with levels in asthmatic controls. If levels are greater than two times those of controls, ABPA can be diagnosed. CT scan of chest should be performed to assess the presence of bronchiectasis.

Corticosteroids are the treatment of choice to decrease the airway inflammation and subsequently create a less favorable environment for the spores to flourish. Treatment includes prednisone (40–60 mg a day), with gradual tapering based on clinical response, and reduction of total IgE levels. In light of the central role of chronic antigenic stimulation by *A. fumigatus*, itraconazole in corticosteroid-dependent ABPA patients has been shown to improve the immunologic and physiologic parameters, as well as having a steroid-sparing effect. Management of ABPA should include environmental control to decrease exposure to molds and optimize treatment of the coexisting disease (asthma, cystic fibrosis).

The present patient's chest radiograph showed a left-sided pneumothorax. He had a good response to chest tube thoracostomy. High-resolution CT revealed extensive bullous disease and interstitial fibrosis. In the subsequent 2 years, he experienced multiple exacerbations of asthma, but now is well controlled on 20 mg of prednisone every other day and inhaled salmeterol and fluticasone.

Clinical Pearls

1. ABPA occurs in 7–37% of corticosteroid-dependent asthmatics. Although *Aspergillus* colonizes 40–57% of cystic fibrosis patients, only 6–10% manifest the typical features of ABPA.

2. Severe bullous disease, mucus plugging acting as a "ball valve," and perforation of a pseudocavity are the described mechanisms causing pneumothorax in ABPA.

3. Misdiagnosed or untreated ABPA progresses to irreversible end-stage fibrosis.

4. Central bronchiectasis with normal peripheral bronchi is *only* seen in ABPA and cystic fibrosis.

5. Corticosteroid-dependent ABPA patients benefit from concurrent itraconazole therapy by reducing the corticosteroid dose used and improving immunologic and physiologic parameters.

REFERENCES

1. Basisch JE, Graves TS, Nasir Baz M, et al: Allergic bronchopulmonary aspergillosis in corticosteroid-dependent asthmatics. J Allergy Clin Immunol 1981;68:98–102.
2. Patterson R, Greenberger PA, Radin RC, Roberts M: Allergic bronchopulmonary aspergillosis: Staging as an aid to management. Ann Intern Med 1982;96:256–291.
3. Ricketti AJ, Greenberger PA, Glassroth J: Spontaneous pneumothorax in allergic bronchopulmonary aspergillosis. Arch Int Med 1984;144:151–152.
4. Patterson R, Greenberger PA, Halwig JM, et al: Allergic bronchopulmonary aspergillosis: Natural history and classification of early disease by serologic and roentgenographic studies. Arch Intern Med 1986;146:916–918.
5. Greenberger PA, Patterson R: Allergic bronchopulmonary aspergillosis: Model of bronchopulmonary disease with defined serologic, radiologic, pathologic, and clinical findings from asthma to fatal destructive lung disease. Chest 1987;91:Suppl:165S–171S.
6. Schwartz HJ, Greenberger PA: The prevalence of allergic bronchopulmonary aspergillosis in patients with asthma, determined by serologic and radiologic criteria in patients at risk. J Lab Clin Med 1991;117:138–142.
7. Reich JM: Pneumothorax due to pleural perforation of a pseudocavity containing aspergillomas in a patient with allergic bronchopulmonary aspergillosis. Chest 1992;102(2):652–653.
8. Judson MA, Marshall C, Beale G, Holt JB: Pneumothorax and bronchopleural fistula during treatment of allergic bronchopulmonary aspergillosis. Southern Medical J 1993;86(9):1061–1063.
9. Mroueh S, Spock A: Allergic bronchopulmonary aspergillosis in patients with cystic fibrosis. Chest 1994;105:32–36.
10. Kurup VP, Grunig G, Knutsen AP, Murali PS: Cytokines in allergic bronchopulmonary aspergillosis. Research Immunol 1998;149(4–5):466–477.
11. Stevens DA, Schwartz HJ, Lee JY, et al: A randomized trial of itraconazole in allergic bronchopulmonary aspergillosis. N Engl J Med 2000;342:756–762.

Wayne Katon, MD

PATIENT 39

A 35-year-old woman with chest pain and labile hypertension

A 35-year-old woman, with a history of migraine headaches and irritable bowel syndrome, presents to her primary care physician with a 1-month history of chest pain and palpitations. These episodes of chest pain and rapid heartbeat are frightening to her and she wonders whether something is wrong with her heart. She has become more fearful of crowds and has been having problems giving oral presentations at work. Her physician orders blood tests (WBC, hematocrit, and thyroid stimulating hormone), and refers her for a treadmill exam and echocardiogram.

Physical Examination: Temperature 36.9°, pulse 90, respiration 20. Blood pressure initially 150/100, but decreased to 130/80 after 10 minutes. General: normal weight (5 feet 6 inches, 130 pounds). HEENT: unremarkable. Cardiac: rate of 90 to 95 with a midsystolic click and murmur. Chest: normal. Abdomen: soft; mild tenderness in left lower quadrant; positive bowel sounds. Extremities: no edema or rash.

Laboratory Findings: WBC 8000/µl, Hct 39%, TSH within normal range. EKG: slight increased pulse at 100 but no other abnormalities, treadmill normal (no sign of ischemia). Echocardiogram: mild mitral valve prolapse with no sign of thickening of mitral valve.

Question: What condition explains this patient's symptoms?

Diagnosis: Panic disorder, with mild agoraphobia.

Discussion: Panic disorder is one of the most prevalent anxiety disorders in primary care populations, occurring in 3–8% of patients. It is twice as common in women. About one-third of patients with panic disorder present with cardiologic symptoms of chest pain and palpitations, one third with neurologic complaints such as dizziness or headaches, and one third with gastrointestinal symptoms such as abdominal pain or diarrhea. Panic disorder is a relapsing remitting illness. Studies have shown there is a genetic component with higher concordance in monozygotic compared to dizygotic twins. Life stressors are also important in precipitating a new episode or relapse of this anxiety disorder.

Like the woman in the case example, patients with panic disorder are more likely to have labile hypertension and mitral valve prolapse compared to primary care controls. Because of these cardiac signs, beta-blockers or calcium channel blockers are often started in these patients, but are not more effective than placebo in alleviating panic attacks. In the Framingham study, about 10% of community respondents met criteria for mitral valve prolapse (MVP) on echocardiogram, but had no more physical symptoms than respondents without MVP. These data suggest that when patients have comorbid panic and MVP, cardiologic symptoms are likely to be due to panic disorder. In patients with chest pain who are referred to treadmill or angiogram, those with negative tests have been found to have a 40–50% prevalence rate of panic disorder versus approximately 5% in those with coronary artery disease.

Patients with migraine headaches and irritable bowel syndrome have also been found to have elevated rates of panic disorder compared to controls. Patients with panic frequently have comorbid problems with major depression (50%), alcohol or substance abuse (25–30%), and agoraphobia. Once panic attacks begin, patients with panic often develop fears of social situations, such as crowds, as well as situations where they feel they are the center of attention, such as public speaking.

Since most patients with panic disorder present with one or two of the most frightening physical complaints, such as chest pain, physicians need to screen for the other 10 autonomic symptoms (e.g., rapid heartbeat, dizziness, shortness of breath, sweatiness, shakiness or nausea). If four or more of these are present, it is helpful to inquire about avoidance of social situations since the attacks have begun. Since depression co-occurs in about 50% of patients, questioning the patient about the nine symptoms of major depression is also helpful.

Once the diagnosis of panic disorder is established, it is essential to understand the patient's fears (e.g., having a heart attack or stroke) and to carefully explain how a brain disorder can provoke frightening physical symptoms. Describe the fact that humans have an alarm system or flight-or-fight response built into the biologic hardware of their brain. Dangerous situations such as a near-auto accident will understandably provoke these flight-or-fight responses. Panic attacks occur when this alarm system is set at too low a threshold, when there is no apparent danger.

This biologic description leads logically to a description of a medication treatment to better regulate this alarm system. The first line of treatment should be **selective serotonin reuptake inhibitors**. Since these can cause transient jitteriness, start at a lower dosage than in depression (fluoxetine 5 mg, paroxetine and citilapram 10 mg, and sertraline 25 mg). However, titer them up to dosages used in depression (fluoxetine, paroxetine, and citilapram 20–40 mg, and sertraline 75–200 mg). Dosages should be increased until panic attacks have stopped completely. **Tricyclic antidepressants** are also effective, with starting dosages of 25 mg of imipramine or nortriptyline. Patients usually need to be titered up to 100–250 mg of imipramine or 75–125 mg of nortriptyline. **Benzodiazepines** have been shown to be effective in double-blind trials. A starting dosage of 0.25 PO TID of clonazepam, alprazolam, or lorazepam can be gradually titered upward, with panic attacks usually going away at a dosage of 1.5–3 mg.

A specific, structured, short-term psychotherapy has been found to be as effective as medication in patients with panic disorder. **Cognitive behavioral therapy** (CBT) emphasizes extensive education about the origin of the physical sensations patients with panic experience and the ability of specific thought patterns to provoke and worsen attacks. A key component of this therapy is to expose patients to feared physical symptoms in the office and teach them to combat catastrophic thoughts regarding these sensations. For instance, if the patient fears that cardiac symptoms such as rapid heart beat are a precursor to having a heart attack, the therapist may provoke these symptoms by having the patient run in place and then help them replace the catastrophic thoughts (e.g., I'm going to have a heart attack) with more realistic ones.

The present patient was started on a selective reuptake inhibitor, with a good clinical response.

Clinical Pearls

1. Primary care patients with panic disorder tend to present with cardiac (chest pain, palpitations), neurologic (dizziness, tingling and headache), and gastrointestinal (abdominal pain, diarrhea) symptoms.

2. Patients with panic disorder have a high prevalence of labile hypertension, migraine headaches, and mitral valve prolapse.

3. Selective serotonin reuptake inhibitors are very effective in the treatment of panic disorder and should be the first-line medication treatment.

REFERENCES

1. Zaubler T, Katon W: Panic disorder in the general medical setting. J Psychosom Research 1998;44:25–42.
2. Katon W: Panic Disorder in the Medical Setting. National Institute of Mental Health. DHHS Pub. No. (ADM) 89-1629. Washington, DC. U.S. Government Printing Office, 1989.
3. Ciechanowski P, Katon W: Overview of anxiety disorders. In Rose BD (ed): UpToDate. Wellsley, MA, Up To Date, Inc., 2000.

Mahesh S. Mokhashi, MD
Michael B. Wallace, MD, MPH

PATIENT 40

A 74-year-old man with abdominal pain, jaundice, and fever

A 74-year-old man is referred for evaluation of recurrent right upper quadrant (RUQ) abdominal pain, jaundice, and fever. He first experienced intermittent RUQ abdominal discomfort 2 years ago and underwent laparoscopic cholecystectomy for gallstones. Six months later, the pain returned acutely, and fever and jaundice developed. An ultrasound examination revealed dilation of the common bile duct (CBD). An ERCP (see below) revealed a stricture of the distal CBD with a normal pancreatogram. Cytological brushings of the stricture showed reactive epithelial cells. A stent was placed in the CBD. Contrast-enhanced CT scan of the abdomen showed a dilated bile duct, but no mass or pancreatic duct dilation.

During the next 18 months, the patient had 5 episodes of cholangitis. In each case, an ERCP revealed an occluded stent and stricture. Cytological brushings at each ERCP showed only inflammatory epithelium. Other than intermittent pruritus, anorexia, and a 5-lb. weight loss, the patient is now asymptomatic. There is no history of alcohol or recreational drug use. He denies any prior liver problems, diarrhea, or foreign travel. A screening colonoscopy done 3 years ago was normal, without any evidence of colitis.

Physical Examination: General: comfortable, no peripheral stigmata of chronic liver disease. Vital signs: normal. Skin: mild jaundice. Chest: normal. Cardiac: grade 2/6 systolic ejection murmur at the left lower sternal border. Abdomen: soft, nontender, no organomegaly nor masses palpable.

Laboratory Findings: CBC: normal, total bilirubin 4.3 mg/dl, direct bilirubin 2.0 mg/dl, AST 177 IU/L, ALT 149 IU/L, alkaline phosphatase 533 IU/L, albumin 2.7 g/dl, CEA and CA 19-9 levels: normal. Abdominal MRI scan: minimal dilation of distal CBD.

Question: The above clinical and laboratory features are typical of what condition?

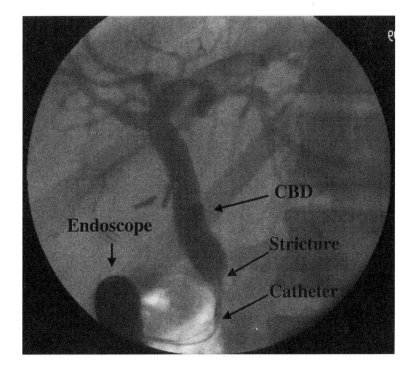

Diagnosis: Extrahepatic bile duct adenocarcinoma (EBDA).

Discussion: Although all bile duct carcinomas are commonly referred to as cholangiocarcinomas, only those arising from the *intrahepatic* portion of the bile ducts are true cholangiocarcinomas. Bile duct adenocarcinomas arising outside the liver are termed *extrahepatic* bile duct adenocarcinomas. This distinction is important, as neoplasia originating from different parts of the biliary tree (1) differ in their clinical presentation, (2) differ in their biological behavior, and (3) harbor different gene mutations. EBDA is a rare disease, with 2500 cases diagnosed annually in the US, mainly between the ages of 50 and 70 years.

Cholangiocarcinoma and EBDA should be considered in the differential diagnosis (table) of any patient with obstructive jaundice and a CBD stricture. Bile duct strictures in elderly patients without ulcerative colitis should be considered malignant until proven otherwise. In this patient, the prior cholecystectomy made surgical injury a distinct possibility, although the site of stricture in the distal CBD is lower than typically seen for surgical injury, which usually occurs in the mid CBD.

Differential Diagnosis of Bile Duct Strictures

Pancreas carcinoma
Ampullary carcinoma
Gall bladder carcinoma
Hepatoma
Metastatic carcinoma to liver or hilar lymph nodes
   (colon, breast, lung, ovarian, renal)
Primary sclerosing cholangitis
Traumatic or post surgical
Chronic pancreatitis
Mirrizzi's syndrome

Risk factors for these adenocarcinomas include primary sclerosing cholangitis (PSC), choledocholithiasis, choledochal cysts, chronic biliary infestation with liver flukes, and anomalous pancreatobiliary ductal union. The relative risk of getting cholangiocarcinoma with PSC is 20 to 30 times higher than in the non-PSC population. Patients with ulcerative colitis in the absence of associated PSC are *not* at increased risk of EBDA.

The most prominent clinical feature of EBDA is **jaundice**, which is present in 90–98% of all patients. Because jaundice may be absent in the early stages, and complete lobar obstruction may occur without overt signs of jaundice, confirm biliary obstruction with biochemical tests. High levels of serum alkaline phosphatase, which is the most sensitive biochemical parameter for biliary obstruction, is a good indicator for further investigation of the biliary tract. Other clinical features include weight loss, abdominal pain, abdominal mass, and fever. Bacteremia and cholangitis frequently are presenting symptoms of cholangiocarcinoma, especially due to *Escherichia coli*, *Streptococcus faecalis*, and *Klebsiella aerogenes*.

Ultrasonography and contrast-enhanced CT scan are useful diagnostic tools to locate an obstruction and evaluate the extent of spread. Ultrasound of patients presenting with jaundice is cost effective and is 85–90% sensitive in detecting bile duct dilation. CT scan is 90–95% sensitive in detecting dilated bile ducts and is more accurate than ultrasound in determining the level and etiology of the obstruction. Note that contrast-enhanced CT scan of the abdomen may be negative if scanning is done immediately after injecting IV contrast. Because of delayed venous drainage, repeat CT images 30 seconds after injection of contrast may facilitate imaging of some cholangiocarcinomas. The suspicion of cancer should be mentioned to the radiologist so that delayed images will be obtained.

Endoscopic ultrasound examination (EUS) uses an endoscope mounted with an ultrasound probe at the tip to image the distal CBD, pancreas, and surrounding region by placing the probe very close to the area of interest. It is also possible to perform fine-needle aspiration (FNA) to make a tissue diagnosis, by passing a needle through the endoscope channel. This technology, which is now available at most tertiary centers in the U.S., is very sensitive in diagnosing abnormalities of the pancreatic head and distal CBD region.

ERCP is useful to locate strictures and exclude other causes of jaundice, but ERCP brushings and biopsy have poor sensitivity (50–70%) for malignancy. Tumor markers (CEA, CA19-9), which were normal in our patient, are helpful if elevated, but have a limited sensitivity (70%) and specificity. More than 50% of EBDA cases occur in the upper one-third of the duct. Direct extension to the liver, portal vein, and pancreas is the most frequent route of spread. Lymph node metastases occur in 40% of all patients. Distant metastases are rare. Along with the above-mentioned tests, mesenteric angiography and laparoscopy are occasionally needed to determine the resectability of the tumor.

Unfortunately, only 20–40% of these tumors are resectable at diagnosis. The average survival from the time of diagnosis is 12 months. Most of these tumors are very slow growing and hence difficult to detect early, when operable. At this time, there is no way of identifying patients with PSC who might develop cholangiocarcinoma. Clinical or radiologic deterioration after a long period of stability with PSC is an ominous sign.

The only option for cure is surgical resection. **Endoscopic stenting** is now the first-line therapy for palliation of malignant biliary obstruction. Conclusive evidence of the benefits of chemotherapy, radiotherapy, and photodynamic therapy is lacking, and patients should be offered the opportunity to participate in clinical trials.

The present patient underwent an EUS of the distal CBD stricture, which revealed a 25 mm × 15 mm hypoechoic mass in the distal CBD (see below). Fine-needle aspirate was positive for adenocarcinoma. No regional lymphadenopathy was seen, and the patient was determined to have a T3N0M0 EBDA, which was resectable. Advanced coronary artery disease made our patient a higher surgical risk, which he was unwilling to accept. He had a self-expanding metal stent placed endoscopically for palliation of his malignant biliary obstruction. The median duration of patency of these metal stents is approximately a year, thus obviating the need for frequent biliary stent exchanges.

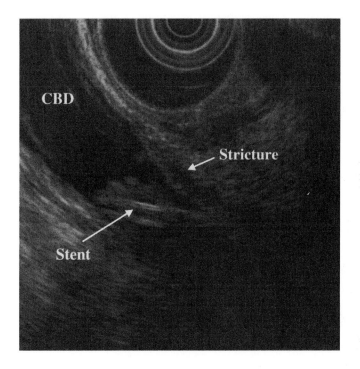

Clinical Pearls

1. Patients presenting with pancreatobiliary problems for the first time in late life should undergo evaluation for an underlying malignancy.

2. Biliary brushings and biopsies obtained at the time of ERCP have poor sensitivity. A negative result should prompt further investigation with techniques such as EUS-FNA, or surgical exploration in highly suspicious cases.

3. EUS is a highly sensitive method for detecting and staging malignancies in the head of the pancreas and the distal bile duct.

REFERENCES

1. Colombari R, Tsui WM: Biliary tumors of the liver. Semin Liver Dis 1995;15:402–413.
2. Lee CK, Barrios BR, Bjarnason H: Biliary tree malignancies: The University of Minnesota experience. J Surg Oncol 1997; 65:298–305.
3. Erickson BA, Nag S: Biliary tree malignancies. J Surg Oncol 1998;67:203–210.
4. Hejna M, Pruckmayer M, Raderer M: The role of chemotherapy and radiation in the management of biliary cancer: A review of the literature. Eur J Cancer 1998;34:977–986.
5. Baillie J: Tumors of the gallbladder and bile ducts. J Clin Gastroenterol 1999;29:14–21.
6. Chen MF: Peripheral cholangiocarcinoma (cholangiocellular carcinoma): Clinical features, diagnosis, and treatment. J Gastroenterol Hepatol 1999;14:1144–1149.

Emile R. Mohler III, MD
Muredach P. Reilly, MB

PATIENT 41

A 68-year-old man with a history of visual disturbance and hypertension

A 68-year-old man with a 15-year history of hypertension presents to the outpatient clinic with visual disturbance described as a transient shadow briefly in front of the left eye. He has a 40-pack-year history of smoking, but quit 10 years previously.

Physical Examination: Blood pressure 150/90 bilaterally, pulse 78, respiration 18. General: thin and comfortable appearing. HEENT: no carotid bruits, carotid upstroke right > left. Funduscopic exam: venous tapering at A-V crossing, but no evidence of cholesterol emboli (Hollenhorst plaque). Cardiac: regular rate and rhythm with an S_4 gallop. Chest: clear. Abdomen: soft, nontender, normal active bowel sounds, no bruits or masses. Extremities: no edema or rash; both upper and lower extremity pulses 2+. Neurologic: normal.

Laboratory Findings: Lipid profile: total cholesterol 220 mg/dl, HDL 35, calculated LDL 160, Lp(a) 80. Complete blood count: within normal limits. Chemistry panel: unremarkable, except for creatinine 2.0. Erythrocyte sedimentation rate: normal. Duplex Doppler ultrasound study: see below.

Question: What clinical condition explains this patient's symptoms?

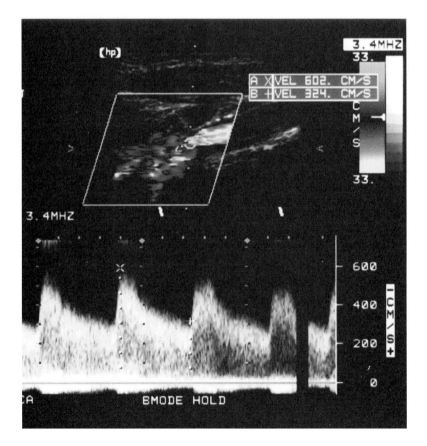

Diagnosis: Embolization from an atherosclerotic internal carotid artery to the ophthalmic artery.

Discussion: Carotid atherosclerosis is a condition that can result in thrombus embolization to the ophthalmic artery from the internal carotid artery, as occurred in this case. Some patients may have embolization of atherosclerotic debris to the eye (Hollenhorst plaque), although this was not observed in this patient. Stroke, the third most common cause of mortality in the United States, can be the result of embolus to the middle cerebral artery arising from the internal carotid artery. The external carotid artery supplies blood flow to the facial region and is usually not associated with stroke. Other causes of stroke include small vessel, cardiac, and an aortic arch atherosclerosis.

The results from the Framingham study indicate that a carotid bruit doubles the risk of stroke. However, a carotid bruit is a relatively poor predictor of underlying stenosis, as only 35% of patients have a carotid stenosis > 70%. It is estimated that among patients with a hemodynamically significant stenosis, only half have a carotid bruit. The vascular examination of the head and neck region should include auscultation of the neck, which is best done with the bell of the stethoscope, to listen for low rumbling bruits. Palpation of the carotid artery is also important, but should be done with a gentle touch so as not to create a false bruit or bradycardia, or dislodge plaque.

The initial diagnostic evaluation of the patient with a suspected carotid artery lesion is ultrasound imaging, which can reliably screen both the intracranial and extracranial arteries. Indications for duplex Doppler ultrasound imaging of the carotid arteries include transient ischemic attack, stroke, visual disturbance, or dizziness. The percent stenosis is usually determined from the velocity on duplex ultrasound. Plaques of less than 50% can also be quantified on B-mode ultrasound image. The patient in this study demonstrated a systolic velocity of > 220 cm/sec and a diastolic velocity of > 120 cm/sec, which in most vascular laboratories indicates a stenosis of > 75%.

The medical treatment of carotid atherosclerosis disease includes cardiovascular risk reduction involving smoking cessation and strict control of hypertension and diabetes mellitus. Low-density lipoprotein cholesterol was not previously thought an important target for stroke risk, but is now considered an important target given the results of recent studies with HMG-CoA reductase inhibitors in reducing the risk of stroke. Patients with symptoms of cerebrovascular ischemia and a hemodynamically significant stenosis of the internal carotid artery should be referred for possible carotid endarterectomy.

The present patient presented with a visual disturbance in a clinical setting that suggested an ophthalmic embolization. The Duplex Doppler ultrasound image of an internal carotid artery showed a peak systolic velocity of 600 cm/sec, consistent with a stenosis of > 70%. He was referred for consideration of carotid endarterectomy.

Clinical Pearls

1. A visual disturbance may be secondary to embolization from an atherosclerotic internal carotid artery to the ophthalmic artery.

2. Among patients with a hemodynamically significant lesion, about half have a carotid bruit on physical examination. The absence of a carotid bruit does not necessarily indicate that a significant stenosis is not present.

3. The initial diagnostic test in patients with suspected carotid artery disease is duplex Doppler ultrasound.

REFERENCES
1. Wolf PA, Kannel WB, Sorlie P, McNamara P: Asymptomatic carotid bruit and risk of stroke. The Framingham study. JAMA 1981;245(14):1442–1445.
2. Silvestry FE, Tarka EA, Mohler ER: Echocardiographic and vascular ultrasound evaluation of cerebrovascular ischemic events. ACC Current Journal Review 1998;6:79–81.
3. Mohler ER, III, Delanty N, Rader DJ, Raps EC: Statins and cerebrovascular disease: Plaque attack to prevent brain attack. Vasc Med 1999;4(4):269–272.

Nicholas A. Smyrnios, MD
Richard S. Irwin, MD

PATIENT 42

A 54-year-old woman with a persistent cough

A 54-year-old woman presents with a chief complaint of cough productive of 30 ml white sputum daily for the last 18 months. She denies fevers, chills, dyspnea, and exercise limitations. She also denies nasal congestion, gastrointestinal complaints, purulent nasal discharge, and any sensation of a postnasal drip, but does complain of hoarseness and frequent throat clearing. She has never had a persistent cough and only noted brief episodes of coughing associated with upper respiratory infections. She has no history of environmental allergies, allergic rhinitis, or smoking. During the preceding 18 months, she has received multiple courses of antibiotics for "bronchitis," including 2 weeks each of clarithromycin, trimethoprim-sulfamethoxazole, amoxicillin-clauvulanate, and ciprofloxacin—all without success. Her only medication is metoprolol 50 mg twice a day for mild hypertension.

Physical Examination: Vital signs: normal. General: healthy appearing with frequent coughing. HEENT: mild erythema of the oropharynx. Cardiac: normal. Chest: expiratory wheeze at the end of a salvo of coughing; no crackles or dullness. Abdomen: nontender without organomegaly. Extremities: no cyanosis, clubbing, or edema.

Laboratory Findings: Chest radiograph: normal. Four-view roentgenograms of sinuses: normal. Pulmonary function tests: normal spirometry. Bronchoprovocation challenge testing with methacholine: negative. Barium swallow: normal.

Course: The patient failed to respond to a 2-week course of a combination antihistamine/decongestant tablet (dexbrompheniramine maleate 6 mg and pseudoephedrine 120 mg) every 12 hours and a 2-week course of prednisone.

Question: What therapeutic intervention is likely to be beneficial at this time?

Diagnosis: Gastroesophageal reflux disease (GERD)

Discussion: Gastrointestinal reflux is a common cause of persistent coughing. This patient fits a clinical profile that is characterized by: (**1**) a cough that has been persistent for months; (**2**) a normal or near normal and stable chest radiograph; (**3**) absence of use of an angiotensin converting enzyme inhibitor (ACEI); (**4**) absence of exposure to environmental irritants, such as cigarette smoke; (**5**) a negative methacholine challenge test; (**6**) failure to improve with treatment for postnasal drip syndrome that includes an oral antihistamine *with* anticholinergic properties; and (**7**) failure to improve after a course of systemic corticosteroids for eosinophilic bronchitis.

Several clues may exist in the history and physical examination in support of a diagnosis of GERD. Patients may complain of hoarseness and frequent throat clearing, both of which can result from GERD. Also, the mild erythema of the oropharynx may signify chronic GERD, which can produce irritation and inflammation of the upper gastrointestinal tract and airway. While the presence of symptoms classically attributed to GERD (heartburn, regurgitation, globus sensation, indigestion) is helpful in suggesting the diagnosis, it does not *prove* the diagnosis, and the absence of these symptoms does not preclude it since chronic cough has been shown to exist as the sole presenting manifestation of GERD. The presence of sputum production does not make any cause of chronic cough more or less likely, nor do the character, timing, or acoustics of the cough.

Treatment of cough due to GERD may be medical or surgical. Medical therapy consists of: (**1**) a high-protein, low-fat (45 gram) anti-reflux diet (i.e., avoiding substances that have the potential of relaxing the lower esophageal sphincter or irritating the esophagus); (**2**) acid suppressing medications such as the proton pump inhibitors; (**3**) a prokinetic agent such as metoclopramide; (**4**) elevation of the head of the bed; (**5**) eating three meals a day without snacking; and (**6**) not eating or drinking, except for taking medicines, for the 2–3 hours prior to lying down. Medical therapy may not start to improve cough for 2–3 months and, on average, can take up to 5.5 months to be completely effective.

When medical therapy is ineffective, surgical treatment such as laparoscopic fundoplication may offer relief. In preparation for such a procedure, additional studies to confirm and characterize the components of the problem usually are performed. These studies include 24-hour esophageal pH probe monitoring with correlation of reflux events with the timing of cough (performed while on maximal medical therapy); upper gastrointestinal endoscopy; radionuclide gastric emptying studies; and esophageal manometry. The use of 24-hour esophageal pH monitoring on treatment confirms that medical therapy has failed to control GERD, and the other studies help the surgeon determine which fundoplication procedure to perform and whether additional procedures, such as a gastric emptying procedure, may improve the result.

It is not generally appreciated that a **cough-phlegm syndrome** (CPS) frequently is due to conditions other than "bronchitis." Because of this, physicians have a tendency to over-diagnose a CPS as bronchitis and prescribe antibiotics because they believe that the bronchitis is bacterial in etiology. Postnasal drip syndrome from a variety of rhinosinus conditions, asthma, and GERD is a common cause of CPS. Therefore, do not diagnose bronchitis in patients with a CPS unless other causes of CPS have been ruled out and unless there is an exposure to irritants. *In the absence of exposure to irritants, the diagnosis of chronic bronchitis is untenable, even if the cough is productive.*

The present patient improved after initiation of medical management.

Clinical Pearls

1. Chronic cough may be the sole presenting manifestation of GERD.

2. Medical therapy for GERD with acid suppression, prokinetic agents, and intensive diet and lifestyle changes may take up to 5–6 months to be completely effective. When it is ineffective, surgical therapy with fundoplication can eliminate cough in properly selected patients.

3. The cause of cough cannot be determined from the presence or absence of sputum or from the character, timing, or acoustics of the cough.

4. Bronchitis is overdiagnosed, and antibiotics are prescribed too often for CPS. Antibiotics should be prescribed for acute exacerbations of COPD and in limited other circumstances (e.g., infection with *Bordetella pertussis*), but otherwise should be used infrequently for cough-phlegm syndromes.

REFERENCES

1. Irwin RS, Zawacki JK, Curley FJ, et al: Chronic cough as the sole presenting manifestation of gastroesophageal reflux. Am Rev Respir Dis 1989;140:1294–1300.
2. Irwin RS, Curley FJ, French CL: Chronic cough. The spectrum and frequency of causes, key components of the diagnostic evaluation and outcome of specific therapy. Am Rev Respir Dis 1990;141:640–647.
3. Smyrnios NA, Irwin RS, Curley FJ: Chronic cough with a history of excessive sputum production: The spectrum and frequency of causes, key components of the diagnostic evaluation, and outcome of specific therapy. Chest 1995;108:991–997.
4. Mello CJ, Irwin RS, Curley FJ: Predictive values of the character, timing, and complications of chronic cough in diagnosing its cause. Arch Intern Med 1996;156:997–1003.

Navid Madani, MD
Paul Schroy, III, MD, MPH

PATIENT 43

A 74-year-old man with epigastric pain, early satiety, and an abnormal UGI series

A 74-year-old man with a past history of polycythemia vera evolving into myelofibrosis and myeloid metaplasia presents with a several-month history of epigastric pain, early satiety, and recent weight loss.

Physical Examination: Vital signs: normal. General: mild cachexia. Abdomen: epigastric tenderness and splenomegaly. Remainder of examination: normal.

Laboratory Findings: Barium upper GI-series: constriction of the distal stomach and duodenal bulb with apparent ulceration, suggesting a circumferential mass (see figure, *right*). Upper endoscopy: large, circumferential, obstructing mass of the antrum (see figure, *left*). Multiple biopsies: acute and chronic inflammation with ulceration and a monotonous, large cell infiltrate; positive Giemsa stain for *Helicobacter pylori*.

Question: What diagnosis would explain this patient's clinical presentation?

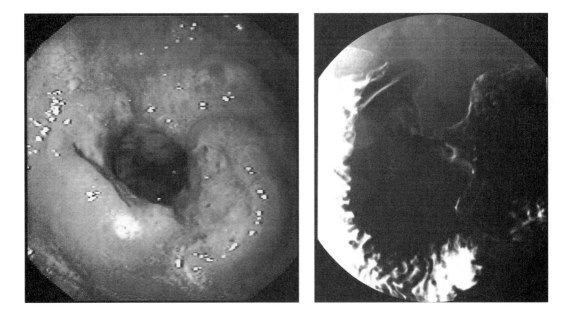

Diagnosis: High-grade non-Hodgkin's lymphoma (MALT-type) and *Helicobacter pylori* infection.

Discussion: The gastrointestinal (GI) tract is the predominant site of extranodal non-Hodgkin's lymphomas (NHLs). **Primary gastrointestinal NHLs** are relatively rare, accounting for 1–4% of GI malignancies. **Secondary GI involvement**, however, is relatively common and may be seen in approximately 10% of patients with limited stage, high-grade NHLs at the time of diagnosis and in up to 60% of those dying from NHL. Most primary GI lymphomas arise from pre-existing mucosa-associated lymphoid tissue and hence are referred to as "MALT-type" lymphomas. MALT lymphomas are of B-cell origin and may involve the stomach, small intestine, colon, and esophagus. Immunoproliferative small intestinal disease (IPSID) is a specialized type of MALT lymphoma that occurs almost exclusively in the Middle East and is characterized by the synthesis of alpha heavy chain paraprotein. With the exception of IPSID, which tends to be a disease of young adults, MALT lymphomas have a predilection for individuals over the age 50 and exhibit a slight male predominance.

Epidemiologic studies support a strong association between MALT-type gastric lymphomas and chronic *H. pylori* infection. Microbial colonization also appears to be an important etiologic factor in IPSID. MALT-type lymphomas also are associated with various autoimmune and immunodeficiency syndromes, inflammatory bowel disease, and nodular lymphoid hyperplasia.

Grossly, MALT lymphomas may present as (1) unifocal masses with ulceration, (2) or without ulceration (both of which mimic other malignancies), or as (3) diffuse infiltrating lesions. Histologically, they can be subdivided into low- and high-grade types. **Low-grade MALT lymphomas** are characterized by the presence of non-neoplastic reactive lymphoid follicles surrounded by small- to medium-sized "centrocyte-like" tumor cells that extend into the surrounding tissue and invade individual gastric glands to form so-called lymphoepithelial complexes. **High-grade MALT lymphomas** are characterized by the presence of confluent sheets or clusters of centroblastic (large, noncleaved) or plasmablastic tumor cells outside of colonized follicles.

Gastric lymphomas typically present with epigastric pain or discomfort, anorexia, weight loss, nausea and/or vomiting, occult or gross gastrointestinal bleeding, and early satiety. Physical examination often is normal. Occasionally, with advanced disease, an abdominal mass is palpable. Clinical features of small intestinal lymphoma include abdominal pain, occult or frank bleeding, bowel obstruction, intussusception, weight loss, and malabsorption. Rarely, perforation occurs.

Other unusual presentations include lactose-intolerance, enteroenteric fistula, ascites, fever, and hepatosplenomegaly. Colorectal lesions may present with pain, bleeding, altered bowel habits, or obstruction. Regardless of the site of involvement, laboratory findings are nonspecific and may include anemia or elevated ESR.

Upper endoscopy and upper GI series are the mainstay of diagnosis of gastric lymphoma. Contrast radiography tends to be the initial diagnostic modality of choice for detecting small bowel lymphomas. Endoscopic approaches may be feasible depending on the site of involvement: proximal lesions may be detected by "push" enteroscopy, whereas intubation of the terminal ileum during colonoscopy may detect distal lesions. Exploratory laparotomy is indicated for lesions not amenable to endoscopic access. Barium enema and colonoscopy are the principle diagnostic modalities for colorectal lymphomas. Obtain computed tomography (CT) scans of the abdomen, pelvis, and chest for staging once the diagnosis is confirmed. In the case of gastric lymphomas, endoscopic ultrasound (EUS) is useful for determining depth of mural involvement and local lymph node status, especially if combined with fine needle aspiration. The gold standard for staging remains laparotomy; employ it for all patients with equivocal imaging studies.

Histologic grade and disease stage dictate the treatment of gastric lymphomas. Eradication of *H. pylori* is the treatment of choice for early stage (IE, IIE), low-grade lymphomas, with complete regression rates in the range of 70%. Patients who do not respond or relapse still have a high rate of cure, with 5-year survival rates of 80–90% following chemotherapy or radiation therapy. Optimal treatment for early-stage, high-grade gastric lymphomas remains controversial, but might include surgery, radiation therapy, and/or chemotherapy. CHOP (cyclophosphamide, doxorubicin, vincristine, and prednisone) chemotherapy remains the treatment of choice for both low-grade and high-grade as well as stage IIIE and IV disease. Overall survival for high-grade gastric lymphomas is approximately 45%.

Optimal treatment of primary intestinal lymphomas depends on extent of involvement, stage, and, to a lesser degree, type. Broad-spectrum antibiotics (e.g., tetracycline), alone or in combination with corticosteroids, are recommended for the treatment of early (prelymphomatous) stage IPSID, with response rates of 33–71%. Regardless of type, surgical resection is indicated for localized lymphomas confined to the bowel wall (stage IE) or involving contiguous nodes only (stage IIE). The role of adjuvant radiation therapy or chemotherapy following curative resection is controversial. Consider resection for more advanced segmental disease, in hope of reducing tumor burden, relieving symptoms (e.g., obstruction), and obviating the risk of bleeding or perforation induced by radiation therapy or chemotherapy. Radiation therapy, alone or combined with chemotherapy, is the treatment of choice for patients with diffuse, unresectable small bowel disease. Disseminated disease is usually treated with radiation therapy plus combination chemotherapy. Five-year survival rates are about 50% for "western-type" intestinal MALT lymphomas and 67% for IPSID.

In the present patient, the diagnosis was suspected because of his immunocompromised state and confirmed by histologic assessment of endoscopic biopsies. Despite the presence of *H. pylori* infection, he was not a candidate for antibiotic therapy because of high-grade histology. Preoperative evaluation with CT and EUS suggested stage IIE disease. The patient was treated with surgery and radiation therapy and is currently alive and well 2 years later.

Clinical Pearls

1. MALT lymphomas of the GI tract are rare, but should be considered in the differential diagnosis of older individuals presenting with new-onset GI symptoms.

2. High-risk groups include patients with longstanding *H. pylori* infection, autoimmune diseases, immunocompromised states, Crohn's disease, and nodular lymphoid hyperplasia.

3. GI lymphomas may be difficult to diagnose; hence, aggressive diagnostic modalities, including exploratory laparotomy with resection, may be necessary when endoscopic biopsies fail to confirm the diagnosis.

4. Low-grade, early-stage diseases may be amenable to antibiotic therapy, whereas more aggressive treatments, including surgery, chemotherapy, and/or radiation therapy may be indicated for higher-grade, and advanced-stage disease. Following treatment, all patients should undergo periodic surveillance because of the risk of recurrent disease.

REFERENCES

1. Isaacson PG, Wright DH: Malignant lymphoma of mucosa associated lymphoid tissue. A distinctive type of B-cell lymphoma. Cancer 1983;52:1410.
2. Fork FT, Haglund U, Hogstrom H, et al: Primary gastric lymphoma versus gastric cancer. An endoscopic and radiographic study of differential diagnostic possibilities. Endoscopy 1985;17:5.
3. Gobbi P, Dionigi P, Barbieri F, et al: The role of surgery in the multimodal treatment of primary gastric non-Hodgkin's lymphomas: A report of 76 cases and review of the literature. Cancer 1990;65:2528.
4. Cogliatti SB, Schmid V, Schmacher U, et al: Primary B-cell gastric lymphoma: A clinicopathologic study of 145 patients. Gastroenterology 1991; 101:1159.
5. Radaszkiewicz T, Dragosics B, Bauer P: Gastrointestinal malignant lymphomas of mucosa-associated lymphoid tissue: Factors relevant to prognosis. Gastroenterology 1992;102: 1628.
6. Fisher RI, Gaynor ER, Dahlberg S, et al: Comparison of CHOP vs. m-BACOD vs. PROMACE-CytaBOM vs. MACOP-B in patients with intermediate or high-grade non-Hodgkin's lymphoma. New Eng J Med 1993;328:1002.
7. Parsonnet J, Jansen S, Rodriguez L, et al: *Helicobacter pylori* infection and gastric lymphoma. N Engl J Med 1994;330:1267.
8. Wiersema MJ, Gatzimos K, Nisi R, Wiersema LM: Staging of non-Hodgkin's lymphoma with endosonography-guided fine-needle aspiration biopsy and flow cytometry. Gastrointest Endosc 1996;44:734.
9. Coiffier B, Salles G: Does surgery belong to medical history for gastric lymphomas? Ann Oncol 1997;8:419.
10. Fine, KD, Stone MJ: Alpha-heavy chain disease, Mediterranean lymphoma, and immunoproliferative small intestinal disease: A review of clinicopathological features, pathogenesis, and differential diagnosis. Am J Gastroenterol 1999;94:1139.
11. Steinbach, G, Ford, R, Glober, G, et al: Antibiotic treatment of gastric lymphoma of mucosa-associated lymphoid tissue. Ann Intern Med 1999;131:88.

Loutfi S. Aboussouan, MD

PATIENT 44

A 45-year-old woman with HIV infection and slowly progressive dyspnea

A 45-year-old woman with a history of HIV infection (diagnosed 12 years earlier) presents to the clinic with dyspnea on exertion. The dyspnea has been progressively worsening over 10 years. She currently reports difficulty going up one flight of stairs. She is an active smoker with a 30-pack-year smoking history, and past history of intravenous drug use. Her past history is also significant for *Pneumocystis carinii* pneumonia 7 years earlier. She is compliant with antiretroviral therapy and Bactrim prophylaxis.

Physical Examination: Temperature 36.5° C; pulse 75; respiration 22; blood pressure 125/75. General: no apparent respiratory discomfort. HEENT: unremarkable. Chest: hyperresonant with diminished air entry bilaterally; no wheezing. Cardiac: regular rate; no murmurs or rubs. Abdomen: soft; active bowel sounds. Extremities: no edema.

Laboratory Findings: CD4 count: 650/μl (normal). HIV1 quantitation by PCR: no HIV1 (< 200 RNA copies/ml). Arterial blood gas (room air): pH 7.39, PaO_2 51 mmHg, $PaCO_2$ 48 mmHg. Current pulmonary function tests: see table. Computed tomography of the chest done 10 years earlier: bilateral bullous changes as well as coalescing noncystic and avascular areas (see figure).

	Predicted	Measured	% Predicted
FVC (liters)	3.04	2.38	78
FEV_1 (liters)	2.32	1.95	84
FEV_1/FVC	0.76	0.82	—
TLC (liters)	4.40	3.97	90
DLCO (ml/mmHg/min)	21.8	7.9	36

Question: What condition may explain the patient's presentation?

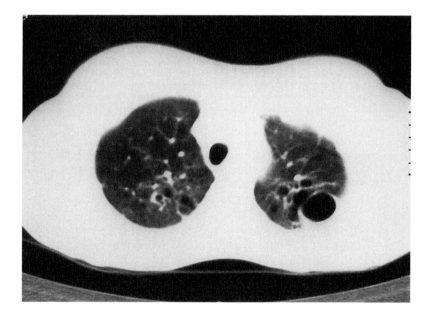

Diagnosis: Emphysema-like disease in HIV.

Discussion: Several reports describe emphysema-like findings in patients with HIV infection. These findings include radiographic demonstration of cystic lesions, decreased diffusion capacity and airway obstruction on pulmonary function tests, and post-mortem documentation of emphysema and bullous lesions—particularly in patients with prior *Pneumocystis carinii* pneumonia (PCP). While these findings may relate to intravenous drug use, prior infections, or smoking history, there also is evidence for a direct role of HIV infection in the pathogenesis of emphysema-like disease.

Intravenous drug use has been implicated in the development of emphysema-like lesions. For instance, bullous cysts are reported in association with talc granulomatosis and intravenous methylphenidate or methadone. The emphysema in case of intravenous methylphenidate or methadone is predominantly basilar, and therefore similar in distribution to that seen in severe alpha-1 antitrypsin deficiency.

Repeated infections, particularly with *P. carinii*, also are associated with the development of emphysema-like changes in both HIV-seropositive individuals and immunocompromised patients with no HIV infection. For instance, radiographic evidence of reversible pneumatoceles can be found in 10–20% of patients with PCP. Also, characteristic pathologic changes of emphysema, including lung parenchymal destruction and bullae, are described in the setting of PCP.

Other studies suggest a direct pathogenetic **role for HIV** in the development of emphysema-like lung changes. CT studies reveal emphysema in 15% of HIV-seropositive patients with no prior history of PCP or other AIDS-related pulmonary complications. The prevalence of emphysema increases to 37% with concomitant smoking history. Similarly, CT shows pulmonary bullous damage in over 40% of patients with AIDS. These bullous changes are not related to an immunocompromised state, smoking history, or prior intravenous drug abuse, and 13% of those patients have no evidence of prior pulmonary infection.

Pulmonary function studies in patients with AIDS document a 33% prevalence of low forced-expiratory flow rates, and a 31% prevalence of improvement in airflow rates after bronchodilators. Similarly, other studies in patients with HIV but no prior AIDS-related pulmonary illness report features suggestive of emphysema with hyperinflation, air trapping, and a corresponding decrease in the diffusion capacity. Recent evidence demonstrates that the reduced diffusion capacity is not associated with a decrease in total lung capacity or with interstitial lung disease, but is correlated with an emphysema score derived from CT evaluation.

Despite radiographic and physiologic findings supportive of a diagnosis of emphysema in such patients, some caveats remain. For instance, most studies usually do not demonstrate significant airway obstruction. This has been suggested to reflect the peripheral location of the changes identified on radiographic examinations. Further, while there is usually a good correlation between CT scanning or diffusion capacity and pathologic examination of emphysematous lungs, definitive confirmation of emphysema rests on pathologic examination. To date, pathologic evidence is available only in HIV-seropositive patients with prior history of intravenous drug use or PCP.

The exact mechanism for the development of emphysema-like disease in HIV is unclear, but may relate to malnutrition, a direct cytotoxic effect of HIV, an increase in pulmonary cytotoxic lymphocytes, or repeated and possibly unrecognized pulmonary infections.

The evaluation and management of patients with suspected emphysema-like disease in the setting of HIV infection includes a careful and thorough evaluation for potential confounding factors such as unrecognized smoking, intravenous drug use, or associated infections. Since smoking appears to be associated with greatly increased susceptibility to the development of emphysema in patients with HIV infection, smoking cessation and counseling are important preventive measures. Evaluation for possible infections may need to include bronchoscopy and bronchoalveolar lavage if clinically indicated. Oxygen therapy should be prescribed when appropriate and may confer the same advantages as in classical COPD. Finally, since the prevalence of bronchodilator responsiveness is high in such patients, conventional and more specific therapy, particularly with ipratropium and albuterol, may be of use.

The present HIV-seropositive patient displays several risk factors for the development of emphysema-like disease. The most striking feature of her presentation is the onset of symptoms of emphysema-like changes at a young age, likely due to a combination of HIV infection and smoking. Other potential contributors include the effects of intravenous drug use and possible lung infections. With adequate control of HIV disease with antiretroviral therapy, allowing long-term survival, her most prominent symptom is now progressive shortness of breath. The diagnosis of emphysema-like disease is supported by the progressive nature of her symptoms, absence of infection on evaluation, marked decrease in diffusion capacity, and chest CT findings of bullous changes and avascular areas with no interstitial lung disease (see figure). In accord with published studies, her pulmonary function tests do not demonstrate significant airway obstruction. She did, however, improve after treatment with bronchodilators and oxygen supplementation.

Clinical Pearls

1. Patients with HIV infection have an increased susceptibility to the development of early-onset emphysema-like disease, particularly with concomitant smoking.

2. Other risk factors that may predispose to emphysema-like changes in HIV include intravenous drug use and history of *Pneumocystis carinii* pneumonia.

3. The diffusion capacity in patients with emphysema-like disease in HIV is reduced and correlates with the degree of emphysema on chest CT studies.

4. Unlike classical emphysema, emphysema-like disease in the setting of HIV infection often is *not* associated with significant airflow obstruction.

5. Prevalence of improved airflow rates after inhaled bronchodilators is > 30% in patients with AIDS.

REFERENCES

1. O'Donnell CR, Bader MB, Zibrak JD, et al: Abnormal airway function in individuals with the AIDS. Chest 1988;94:945–948.
2. Gurney JW, Bates FT: Pulmonary cystic disease: Comparison of *Pneumocystis carinii* pneumatocoeles and bullous emphysema due to intravenous drug abuse. Radiology 1989;173:27–31.
3. Kuhlman JE, Knowles MC, Fishman EK, Siegelman SS: Premature bullous pulmonary damage in AIDS: CT diagnosis. Radiology 1989;173:23–26.
4. Sahebjami H, Domino M: Effects of starvation and refeeding on elastase-induced emphysema. J Appl Physiol 1989;66: 2611–2616.
5. Sandhu JS, Goodman PC: Pulmonary cysts associated with *Pneumocystis carinii* pneumonia in patients with AIDS. Radiology 1989;173:33–35.
6. Diaz PT, Clanton TL, Pacht ER: Emphysema-like pulmonary disease associated with HIV infection. Ann Intern Med 1992;116:124–128.
7. Stern EJ, Frank MS, Schmutz JF, et al: Panlobular pulmonary emphysema caused by IV injection of methylphenidate (ritalin): Findings on chest radiographs and CT scans. AJR 1994;162:555–560.
8. Diaz PT, King MA, Pacht ER, et al: The pathophysiology of pulmonary diffusion impairment in HIV infection. Am J Respir Crit Care Med 1999;160:272–277.
9. Diaz PT, King MA, Pacht ER, et al: Increased susceptibility to pulmonary emphysema among HIV-seropositive smokers. Ann Intern Med 2000;132:369–372.

David K. McCulloch, MD

PATIENT 45

A 76-year-old man with diabetes and stroke

A 76-year-old, retired military man presents to the emergency department with a left hemiplegia. Four weeks ago, he presented with an 8-pound weight loss, thirst, polyuria, and tiredness following an episode of "the flu." He was told at that time to cut out all sugar and eat a high-fiber, high-carbohydrate, low-fat diet (1500 KCal). Glyburide was started, 5 mg twice daily. The patient's past medical history includes an anterior myocardial infarction 6 years ago, with residual poor left ventricular function. He is taking 80 mg of furosemide daily, along with supplements of potassium chloride.

Physical Examination: Pulse 110, respirations 18, blood pressure 185/100. General: drowsy and agitated, with diaphoresis. HEENT: normal; no bruits in neck. Chest: clear. Cardiac: no murmurs. Extremities: right femoral bruit. Neurologic: left hemiplegia.

Laboratory Findings: Glucose 435 mg/dl (24.2 mmol/L), BUN 45 mg/dl, creatinine 1.4 mg/dl, Na 136 mEq/L, K 4.4 mEq/L, CO_2 23 mEq/L. Chest radiograph: cardiomegaly with mild pulmonary congestion.

Question: What tests and treatment should be carried out in the emergency department?

Answer: Check plasma glucose; if < 70 mg/dl, administer glucose infusion.

Discussion: The biological half-life of glyburide often is longer than 24 hours in elderly patients, partly because the metabolites of glyburide have hypoglycemic activity. In addition, patients with poor left ventricular function and reduced renal perfusion can develop toxic levels of glyburide and its metabolites. This patient, who followed all of his medical instructions to the letter, suffered profound and prolonged hypoglycemia.

In a patient with generalized atheroclerosis and inadequate cerebral perfusion, prolonged hypoglycemia may present as hemiplegia, which will resolve completely if the underlying hypoglycemia is recognized and treated promptly. Glucose infusions may have to be continued for several days until the sulfonylurea and its metabolites are cleared from the body. A shorter-acting sulfonylurea (such as glipizide or tolbutamide) is a better option for treatment in this gentleman.

Patients with a past history of myocardial infarction, as well as evidence of generalized atherosclerosis and hypertension, should be started on an angiotensin-converting enzyme (ACE) inhibitor (such as ramipril). The Heart Outcomes Prevention Evaluation (HOPE) trial showed that the risks of future myocardial infarction, stroke, or sudden death were reduced by 20–40% over a 5-year period in diabetic patients over age 55 years of age who had any other risk factor for heart disease. Whether this beneficial effect is specific to ramipril (the ACE inhibitor used in the trial) or is a class effect of all ACE inhibitors is unclear.

In the present patient, a plasma glucose taken in the emergency department was 24 mg/dl. A bolus of 50% dextrose was given, followed by a 10% glucose infusion for the next 4 days. His hemiplegia resolved completely. At the time of discharge, he was receiving 2.5 mg glipizide twice daily and 10 mg ramipril once daily, in addition to his furosemide and potassium chloride.

Clinical Pearls

1 Glyburide can cause profound and prolonged hypoglycemia in elderly patients.
2. Hypoglycemia may present as a hemiplegia in the elderly.
3. ACE-inhibitor treatment should be considered in all diabetic patients aged 55 years and above who have any other risk factor for heart disease.

REFERENCES

1. Rydberg T, Jönsson A, Roder M, Melander A: Hypoglycemic activity of glyburide (glibenclamide) metabolites in humans. Diabetes Care 1994;17:1026–1030.
2. Shorr RI, Ray WA, Daugherty JR, Griffin MR: Individual sulfonylureas and serious hypoglycemia in older people. J Am Geriatr Soc 1996; 44:751–755.
3. The Heart Outcomes Prevention Evaluation Study Investigators: Effect of an angiotensin-converting-enzyme inhibitor, ramipril, on cardiovascular events in high-risk patients. N Engl J Med 2000;342:145–153.

Scott Choi, MD
Arun J. Sanyal, MD

PATIENT 46

A 50-year-old man with cirrhosis of the liver

A 50-year-old man is discovered to have elevated liver enzymes during a routine examination. He has a history of intravenous drug abuse when he was in his teens. He denies history of melena, hematemesis, and hematochezia.

Physical Examination: Vital signs: normal. Skin: anicteric. Chest: normal. Cardiac: normal. Abdomen: palpable splenomegaly. Extremities: no edema. Neurologic: no asterixis.

Laboratory Findings: Hemoglobin 14 g/dl, platelets 75,000/μl. PT 16 (PT control 12). Na$^+$ 132 mEq/L, K$^+$ 3.5 mEq/L, BUN 10 mg/dl, Cr 1.0 mg/dl. Alkaline phosphatase 60 (60–100 normal), AST 30 (0–60), ALT 45 (0–60), bilirubin 3.5 mg/dl (2.5 conjugated), albumin 2.5 g/L. Hepatitis C antibody: positive. Liver biopsy: active cirrhosis.

Questions: How would you assess this patient's risk of gastrointestinal bleeding? What can you do to prevent it?

Answer: Endoscopy should be performed. Bleeding can be prevented with nonselective beta blockers.

Discussion: Variceal hemorrhage is a major cause of morbidity and mortality in patients with cirrhosis. Consequently, the prevention and treatment of variceal hemorrhage is a major objective in patients who present with cirrhotic liver disease.

The annual rate of development of esophageal varices is about 2–4%. Varices develop when the portal pressures, as measured by the hepatic venous pressure gradient (HVPG), exceed 12 mmHg. However, only a third of subjects with varices will experience variceal hemorrhage in their lifetime. It is therefore important for the practicing physician to stratify the risk of variceal hemorrhage in any patient known to have cirrhosis, and to provide therapy for those at risk.

The risk factors for development of variceal hemorrhage include variceal size, degree of hepatic failure, severity of ascites, and several features described on endoscopic examination as **red signs**. The latter represent partial disruption and thinning of the mucosa overlying the varices, allowing the underlying blood stream to be visualized as red streaks (red wale signs) or blood blisters (hematocystic spots). Of all risk factors, the **sizes of the varices** are the most important predictors of hemorrhage.

In a given patient, many permutations of the above-mentioned risk factors can occur. Thus, the risk of bleeding varies accordingly and has been best characterized by an important study by the North Italian Endoscopy Club. A patient with normal liver function, small varices, and absence of red signs would have an approximately 5% risk of bleeding. A patient with Child-Pugh class C cirrhosis, large varices, and red signs would be expected to have an approximately 70% risk of bleeding (see table). This risk is greatest in the first two years after initial detection of varices. *Since endoscopic examination of the varices is essential for risk-stratification, it is recommended that a diagnostic endoscopy be performed in all patients with established cirrhosis.*

In general, those with either normal liver function and medium-to-large varices or liver failure with varices of any size—especially if red signs are present—should be considered for primary prophylaxis of variceal hemorrhage. Based on the laboratory evidence of hepatic synthetic failure, this patient should be considered for primary prophylaxis of variceal hemorrhage if he has varices.

The mainstay of prevention of the index variceal bleed is pharmacologic treatment with **nonselective beta blockers**, e.g., propranolol or nadolol. These agents act by blocking the vasodilatory β adrenergic effects in the mesenteric arterioles, thereby allowing unopposed α adrenergic vasoconstriction. This decreases inflow to the portal vein and decreases portal pressures. A large number of studies have examined the efficacy of nonselective β blockers for primary prophylaxis of variceal hemorrhage. Meta-analyses of the data indicate that these agents decrease the risk of variceal hemorrhage by about 50% and also decrease bleeding-related mortality. However, these do not translate into an overall improvement in long-term survival. Also, up to 20% of subjects are unable to tolerate these agents, which cause tiredness, sexual dysfunction, and bronchoconstriction and worsen heart failure.

Virtually all studies have titrated the dose of the β blockers to achieve a resting heart rate of about 55–60 beats/minute, i.e., maximally-tolerated doses. Unfortunately, the portal hypotensive effects of β blockers do not correlate with heart rate. Those with a sustained drop in HVPG of > 25% or below 12 mmHg almost never bleed while on long-term β blocker therapy. It has been proposed that serial measurements of HVPG be used to monitor

Estimated 1-Year Percentage Probability of Bleeding as a Function of All Possible Combinations of the Endoscopic Variables Form (F) and Red Wale Markings in Child's Class A, B, and C Patients

	Child's Class								
	A			B			C		
	F1	F2	F3	F1	F2	F3	F1	F2	F3
Red wale markings									
	6	10	15	10	16	26	20	30	42
+	8	12	19	15	23	33	28	38	54
++	12	16	24	20	30	42	36	48	64
+++	16	23	34	28	40	52	44	60	76

Adapted from North Italian Endoscopic Club for the Study and Treatment of Esophageal Varices: Prediction of the first variceal hemorrhage in patients with cirrhosis of the liver and esophagel varices. New Engl J Med 319:983, 1988; with permission.

long-term β blocker use for portal hypertension. Also, recently, the measurement of intravariceal pressure by endoscopic methods have been shown to accurately predict the risk of variceal hemorrhage. However, the cost-effectiveness of these approaches remains to be proven, and facilities for HVPG measurements are not routinely available in many hospitals. Thus, the standard-of-care remains titration of the dose to heart rate or to development of side effects.

An important cause of failure of β blockers is an increase in porto-collateral resistance, which negates the benefits of decreased portal inflow on portal pressures. Orally administered nitrates decrease porto-collateral resistance and decrease portal pressure. Used as monotherapy for primary prophylaxis of variceal hemorrhage, they are less effective than β blockers and are associated with a higher mortality in those over the age of 50 years. However, used in combination with β blockers, they have a sustained synergistic lowering effect on portal pressures. In a recent study, a combination of isosorbide mononitrate (20 mg po q daily) and nadolol was superior to nadolol for prevention of the index variceal bleed, but did not produce a significant improvement in survival (see figure). These data await corroboration in additional trials.

Several clinical trials of **endoscopic sclerotherapy** for primary prophylaxis of variceal hemorrhage have been performed. The results are variable, and one large study was terminated prematurely because of a higher mortality in those undergoing sclerotherapy. It is therefore not used for primary prophylaxis. Recently, **endoscopic band ligation** (EBL) has been used for this indication. Clinical trials, performed in Asia, indicate that EBL is superior to no treatment both in terms of prevention of the index bleed and in improving survival. A single study reported that EBL was superior to propranolol for prevention of the index bleed, although survival was not affected. However, the bleeding rates in this trial were very high for those on propranolol, and this study needs corroboration in other trials before these data can be used to change the standard-of-care. At this time, EBL may be considered for primary prophylaxis in those patients who are intolerant of β blockers and are considered to be at moderate or high risk of bleeding.

The present patient underwent endoscopy and was found to be at low risk for variceal hemorrhage.

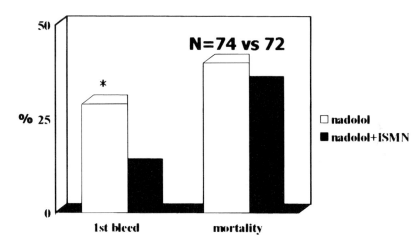

The long-term efficacy of nadolol vs. nadolol + isosorbide mononitrate for the primary prophylaxis of variceal hemorrhage. Combination therapy was superior in terms of preventing the index variceal bleed, but did not improve overall survival. (Figure drawn from data presented in Merkel C, et al: Long-term results of a clinical trial of nadolol with or without isosorbid mononitrate for primary prophylaxis of variceal bleeding in cirrhosis. Hepatology 2000;31(2):324–329.)

Clinical Pearls

1. Clinical predictors of first esophageal variceal bleed include variceal size, Child's class, and the presence of "red wale" signs. Endoscopy is essential to assess the risk of variceal hemorrhage in patients with cirrhosis of the liver.

2. Primary prophylactic measures with proven efficacy consist of nonselective beta-blockers with or without isosorbide mononitrate. Esophageal variceal ligation may be used in those at high risk who are unable to tolerate beta blockers.

3. Measurements of HVPG and variceal pressure are newer modalities that may allow physicians to predict the risk of initial variceal bleed and titrate the pharmacologic prevention of the index variceal bleed.

REFERENCES

1. deFranchis R and the Northern Italian Endoscopy Club: Prediction of the first variceal hemorrhage in patients with cirrhosis of the liver and esophageal varices. New Engl J Med 1988;319:983–989.
2. Groszmann RJ, Bosch J, Grace ND, et al: Hemodynamic events in a prospective randomized trial of propranolol versus placebo in the prevention of a first variceal hemorrhage. Gastroenterol 1990;99:1401–1407.
3. Poynard T, Cales P, Pasta L, et al: Beta-adrenergic antagonist drugs in the prevention of gastrointestinal bleeding in patients with cirrhosis and esophageal varices, an analysis of data and prognostic factors in 589 patients from four randomized clinical trials. New Engl J Med 1991;324:1532–1538.
4. Nevens F, Bustami R, Scheyes I, Lesaffre E, Fevery J: Measurement of variceal pressure with an endoscopic pressure sensitive gauge: Validation and effect of propranolol therapy in chronic conditions. J Hepatol 1996;24:66–73.
5. Angelico M, Carli L, Piat C, et al: Effects of isosorbide mononitrate compared to propranolol on first bleeding and long-term survival in cirrhosis. Gastroenterology 1997;113:1632–1639.
6. Grace ND: Diagnosis and treatment of gastrointestinal bleeding secondary to portal hypertension. American College of Gastroenterology Practice Parameters Committee. Am J Gastroenterol 1997;92:1081–1091.
7. Sarin SK, Lamba GS, Kumar M, et al: Comparison of endoscopic ligation and propranolol for the primary prevention of variceal bleeding. New Engl J Med 1999;340:988–993.
8. Merkel C, Marin R, Sacerdoti D, et al: Long-term results of a clinical trial of nadolol with or without isosorbide mononitrate for primary prophylaxis of variceal bleeding in cirrhosis. Hepatology 2000;31(2):324–329.

Amal Jubran, MD

PATIENT 47

A 60-year-old man with difficulty weaning from mechanical ventilation

A 60-year-old man with a history of chronic obstructive pulmonary disease and hypertension required mechanical ventilation for management of hypoxemic respiratory failure resulting from pneumonia and pulmonary edema. Oxygenation and clinical status of the patient improved with antibiotics and diuretics. Arterial blood gas (ABG) values after a few days of therapy are pH 7.41, $PaCO_2$ 44 mmHg, and PaO_2 72 mmHg on ventilatory settings of assist control ventilation, tidal volume 600 ml, respiratory rate 12, fractional inspired oxygen concentration (FiO_2) 0.40, and positive end-expiratory pressure (PEEP) 5 cm H_2O. Recordings with pulmonary artery catheter (PAC) during mechanical ventilation reveal a pulmonary artery occlusion pressure (PAOP) of 10 mmHg, mean pulmonary artery pressure (MPAP) of 35 mmHg, mean arterial pressure of 88 mmHg, and a cardiac index of 3.6 L/min/m². The patient undergoes a weaning trial using a T-tube circuit with an FiO_2 of 0.40. After 20 minutes of spontaneous breathing, he becomes agitated and diaphoretic.

Physical Examination: Blood pressure 160/73; pulse 100; respiratory rate 35. General: increased activity of sternomastoid and abdominal muscles. Chest: bibasilar crackles. Cardiac: normal.

Laboratory Findings: ABG at end of trial: pH 7.40, $PaCO_2$ 50 mmHg, PaO_2 46 mmHg. PAC and esophageal catheter recordings at start and end of T-piece trial: see below.

Question: Why did the patient become hypoxemic and fail the trial of spontaneous breathing?

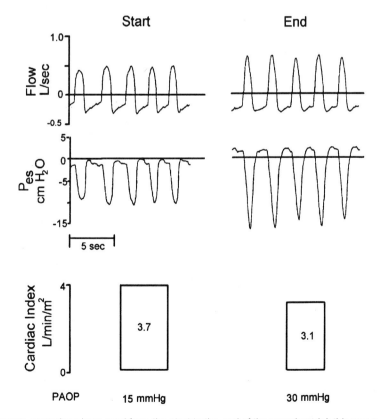

Esophageal pressure excursions increased from the start to the end of the weaning trial; this was accompanied by increases in PAOP, MPAP, and mean arterial pressure and a decrease in the cardiac index.

Answer: Acute cardiac dysfunction during weaning trial.

Discussion: Discontinuation of mechanical ventilation is difficult in about one-third of patients. The most common cause of failure to wean from mechanical ventilation is failure of the respiratory muscle pump. Such alterations in respiratory muscle function can have detrimental effects on cardiovascular performance and cause a decreased supply of oxygen to the respiratory muscles.

The most characteristic finding in patients who fail a weaning trial is that they develop rapid shallow breathing immediately upon discontinuation of mechanical ventilation. Within the first minute of spontaneous breathing, tidal volume decreases and respiratory frequency increases. The increase in frequency is commonly associated with dynamic hyperinflation, which has numerous adverse effects on respiratory muscle function. An increase in lung volume can also have detrimental effects on pulmonary vascular resistance. As lung volume increases from residual volume to total lung capacity, resistance of the alveolar vessels increases while the resistance of extra-alveolar vessels decreases. However, the net effect of increasing lung volume is to increase pulmonary vascular resistance, which, in turn, causes a decrease in cardiac index.

The major mechanical effect of switching from positive pressure to spontaneous breathing is a decrease in pleural pressure. The swings in **esophageal pressure** (Pes), an indirect measure of pleural pressure, are greater in patients who fail a weaning trial than in those who are successfully extubated, as a result of increases in inspiratory resistance, dynamic elastance, and intrinsic PEEP. The large swings in Pes cause an increase in left-ventricular afterload, which, in turn, causes an increase in PAOP.

Mixed venous oxygen saturation (SvO$_2$), a surrogate measure of tissue oxygenation, is another important determinant of weaning outcome. Immediately before a weaning trial, SvO$_2$ is similar in weaning failure and weaning success patients. During spontaneous breathing, SvO$_2$ falls progressively in patients who fail a weaning trial, whereas it remains unchanged in weaning success patients. O$_2$ demand is similar in the two patient groups during a weaning trial, but the manner in which it is met differs. The success patients meet their O$_2$ demand by increasing O$_2$ transport. In contrast, O$_2$ transport does not change in the failure patients. The manner in which weaning failure patients meet their increase in O$_2$ demand is by increasing O$_2$ extraction by the tissues—presumably the respiratory muscles—which together with a relative decrease in O$_2$ transport results in a decrease in SvO$_2$.

The difference in O$_2$ transport responses during weaning is mostly due to changes in **cardiac index**, which increases in the success group, but does not change in the failure group. An increase in cardiac index is the anticipated response to discontinuation of mechanical ventilation in patients with intact cardiovascular function and is largely mediated by an increase in preload. Several mechanisms contribute to the relative decrease in cardiac index in failure patients. Impairment in cardiac contractility secondary to respiratory acidosis and hypoxemia that occurs in weaning failure patients can decrease cardiac index. Myocardial ischemia during a weaning trial can also contribute to a decrease in cardiac index, especially in patients with documented coronary artery disease. Finally, an increase in right and left-ventricular afterload, because of more negative swings in pleural pressure, can lead to a decrease in cardiac index.

The present patient experienced worsening cardiac function during a weaning trial due to negative swings in pleural pressures (figure, previous page). Mechanical ventilation was reinstituted in the present patient for an additional 2 days. Bronchodilators were given to reduce airway resistance and minimize patient effort. In addition, diuretics and inotropic agents were maximized to improve cardiac function. Subsequently, the patient tolerated a trial of spontaneous breathing and was successfully extubated.

Clinical Pearls

1. Cardiac dysfunction is an under-appreciated cause of weaning failure.
2. Increase in patient effort during a weaning trial can have detrimental effect on cardiovascular performance.
3. Decrease in intrathoracic pressure during weaning may impair O_2 transport through an increase in biventricular afterload.
4. An increase in O_2 extraction by the tissues together with a relative decrease in O_2 transport can impair tissue oxygenation in patients who fail a weaning trial.

REFERENCES

1. Lemaire F, Teboul JL, Cinotti L, et al: Acute left ventricular dysfunction during unsuccessful weaning from mechanical ventilation. Anesthesiology 1988;67:171–179.
2. Yang K, Tobin MJ: A prospective study of indexes predicting outcome of trials of weaning from mechanical ventilation. N Engl J Med 1991;324:1445–1450.
3. Brochard L, Rauss A, Benito S, et al: Comparison of three methods of gradual withdrawal from ventilatory support during weaning from mechanical ventilation. Am J Respir Crit Care Med 1994;150:896–903.
4. Esteban A, Frutos F, Tobin MJ, et al: A comparison of four methods of weaning patients from mechanical ventilation. N Engl J Med 1995;332:345–350.
5. Jubran A, Tobin MJ: Pathophysiological basis of acute respiratory distress in patients who fail a trial of weaning from mechanical ventilation. Am J Respir Crit Care Med 1997;155:906–915.
6. Jubran A, Mathru M, Dries D, Tobin MJ: Continuous recordings of mixed venous oxygen saturation during weaning from mechanical ventilation and the ramifications thereof. Am J Respir Crit Care Med 1998;158(6):1763–1769.

Graham F. Pineo, MD
Russell D. Hull, MBBS, MSc

PATIENT 48

A 32-year-old woman with invasive adenocarcinoma of the cervix and a swollen leg

A 32-year-old woman presents with a 1-week history of swelling of her left leg and pain in the left calf. She was diagnosed 5 years ago with invasive adenocarcinoma of the cervix with positive lymph nodes in the left pelvic wall. She underwent a hysterectomy with resection of involved lymph nodes without additional therapy. Six months ago, 4.5 years after surgery, she presented with left leg pain and weakness. An MRI study demonstrated nerve root thickening at the L3 to L4 level and a destructive lesion in the left sacrum with nerve impingement. Biopsy of the lesion at L4 revealed metastatic adenocarcinoma similar to her primary cervical tumor. She underwent abdominal radiotherapy and therapy with cis-platinum.

Physical Examination: Vital signs: normal. General: no acute distress. Chest: clear. Cardiac: normal heart sounds. Abdominal: well-healed surgical scars, no organomegaly. Extremities: swelling in the left leg extending proximally to the groin. Neurologic: normal.

Laboratory Findings: CBC: normal. PTT 27 sec, INR 1.0. Ultrasound lower extremities: focal thrombus in the left common femoral vein.

Clinical Course: The patient is treated with intravenous unfractionated heparin and coumadin begun on the first hospital day. The PTT quickly rises to a range of 71 to 150 sec, which is maintained for 7 days. The INR on day three is 2.2 and remains between 2.0 to 4.4. The patient is discharged on coumadin, but presents 2 weeks later with increasing pain and swelling in her left leg and an INR of 2.3. An ultrasound study demonstrates thrombus extending from the popliteal fossa to the iliac vessels. An MRI demonstrates enlarged lymph nodes compressing the left common and external iliac veins (see below).

Question: How would you approach this patient's care?

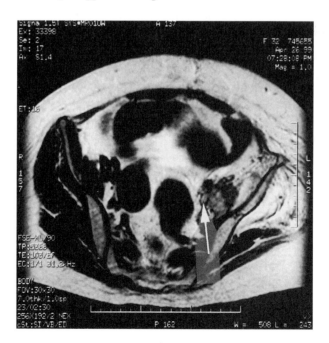

Diagnosis: Recurrent venous thrombosis with an underlying adenocarcinoma.

Discussion: Multiple factors underlie the long-recognized association of venous thromboembolism with the presence of cancer. These include the release of thrombogenic material into the circulation, abnormalities of the coagulation factors that promote and inhibit thrombosis, and local tumor growth. Moreover, a variety of chemotherapeutic drugs promote thrombotic events in patients with cancer.

Anticoagulants in the form of heparin and coumadin have demonstrated utility in the care of cancer patients with thrombotic events. Anticoagulants also have beneficial effects for patients with cancer even in the absence of venous thrombosis. These benefits include the inhibition of tumor growth and improved overall survival.

Although anticoagulants are the first line of therapy for venous thrombosis complicating cancer, management of these patients can be extremely difficult and frustrating. Patients with cancer-associated thrombophilia may not respond as well to anticoagulation as patients without underlying malignancies. Also, bulky tumor deposits can obstruct venous vessels and produce secondary thrombosis that fails to respond to systemic anticoagulation. Clinical trials are now underway to assess the efficacy of low-molecular-weight (LMW) heparin in the prevention and treatment of cancer-related deep venous thrombosis. Studies are also evaluating the utility of LMW heparin in improving survival of cancer patients who do not have deep venous thrombosis. At present, it appears that LMW heparin is a suitable substitute for coumadin for long-term outpatient treatment of deep venous thrombosis.

In caring for patients with cancer-associated venous thrombosis, it is important to use a **validated heparin dosing nomogram** to ensure the rapid and safe implementation of anticoagulation. Studies demonstrate that patients who do not achieve prolongation of their PTT values to a therapeutic range within the first 24 hours of care have an increased incidence of recurrent venous thromboembolism in the subsequent 3 months, compared with patients who experience rapid anticoagulation.

As commonly occurs in patients with cancer, this patient experienced a recurrence of deep venous thrombosis despite coumadin therapy, with more extensive propagation of clot than detected at her initial presentation. In such settings, few therapeutic options exist for the clinician. In the past, many experts recommended the routine placement of inferior vena caval (IVC) filters for any cancer patient presenting with deep venous thrombosis because of the risk of propagation despite anticoagulation. No data from clinical trials, however, support this recommendation. Moreover, IVC filters have not been shown to decrease mortality from pulmonary embolism in the short term, and they lead to an increased incidence of recurrent venous thrombosis in the long term. At present, **indications for insertion of an IVC filter** for the management of deep venous thrombosis include: the presence of absolute contraindications to anticoagulation, recurrent thromboembolism in the presence of adequate anticoagulation, complications of anticoagulation such as major bleeding or heparin-induced thrombocytopenia, and emergency surgery in a patient with incompletely treated proximal deep venous thrombosis. If an IVC filter cannot be placed, another option is to increase the INR to a range of 3.0 to 4.0.

The present patient was placed back on intravenous heparin and underwent placement of an IVC filter to prevent pulmonary emboli. She was treated with cis-platinum and vincristine for her underlying malignancy. She underwent placement of a Porta-cath, and her coumadin was discontinued for 3 days before and 2 days after surgery. Within days of surgery, she developed deep venous thrombosis in the right leg, extending from the popliteal trifurcation to the right groin. She was treated with LMW heparin, which was continued as an outpatient. She expired 1 month later due to carcinomatous meningitis.

Clinical Pearls

1. Patients with cancer are prone to develop deep venous thrombosis. Various chemotherapeutic drugs increase this tendency, which can be managed with prophylactic anticoagulation.

2. Low molecular weight (LMW) heparin is gaining an increasingly important role in the prevention and treatment of venous thromboembolism in cancer patients. It may have a positive impact on mortality in these patients.

3. LMW heparin can be safely used in patients on long-term coumadin therapy who require interruption of oral anticoagulation for surgical procedures.

4. Insertion of an IVC filter is a useful adjunct to anticoagulation in patients with recurrent deep venous thrombosis despite anticoagulation. Anticoagulation should be continued in these patients, however, to prevent thrombosis at the site of the filter.

REFERENCES

1. Raschke RA, Reilly BM, Guidry JR, et al: The weight-based heparin dosing nomogram compared with a "standard care" nomogram: A randomized controlled trial. Ann Intern Med 1993;119:874–881.
2. Decousus H, Leizorovicz A, Prent F, et al: A clinical trial of vena caval filters in the prevention of pulmonary embolism in patients with proximal deep-vein thrombosis. N Engl J Med 1998;338:409–415.
3. Hyers TM, Agnelli G, Hull RD, et al: Antithrombotic therapy for venous thromboembolic disease. Chest 1998;114(5): 561s–578s.
4. Kakkar AK, Lorenzo F, Pineo GF, Williamson RCN: Venous thromboembolism and cancer. Balliere's Clin Haematol 1998;11(3):675–687.
5. Monreal M, Roncales FJ, Ruiz J, et al: Secondary prevention of venous thromboembolism: A role for low-molecular-weight heparin. Haemostasis 1998;28(5):236–243.
6. Zacharski LR, Ornstein DL: Heparin and cancer. Thromb Haemost 1998;80(1):10–23.
7. Anand SS, Bates S, Ginsberg JS, et al: Recurrent venous thrombosis and heparin therapy: An evaluation of the importance of early activated partial thromboplastin times. Arch Intern Med 1999;159:2029–2032.
8. Gould MK, Dembitzer AD, Sanders GD, Garber AM: Low-molecular-weight heparins compared with unfractionated heparin for treatment of acute deep venous thrombosis. Ann Intern Med 1999;130:789–799.
9. Johnson J, Turpie AGG: Temporary discontinuation of oral anticoagulants: Role of low molecular weight heparin (dalteparin). Thromb Haemost 1999;Supplement:62–63.

PATIENT 49

A 48-year-old woman with changing thyroid function tests

A 48-year-old woman with a history of rheumatoid arthritis presents with increasing constipation, cold intolerance, and weight gain. She was initially discovered to have subclinical hypothyroidism with a slightly enlarged, smooth, nontender thyromegaly in 1993. In 1995, she experienced mild symptoms of hypothyroidism, and she was noted to have a slightly larger and firmer nontender thyromegaly. She was maintained on L-thyroxine (125 µg/day) after dose adjustments to produce a euthyroid state. In 1998, she was placed on ferrous sulfate therapy by her gynecologist as part of the management for menorrhagia. She is now returning, several months later, with recurrence of mild symptoms of hypothyroidism.

Physical Examination: Vital signs: normal. Skin: vitiligo of hands. HEENT: unremarkable, except for a slightly enlarged, smooth, nontender thyromegaly. Chest: normal. Cardiac: regular rate, without murmurs. Abdomen: normal bowel sounds, no tenderness or masses. Extremities: ulnar deviation of hands, synovial thickening with some wasting of muscles.

Laboratory Findings:

Serial Thyroid Studies

Year	TSH (0.4–4.7 µIU/ml)	FREE T4 (.71–1.85 ng/dl)	T3 (72–160 ng/dl)	
1993	8	.82	120	Phase 1
1995	24	.43	95	Phase 2
• Antimicrosomal (antiperoxidase) and antithyroglobulin antibodies strongly positive; serum cholesterol 245 mg/dl.				
• Treatment-L-thyroxine (125 µg/day)				
1996	2.5	1.24	130	Phase 3
• Ferrous sulfate therapy started in 1998				
1999	15	.80	82	Phase 4
• Increase in L-thyroxine dosage (150 µg/day)				

Question: What clinical condition does this patient have?

Diagnosis: Hashimoto's thyroiditis and interference with L-thyroxine absorption due to ferrous sulfate therapy.

Discussion: When patients present with manifestations of hypothyroidism, it should be recognized that hypothyroidism is only a functional diagnosis. In evaluating such patients, consider several questions: Where is the patient in the clinical spectrum from subclinical hypothyroidism to overt myxedema? Does the patient have primary (high TSH), secondary (normal to low TSH), or tertiary (normal to low TSH) hypothyroidism? What is the cause of the hypothyroidism?

The **presence of an autoimmune condition**, such as the rheumatoid arthritis in the present patient, suggests that autoimmune thyroid disease (Hashimoto's thyroiditis) is the cause of hypothyroidism—especially in a woman, as this condition is relatively common in females. Had tests for antithyroglobulin and antimicrosomal (antiperoxidase) antibodies been performed at her initial presentation, the diagnosis could have been established earlier.

In 1998, the American College of Physicians published guidelines on screening for thyroid disease. Screening for men and women younger than 50 was not recommended. Asymptomatic women older than 50 years of age, however, were considered to benefit from routine screening. Screening in the present patient detected a **mild elevation in TSH** with normal T4 and T3 concentrations, which supported the diagnosis of subclinical hypothyroidism (phase 1). Note, however, that other causes of mildly elevated TSH concentrations exist, including recovery from non-thyroidal illness, metoclopramide and domperidone therapy, and TSH assay variability. Confirm the persistence of a minimal TSH elevation before definitively establishing the diagnosis of subclinical hypothyroidism. In contrast to the care of the present patient, once subclinical hypothyroidism is detected, an underlying etiology should be pursued.

It remains controversial whether all patients with subclinical hypothyroidism should be treated with thyroid replacement therapy. Consensus exists, however, that therapy should be strongly considered if the TSH is > 10 µU/ml, the antithyroid antibody titers are elevated, the patient has a palpable goiter, or nonspecific symptoms of hypothyroidism exist, such as depression, constipation, and fatigue. Women with subclinical hypothyroidism associated with high antithyroid antibody titers develop overt hypothyroidism at a rate of 4.3% per year.

As the thyroid gland continues to fail, patients with subclinical hypothyroidism may develop preferential T3 secretion (phase 2). Failing glands switch to preferential T3 secretion because only three atoms of iodine are needed to produce one molecule of T3, as opposed to four atoms of iodine for one molecule of T4. Moreover, T3 has five times the bioactivity of T4, producing a considerable metabolic gain from the switch to T3. Normally, only 20% of circulating T3 comes from thyroidal secretion, while the remaining 80% comes from peripheral monodeiodination from T4. With a failing gland, more T3 comes from the thyroid itself as preferential T3 secretion occurs. Such patients may experience further increases in serum TSH concentrations with a decreasing T4, but a T3 that remains in the normal range. Maintenance of normal T3 levels allows patients to have only mild or no symptoms of hypothryoidism.

With the detection of hypothyroidism, start patients on levothyroxine, with a slow dose adjustment every 6–8 weeks until they become euthyroid. The average required replacement dose of levothyroxine in adults is 1.6 µg/kg body weight per day (about 112 µg in a 70-kg adult). Note that the range of the optimal replacement dose varies widely—from 50 to 200 µg/day.

The role of T3 as a component of replacement therapy remains controversial. A recent study revealed that partial substitution using 12.5 µg of T3 for 50 µg of T4 per day improves the neuropsychological function of these patients. However, conventional wisdom among endocrinologists is that T3 replacement therapy should be considered only in patients who do not attain adequate "well being" on levothyroxine therapy.

Patients who have become euthyroid on replacement therapy may subsequently experience an increasing TSH level with normal levels of circulating hormone, as occurred in the present patient (phase 4). A plausible explanation is that the patient stopped taking her replacement medication for several months and then restarted levothyroxine 1 or 2 weeks before having her thyroid tests done. This scenario would result in normal circulating T3 and T4 levels with an elevated TSH. In this setting, the interpretation of an elevated TSH in hypothyroidism is similar to that of an elevated hemoglobin A1C in a diabetic. A patient with diabetes can bring the glucose concentration into normal range by taking insulin for several days, while the hemoglobin A1C reflects the glycemic status during a prior period of 2 months. The TSH is comparable in that it takes a prolonged time for TSH levels to fully respond to changes in circulating thyroid hormone levels.

This pattern of thyroid test results can also be seen in patients who fail to absorb their levothyroxine replacement therapy, or who rapidly metabolize the absorbed drug. The medications that interfere with

T4 absorption across the gut include ferrous sulfate, cholestyramine, sucralfate, and aluminum-hydroxide gels. Medications that accelerate metabolism of levothyroxine include phenytoin, carbamazepine, phenobarbital, and rifampin.

In the present patient, the addition of ferrous sulfate interfered with absorption of levothyroxine. Her dose replacement hormone was increased to 150 µg/day, with resolution of her symptoms and return of her serum TSH level to normal.

Clinical Pearls

1. Hypothyroidism is a functional diagnosis, and a complete evaluation as to the site, cause, and temporary or permanent nature of the hypothyroidism needs to be made. Subclinical hypothyroidism is being diagnosed more frequently, and a logical approach to therapy is needed.

2. Progressive failure of the thyroid gland can result in preferential T3 secretion prior to overt hypothyroidism.

3. Combined T4 and T3 therapy for replacement is probably not indicated in most patients.

4. TSH monitoring for optimal levothyroxine replacement in primary hypothyroidism might be analogous to monitoring the hemoglobin A1C in the diabetic patient.

5. An increase in thyroid hormone dosage might be precipitated by concurrent use of other medications that block replacement hormone absorption or increase its catabolism.

REFERENCES

1. Toft AD: Thyroxine therapy. N Engl J Med 1994;331:174.
2. Vanderpump MP, Turnbridge WM, French JM, et al: The incidence of thyroid disorders in the community: A 20-year follow-up of the Whickham survey. Clini Endocrinol (Oxf) 1995;43:55.
3. American College of Physicians: Clinical guideline, Part 1. Screening for thyroid disease. Ann Intern Med 1998;129:141.
4. Bunevicius R, Kazanavicus G, Zalinkevicius R, Prange AJ Jr: Effects of thyroxine as compared with thyroxine plus trioiodothyronine in patients with hypothyroidism. N Engl J Med 1999;340:424.
5. Toft AD: Thyroid hormone replacement—one hormone or two? (Editorial). N Engl J Med 1999;340:469.

Lisa M. Bellini, MD

PATIENT 50

A 54-year-old woman with severe dyspnea and anorexia

A 50-year-old woman is referred for increasing dyspnea on exertion and anorexia. She has an 80-pack-year history of tobacco use, but quit smoking 8 years ago. She notes a 40-pound weight loss over the past 5 years and progressive dyspnea on exertion. The dyspnea limits her activities of daily living, resulting in a sedentary lifestyle. She denies fevers, chills, night sweats, wheezing, cough, or nocturnal awakenings. She admits to having a very poor appetite and denies indigestion, dysphagia, odynophagia, or vomiting. A diet history for the previous 24 hours reveals a slice of toast and glass of juice for breakfast, no lunch, and a can of soup for dinner, which is her usual eating pattern.

Physical Examination: Temperature 37.8; pulse 70; respirations 28; blood pressure 130/72. Weight 75 pounds, height 5 feet 2 inches. General: cachectic with bitemporal wasting and sunken supraclavicular fossea; mild dyspnea with speech. HEENT: dentition in good repair. Cardiac: regular rate without murmur. Chest: decreased, but symmetric expansion bilaterally; decreased breath sounds throughout all lung fields; no egophony, rhonchi, or wheezes. Abdomen: unremarkable. Extremities: no cyanosis, clubbing, or edema.

Laboratory Findings: Hemoglobin 11.5 mg/dl. Creatinine 0.8 mg/dl. Albumin 3.2 g/dl. Transferrin 150 µg/dl (nl 200–400 µg/dl). Liver-associated enzymes: normal. TSH 1.0 uIU/ml (nl 0.5–6.9) Resting oxyhemoglobin saturation on room air: 86%, falling to 80% after ambulating 20 feet. Pulmonary function studies: severe obstruction with air trapping and a moderate diffusion abnormality (see table). Chest radiograph: hyperinflation without signs of active disease.

Question: What explains this patient's malnutrition?

Pulmonary Function Studies

	Actual	Predicted	% Predicted
FEV1	0.36	1.66	21
FVC	1.09	2.07	53
FEV1/FVC	32	80	40
RV	3.17	1.71	186
TLC	4.31	3.85	112

Answer: Pulmonary cachexia syndrome.

Discussion: Malnutrition associated with advanced lung disease has been termed the "pulmonary cachexia syndrome." Of patients with **chronic obstructive pulmonary disease** (COPD), 30–70% have clinical evidence of malnutrition. This syndrome has been associated with an increased mortality and a decline in functional status. The development of the syndrome is a function of many variables, including aging, exercise, metabolism, tissue hypoxia, inflammation, and medications.

During the natural aging process, body composition undergoes a progressive loss of non-fat body mass, primarily of muscle tissue, and a progressive increase in fat mass. The predominant loss of muscle tissue results in a decrease in muscle mass, causing a reduction in muscle strength as well as a reduction in the basal metabolic rate. This translates into limited exercise capacity. Inactive older patients demonstrate significantly greater loss of muscle mass than active age-matched controls. Thus, physical activity seems to be a regulator of muscle protein synthesis. The significant reduction in cardiopulmonary reserve experienced by patients with COPD is likely a significant contributor to muscle wasting. Additionally, the basal metabolism of patients with COPD does not follow the expected age-related decline seen in normal individuals. The increased work of breathing creates a state of hypermetabolism. Activity, inflammatory conditions, and corticosteroids further exacerbate hypermetabolism. All of these factors contribute to increased oxygen demand. In order to meet oxygen demand at the tissue level, cardiac output must be augmented. Given the limited ability to augment cardiac output, especially in emphysema, oxygen delivery is rationed to critical sites like ventilatory muscles, the heart, and the CNS—resulting in an oxygen and nutrient debt for the peripheral tissues. The interplay of all of these factors is important in individuals with COPD and results in the pulmonary cachexia syndrome.

Clinical manifestations of the pulmonary cachexia syndrome include altered sensation of taste due to chronic sputum production, fatigue, and dyspnea (which interfere with food preparation and ingestion), depression, flattening of the diaphragm with resultant pressure on abdominal contents causing early satiety, eating-induced oxyhemoglobin desaturation resulting in dyspnea, and side effects of medication such as nausea and indigestion. Our patient had fatigue, dyspnea, early satiety, and oxyhemoglobin desaturation, and she was minimally active. This case reflects the **multifactorial nature of this syndrome**.

The diagnosis of pulmonary cachexia syndrome can be made in any advanced lung disease patient with an ideal body weight of less than 90% predicted and in whom no other cause of weight loss can be determined. This patient weighed 82 pounds, which is 70% of her ideal body weight. Nutritional status can be further defined through laboratory measures such as albumin and transferrin, which are markers of protein stores and reflective of protein intake. Serum albumin < 2.3 g/dl is indicative of severe malnutrition. This patient had an albumin that was consistent with long-standing malnutrition, along with a slightly low transferrin, suggesting poor recent intake of protein. Serum chemistries are less valuable and should not routinely be ordered unless indicated by other clinical circumstances.

Increasing caloric intake alone is not sufficient to impede the pulmonary cachexia syndrome. All of the above variables need to be assessed on a regular basis, with emphasis on exercise as tolerated, improving oxygen delivery through oxygen therapy and/or augmentation of cardiac output, control of inflammation, and limitation of corticosteroid use. Even with the proper assessment of all of these factors, patients must increase their caloric intake. This can be accomplished by encouraging patients to eat frequent, small meals and to have convenience meals and meal providers available. Increased caloric intake should be accomplished by increasing *protein* intake, not fats or carbohydrates. The use of nutritional supplements should be recommended cautiously to avoid calorie substitution. The goal is to increase caloric intake and not substitute supplements for meals. Additionally, if anorexia is present in addition to weight loss, the use of appetite stimulants like Megace should be considered.

The present patient was diagnosed with severe COPD complicated by the pulmonary cachexia syndrome. She was begun on 2 L of oxygen by nasal cannula. She also was enrolled in a pulmonary rehabilitation program. The patient was instructed to eat five small meals per day and drink two cans of nutritional supplements daily. Three months after her first visit, she returned with little change in weight or appetite. She was begun on Megace 40 mg a day, and the initial set of recommendations was reinforced. When she returned 3 months later, she had gained 8 pounds and noted a significantly improved appetite and increased exercise tolerance, such that she was no longer dyspneic with her activities of daily living.

Clinical Pearls

1. The pulmonary cachexia syndrome is a relatively common complication of severe chronic obstructive pulmonary disease.

2. Encourage increased caloric intake—specifically, protein intake.

3. A daily exercise program is important to maintaining muscle tone and cardiopulmonary conditioning.

4. Appetite stimulants such as Megace are effective when anorexia is also present.

REFERENCES:

1. Donahoe M, Rogers R, Wilson D, et al: Oxygen consumption of respiratory muscles in normal and malnourished patients with chronic obstructive pulmonary disease. Am Rev Respir Dis 1989;140:385.
2. Wilson D, Rogers R, Wright E, et al: Body weight in chronic obstructive pulmonary disease: The National Institutes of Health Intermittent Positive Pressure Breathing Trial. Am Rev Respir Dis 1989;139:1435.
3. Klitgaard H, Mantoni M, Schiaffino S, et al: Function, morphology, and protein expression of aging skeletal muscle: A cross-sectional study of elderly men with different training backgrounds. ACTA Physiol Scand 1990;140:41.
4. Schols A, Soeters P, Mostert R, et al: Energy balance in chronic obstructive pulmonary disease. Am Rev Respir Dis 1991;143:1248.
5. Weiner P, Azgad Y, Weiner M: The effect of corticosteroids on inspiratory muscle performance in humans. Chest 1993;104;1788.
6. Donahoe M: Nutritional support in advanced lung disease. Clin Chest Med 1997;18:547.
7. Thomsen C: Nutritional support in advanced pulmonary disease. Respir Med 1997;91:249.

Liselle Douyon, MD
Douglas Greene, MD

PATIENT 51

A 38-year-old woman with diabetes and foot pain

A 38-year-old woman with depression and an 11-year history of type 1 diabetes mellitus presents to the office with bilateral foot pain. The pain started 2 years ago when she decided to improve her glycemic control. It has progressed to a severe, burning sensation associated with constant numbness of the balls of her feet. It is so severe at night that she cannot sleep. She wears her bedroom slippers to work because her sensitive feet do not tolerate shoes. She smokes two packs of cigarettes daily. She uses Vicodin for pain.

Physical Examination: Blood pressure 110/62, pulse 88, weight 147.8 pounds, height 63 inches. General: alert, oriented, tearful during the interview, complaining of pain in her feet. HEENT: no retinopathy. Neck: thyroid normal. Chest: clear. Cardiac: regular rate, normal heart sounds. Abdomen: benign. Extremities: minimal hair on toes, 2+ pulses, no lesions. Neurological: intact pinprick and light touch sensation.

Laboratory Examination: Glucose 259 mg/dl, hemoglobin A1C 10%. EMG: see below. All other studies normal.

Question: What is the cause of her pain?

EMG of Lower Extremities

Nerve and Site	Latency	Amplitude	Segment	Latency	Distance	Conduction
Peroneal nerve, right						
Ankle	6.8 ms	0.875 mV		ms	mm	m/s
Below fibular head	14.5 ms	0.665 mV	Ankle—below fibular head	7.7 ms	290 mm	38 m/s
Tibial nerve, right						
Ankle	5.1 ms	1.029 mV		ms	mm	m/s
Popliteal fossa	16.4 ms	0.979 mV	Ankle—popliteal fossa	11.3 ms	380 mm	34 m/s
Peroneal nerve, right						
Ankle	6.0 ms	1.164 mV		ms	mm	m/s
Below fibular head	15.2 ms	0.649 mV	Ankle—below fibular head	9.2 ms	290 mm	32 m/s
Superficial peroneal, right	No					
Lower leg	response	µV	Ankle—lower leg	ms	mm	m/s
Superficial peroneal, left	No					
Lower leg	response	µV	Ankle—lower leg	ms	mm	m/s
Sural nerve, right	No					
Lower leg	response	µV	Ankle—lower leg	ms	mm	m/s
Sural nerve, left						
Lower leg	5.2 ms	3.161 µV	Ankle—lower leg	5.2 ms	150 mm	29 m/s

Significant findings on EMG of lower extremities. Monopolar needle examination was normal. Upper half of table represents motor conduction. Lower half of table represents sensory conduction. mm = millimeter, ms = millisecond, µV = microvolt, m/s = minute per second.

Diagnosis: Diabetic polyneuropathy

Discussion: Distal symmetric polyneuropathy is the most common neuropathic complication of diabetes mellitus. When corrections are made for duration of disease, it affects type 1 and type 2 diabetics equally. It is predominantly a sensory loss of peripheral nerve function. As neural function deteriorates, sensory-motor deficits become more prominent and may be accompanied by dysesthesias or paresthesias. Coexistent autonomic neuropathy is frequent.

The exact mechanism of disease remains unclear. Studies support a role for axonal loss and segmental demyelination. The prevailing theory attributes pathology to decreased cellular levels of myoinositol as a result of hyperglycemia-induced changes in the polyol pathway. Neuroprotein glycation, ischemia, lipid and amino acid derangements, and secondary effects of growth factors have also been postulated to play a role in the disease process. However, current experimental animal models have failed to demonstrate all of the observed human pathologic changes.

Many patients present with subclinical disease. They are asymptomatic on history and physical examination, with abnormal results found on nerve function studies or nerve biopsy. Decelerated nerve conduction velocities, decreased nerve action potential amplitude, and delayed F-wave or Hoffman reflex are the nerve function abnormalities seen on electromyography (EMG). **Sural nerve dysfunction**, the most sensitive indicator of disease, correlates best with neuropathology. When clinical neuropathy becomes apparent, nerve degeneration is in far advanced stages. Neuropathy usually affects the most distal anatomic sites first, with progression in a stocking-glove distribution. Although sensory loss correlates well with ongoing neuropathology, pain is a poor predictor of neural dysfunction. Pain may be acute or chronic. It may occur with poor glycemic control or with rapid improvement of glycemic control. Sural nerve biopsies in the former reveal nerve degeneration; in the latter they reveal nerve regeneration. As in this patient, the severity of pain may be out of proportion to the mild neurologic findings on EMG. Anesthesia, foot ulcer, limb deformity, or amputation marks the development of end-stage complications.

Simple techniques are used to screen for neuropathy in the office setting. They include the use of a neuropathy questionnaire to identify symptoms, visual inspection to look for foot deformities and skin abnormalities, a cotton tip to assess light touch, a disposable pin to elicit pain, a 128 mHz tuning fork to test vibration and temperature, a reflex hammer to elicit reflex responses, and a 10-gram monofilament to determine the cutaneous pressure perception threshold. The inability to detect the monofilament pressure is associated with increased risk of foot ulceration and amputation.

This patient has three risk factors for the development of diabetic neuropathy: poor glycemic control, more than 10 years of disease, and active tobacco use. Other factors implicated in the development of disease are height, advanced age, hypertension, dyslipidemia, hypoinsulinemia, low socioeconomic status, renal failure, and high alcohol consumption.

Successful management of diabetic polyneuropathy remains a challenge. *The most effective therapy is prevention.* Improving glycemic control and educating the patient regarding the nature of disease can accomplish this. It is the only strategy that has been shown to alter the course of the disease. Information gleaned from the Diabetes Control and Complications Trial, the United Kingdom Prospective Diabetes Study, and other randomized controlled clinical trials, observational studies, and pathological studies support the conclusion that improved glycemic control decreases the risk of diabetic neuropathy. Nonsteroidal anti-inflammatory drugs, tricyclic antidepressants, anticonvulsants, antiarrhythmic agents, opioids, and topical agents are used to treat diabetic polyneuropathy. Even alternative therapy such as acupuncture has been tried. Its use is supported by at least two short-term studies. Despite the variety of medication options, therapy may be unsuccessful or limited by side effects.

In the present patient, the history, the physical exam, and the EMG provided evidence of a distal symmetrical polyneuropathy. Excluding the other nondiabetic causes of neuropathy, such as metabolic diseases, malignancy, toxic substances, infectious diseases, or iatrogenic causes, made the diagnosis. Her pain was quite debilitating and had not responded well to the Vicodin. It prompted her to call the office on numerous occasions. Measures were taken to improve her glycemic control and to teach her good foot care. She stopped smoking. After several months of unsuccessful trials with nonsteroidal anti-inflammatory agents and tricyclic antidepressants, her painful symptoms responded to gabapentin and capsaicin. Her EMG findings did not change. This underscores the critical need for improved glycemic control in disease prevention.

Clinical Pearls

1. Diabetic polyneuropathy affects patients with type 1 and type 2 diabetes equally.
2. Asymptomatic patients may have subclinical disease.
3. Sural nerve dysfunction is the most sensitive indicator of neuropathology.
4. Pain is not always a poor prognostic sign.
5. The most effective therapy for disease prevention is improved glycemic control.

REFERENCES

1. Diabetes Control and Complications Trial Research Group: The effect of intensive treatment diabetes therapy on the development and progression of diabetic neuropathy in insulin-dependent diabetes mellitus. Ann Intern Med 1995;122:561–568.
2. Partanen J, Niskanen L, Lehtinen J, et al: Natural history of peripheral neuropathy in patients with non-insulin dependent diabetes mellitus. N Engl J Med 1995;333:89–94.
3. Eaton S, Tesfaye S: Clinical manifestations and measurement of somatic neuropathy. Diabetes Reviews 1999;7:312–325.
4. UK Prospective Diabetes Study Group: Intensive blood-glucose control with sulphonylureas or insulin compared with conventional treatment and risk of complications in patients with type 2 diabetes (UKPDS 33). Lancet 1998;352:837–853.

Javier Bogarin, MD
Robert A. Balk, MD

PATIENT 52

A 74-year-old woman with arthritis, dyspnea, and pulmonary infiltrates

A 74-year-old woman presents complaining of 3 months of progressive dyspnea on exertion, cough, and fever. The symptoms failed to respond to a course of macrolide antibiotics prescribed by her physician. She is presently unable to do her laundry and shopping. She has a 35-year history of rheumatoid arthritis and has undergone treatment with multiple drugs. Her past history also includes hypothyroidism, cataract surgery, and bilateral total knee replacements. She is currently taking prednisone 5 mg/d, leflunomide 20 mg/d, levothyroxine, calcium, estrogen, folic acid, and methotrexate (started 8 years ago). She is an ex-smoker and has no pets at home.

Physical Examination: Temperature 100.5° F; pulse 96; respirations 24; blood pressure 110/62 mmHg. General: thin. HEENT: surgical changes left eye. Cardiovascular: regular rhythm, no extra sounds or jugular venous distention. Chest: bibasilar inspiratory crackles, equal fremitus, no dullness to percussion. Abdomen: normal. Extremities: ulnar deviation of digits and joint deformities in both hands, no pitting edema, no clubbing of digits, no active joint inflammation.

Laboratory Findings: WBC 9500/μl with a normal differential. Arterial blood gases (room air): pH 7.44, $PaCO_2$ 32 mmHg, PaO_2 67 mmHg, SaO_2 89%. Sputum Gram stain and culture: normal respiratory flora. Pulmonary function tests: FEV1 67% predicted, FEV1/FVC 84%, TLC 66% of predicted, diffusing capacity 49% of predicted. Chest radiograph: increased interstitial markings at the bases (see figure, *left*). High-resolution chest computed tomography: diffusely thickened interlobular septa most prominent in lung bases, focal area of alveolar infiltrate in right lower lobe (see figure, *right*).

Question: What is the most likely cause of her symptoms and the chest imaging abnormalities?

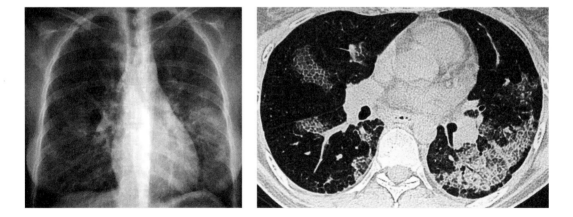

Diagnosis: Acute interstitial pneumonitis due to methotrexate (MTX).

Discussion: Acute interstitial pneumonitis due to MTX occurs predominantly in patients with rheumatoid arthritis (RA) on chronic MTX therapy. Other clinical conditions that are chronically treated with MTX, such as psoriasis and sarcoidosis, may be associated with this form of toxicity. Additional manifestations of chronic low-dose MTX lung toxicity include chronic interstitial fibrosis and hyperreactive airways disease. In addition, high-dose methotrexate treatment has been associated with noncardiogenic pulmonary edema, bronchiolitis obliterans with organizing pneumonia (BOOP), pleuritis, and pleural effusions. Opportunistic infections also can develop as a potential complication of methotrexate treatment..

A majority of the case reports and clinical information concerning methotrexate lung toxicity concern the syndrome of acute interstitial pneumonitis and were derived from case series and cohort studies of patients with RA. The lack of a diagnostic gold standard to definitively make this diagnosis and the difficulty in excluding other confounding conditions, such as infection or rheumatoid lung involvement, complicate the study of this disorder.

Acute pneumonitis has been reported to develop in 0.3–18% of patients treated with methotrexate; it develops in 3–5% of patients when treatment is long-term, typically within the first 2 years of treatment. Risk factors for the development of clinically evident lung toxicity associated with methotrexate treatment include **age > 65, diabetes mellitus, hypoalbuminemia, previous use of disease-modifying antirheumatic drugs**, and the presence of **underlying lung disease**.

The exact pathophysiology of MTX-associated acute pneumonitis is unknown. Despite the frequent use of the term "hypersensitivity pneumonitis secondary to methotrexate," a classical immune-mediated mechanism of injury has not been definitely established. Other potential mechanisms include an idiosyncratic reaction to MTX or a viral infection secondary to the MTX-induced immune suppression. Pathologic features include interstitial pneumonitis, eosinophilia, giant-cell formation, bronchiolitis, and occasional granuloma formation. Desquamation and proliferation of type II pneumocytes are considered most characteristic of MTX-induced injury.

The clinical and laboratory features of methotrexate lung toxicity are nonspecific. Typical symptoms include subacute onset of dry cough, dyspnea, and chest discomfort. Sputum production is most frequently secondary to infection. The physical exam may demonstrate a low-grade fever, tachypnea, and inspiratory crackles. Laboratory data include hypoxemia, mild leukocytosis, and elevation of lactate dehydrogenase. Peripheral blood eosinophilia is present in one-third of cases. Pulmonary function testing typically shows a restrictive pattern, with decreased carbon monoxide diffusion capacity. However, obstructive changes can also occur. Chest radiographs are abnormal in most cases. The most frequent pattern is that of **interstitial infiltrates with basilar predominance**, as seen in the present patient. Alternatively, alveolar opacities, increased interstitial markings, or, less frequently, parenchymal nodules or pleural effusions are present. Chest computed tomography is more sensitive than standard radiographs and may show "ground glass" attenuation with small areas of consolidation (CT scan, previous page). Bronchoscopy is helpful in excluding infectious etiologies. The bronchoalveolar lavage fluid typically reveals a lymphocytosis with a predominance of CD4-positive cells and increased CD4/CD8 ratio. These characteristic features may help distinguish methotrexate pulmonary toxicity from rheumatoid lung involvement.

The diagnosis of MTX pulmonary toxicity should be suspected in any methotrexate-treated patient with new pulmonary symptoms or radiographic abnormalities. The differential diagnosis includes infection (including viral and opportunistic pathogens like *Pneumocystis carinii*) and RA lung involvement. Unfortunately, the diagnosis is one of exclusion. Serial pulmonary function testing has not been useful in the prediction or early identification of methotrexate lung toxicity. Pulmonary histology may be helpful, but is often nonspecific. Diagnostic scoring systems for MTX pneumonitis have been proposed. However, their usefulness is mostly restricted to research studies, and their positive and negative predictive values have not been established.

The management of patients with suspected methotrexate pneumonitis includes immediate discontinuation of MTX and supportive care for the gas exchange abnormalities and other pulmonary symptoms. A diagnostic work-up should be directed toward ruling out an infection. Empiric antibiotic therapy can be instituted until the results of cultures and the infectious work-up are confirmed to be negative. Corticosteroids have been used in published series; however, there are no prospective, randomized, double-blind, placebo-controlled studies documenting their efficacy. Folic acid supplementation has not been shown to prevent or treat lung toxicity due to MTX.

The clinical course depends on the severity of lung involvement, the underlying pulmonary reserve, and the time of recognition of the syndrome. Most patients recover with discontinuation of the drug. The reported case-fatality rate is 1–17% depending on the series.

In the present patient, the subacute nature of her symptoms argues against rheumatoid lung involvement, which is more chronic and insidious in onset. In addition, her age and previous history of treatment with other disease-modifying agents for RA constitute risk factors for MTX-induced pneumonitis. Her rather long-term course of MTX use before the onset of lung toxicity is somewhat atypical, but has been reported. MTX was immediately discontinued, and she underwent a diagnostic fiberoptic bronchoscopy with bronchoalveolar lavage. No infectious agents were identified. She was started on home O_2 therapy and was followed closely as an outpatient. Her clinical condition improved over the course of a couple of weeks. Her radiographic abnormalities completely resolved within 3 weeks of discontinuing MTX, and she no longer required supplemental O_2 therapy. She is currently on an alternative drug regimen for her RA. While some have reported successful rechallenge of patients with MTX without the development of recurrent pulmonary toxicity, in this case it was decided not to tempt fate.

Clinical Pearls

1. MTX lung toxicity can manifest as several different clinical syndromes.

2. The exact pathophysiology responsible for this toxicity has not been definitely established, and a hypersensitivity mechanism has not been conclusively proven.

3. There are no pathognomonic features or gold standards for the diagnosis of MTX lung toxicity. Diagnosis requires a high index of suspicion and elimination of confounding infection.

4. Management centers around early recognition, discontinuation of methotrexate, and provision of supportive therapy.

REFERENCES:
1. Jones G, Mierins E, Karsh J: Methotrexate-induced asthma. Am Rev Respir Dis 1991;143:179–181.
2. Golden MR, Katz RS, Balk RA et al: The relationship of preexisting lung disease to the development of methotrexate pneumonitis in patients with rheumatoid arthritis. J Rheumatol 1995;22:1043–1047.
3. Beyeler C, Jordi CB, Gerber NJ et al: Pulmonary function in rheumatoid arthritis treated with low-dose methotrexate: A longitudinal study. Br J Rheum 1996;35:446–452.
4. Alarcon G, Kremer J, Macaluso M et al: Risk factors for methotrexate-induced lung injury in patients with rheumatoid arthritis. Ann Intern Med 1997;127:356–364.
5. Cannon G: Methotrexate pulmonary toxicity. Rheum Dis Clin North Am 1997;23:917–937.
6. Kremer J, Alarcon G, Weinblatt M et al: Clinical, laboratory, radiographic, and histopathologic features of methotrexate-associated lung injury in patients with rheumatoid arthritis. Arthritis Rheum 1997;40:1829–1837.
7. Salaffi F, Manganelli P, Carotti M et al: Methotrexate-induced pneumonitis in patients with rheumatoid arthritis and psoriatic arthritis: report of five cases and review of the literature. Clin Rheum 1997;16:296–304.
8. Schnabel A, Richter C, Bauerfeind S et al: Bronchoalveolar lavage cell profile in methotrexate induced pneumonitis. Thorax 1997;52:377–379.

Peter F. Malet, MD

PATIENT 53

A 27-year-old man with elevated serum bilirubin

A 27-year-old man is undergoing a physical examination and blood testing prior to starting a residency in internal medicine. He is found to have a total bilirubin of 3.0 mg/dl. He is asymptomatic and has no chronic medical illnesses. He had acute hepatitis A when 7 years old, and he was vaccinated against hepatitis B during medical school. His only medications are occasional (about twice monthly) ibuprofen for headaches or body aches. He is single and jogs about three times weekly. He does not smoke cigarettes. Alcohol consumption averages one or two beverages per week. He has never used IV drugs nor cocaine, and has no tattoos. Further diagnostic testing is ordered.

Physical Examination: Vital signs: normal. Skin: anicteric. Lymph nodes: normal. Abdomen: liver and spleen not palpable; liver span 9–10 cm by percussion; no abdominal tenderness, masses, or ascites.

Laboratory Findings: Total bilirubin 3.0 mg/dl (normal 0.2–1.1), direct bilirubin 0.2 mg/dl, indirect bilirubin 2.8 mg/dl; repeat testing 3 weeks later showed total bilirubin 2.2 mg/dl, direct bilirubin 0.2 mg/dl, indirect bilirubin 2.0 mg/dl. Hct 44%, MCV 92 fl, MCHC 35 g/dl, MCH 30 pg, RDW 12.5%, WBC 7500/μl, platelets 255,000/μl; peripheral blood smear normal. ALT, AST, alkaline phosphatase, GGTP, total protein, albumin, PT, PTT: normal. Serum haptoglobin 55 mg/dl (normal 26–185), reticulocyte count 0.8%. Urinalysis: normal. Hepatitis C antibody negative, HbsAg negative, anti-HBs positive, anti-HBc negative, total anti-HAV positive.

Question: What is the most likely cause for the elevation of serum bilirubin?

Answer: Gilbert's syndrome.

Discussion: Gilbert's syndrome is characterized by mild unconjugated (indirect) hyperbilirubinemia. The physiologic defect responsible is **impaired bilirubin clearance by the liver**.

Two other common causes of unconjugated hyperbilirubinemia in adults are **hemolytic anemia** and **resorption of large hematomas**. Type II Crigler-Najjar syndrome is very rare, and bilirubin levels are higher (5–8 mg/dl), so patients always have jaundice.

Gilbert's syndrome is fairly common; estimates are that up to 5–7% of the population may be affected. Males are more often affected, and the syndrome usually is recognized after puberty. Although many cases are sporadic, there is a familial component to this syndrome.

Normal serum bilirubin levels are variable, but generally in the range of 0.2–1.0 mg/dl. The average level of serum bilirubin in Gilbert's syndrome is 2–3 mg/dl and usually < 4 mg/dl. The level of total bilirubin typically fluctuates and may, at times, enter the normal range, although the indirect fraction remains very high. The proportion of indirect (unconjugated) bilirubin is at least 85–90%. Thus, with hyperbilirubinemia due to various types of chronic liver disease, even proportions of indirect bilirubin in the range of 60–70% are not suggestive of Gilbert's syndrome.

The diagnosis is made by demonstrating the proportion of **indirect bilirubin** to be **> 85–90%** and ensuring that hemolysis is not present. Elevations of the serum transaminases or alkaline phosphatase must prompt a search for underlying liver disease. Since Gilbert's syndrome is common, it may be seen in patients with coexisting, unrelated liver disease. The separation of the Gilbert's component of bilirubin elevation from that potentially caused by the liver disease requires an extensive evaluation, but in these patients, if the proportion of indirect bilirubin is > 85–90%, the elevation can be attributed to Gilbert's.

Although not absolutely necessary for the diagnosis and not totally specific, a 24–48 period of caloric restriction (< 400 Kcal/day) results in about a two-fold increase in total bilirubin in patients with Gilbert's syndrome. In normal patients, this fasting only results in an increase of < 1.0 mg/dl.

There are no specific symptoms that are attributable to Gilbert's syndrome. Physical examination is normal, except for mild icterus in those with bilirubin levels above about 3 mg/dl. All other liver enzymes are normal, as is liver histology.

The unconjugated hyperbilirubinemia is thought to be due to reduced hepatic clearance of bilirubin. There is evidence that the reduced clearance is due to both defective hepatic uptake of bilirubin and also to decreased hepatic conjugation with glucuronic acid. The activity of the enzyme bilirubin-glucuronyl transferase is reduced to about 30–50% of normal. An abnormality in the promoter region ("TATA box") of the bilirubin uridine diphosphate-glucuronyltransferase (UGT-1) gene has been found. Patients have a reduced proportion of bilirubin diglucuronide and an increased proportion of bilirubin monoglucuronide in bile.

Although not thought to be an important component of the pathophysiology, about half of patients with Gilbert's syndrome have a mild decrease in red blood cell survival.

Treatment for Gilbert's syndrome is rarely necessary since there is no long-term harm as a result of the mild hyperbilirubinemia. In unusual instances—for example, if the patient is excessively concerned about the cosmetic appearance of persistent jaundice as a result of an above average bilirubin level that does not spontaneously fluctuate downwards—low doses of phenobarbital will lower the bilirubin level and clear the jaundice.

Research into how the glucuronidation defect may affect therapeutic drug metabolism is ongoing.

This young man had Gilbert's syndrome, based on hyperbilirubinemia with an indirect fraction of 91–93% with normal liver enzymes. He showed past immunity to both hepatitis A and B. Clinical hemolysis was ruled out. He went on to complete his medical residency without any medical problems.

Clinical Pearls

1. Gilbert's syndrome is fairly common, affecting about 5% of the population; it is seen in males more often than females and rarely appears before puberty.

2. Laboratory characteristics of Gilbert's syndrome are serum bilirubin 2–4 mg/dl and proportion of indirect bilirubin > 85–90%.

3. The physiologic defect is impaired hepatic clearance of bilirubin due to both defective uptake and conjugation.

4. Fasting (< 400 Kcal/day) for 24–48 hours approximately doubles bilirubin in those with Gilbert's syndrome; in normal patients, the increase is < 1.0.

REFERENCES

1. Watson KJ, Gollian JL: Gilbert's syndrome. Baillieres Clin Gastroenterol 1989; 3:337–355.
2. Berk PD, Noyer C: Hereditary hyperbilirubinemias. In Haubrick WS, Schaffner F, Berk JE (eds): Bockus Gastroenterology, 5th ed, Vol. 3. Philadelphia, WB Saunders, 1995, pp 1906–1930.
3. Burchell B, Hume R: Molecular genetic basis of Gilbert's syndrome. J Gastroenterol Hepatol 1999; 14:960–966.

Allan S. Jaffe, MD

PATIENT 54

An 80-year-old man with sudden onset of shortness of breath and weakness

An 80-year-old man presents with sudden onset of dyspnea and weakness while attending church. Parishioners gave him sublingual nitroglycerin, which caused him to fall and lose consciousness for a few seconds. His pulse remained strong throughout the episode. In the emergency department, the patient complains of pain in his left thigh, but denies other symptoms. He has otherwise felt well recently.

He has a history of hypertension, a chronic neuropathy, chronic obstructive pulmonary disease, and coronary artery disease. He underwent three-vessel coronary artery bypass grafting after an inferior myocardial infarction 6 years ago. An echocardiogram 2 years ago showed a normal left ventricular ejection fraction with inferior hypokinesis, right ventricular dilatation, and an estimated pulmonary artery (PA) pressure of 46 mmHg. His medications include an angiotensin converting enzyme inhibitor, hydrochlorothiazide, and a beta blocker agent.

Physical Examination: Pulse 72 and regular, respirations 18, blood pressure 150/80. General: mild dyspnea, jugular venous distention to 10 cm. Chest: clear, prolonged expiratory phase. Cardiac: PMI in the fifth intercostal space, midclavicular line, S4, palpable right ventricle, slightly increased P2. Extremities: ecchymoses over the left thigh, slight ankle edema.

Laboratory Findings: Chest radiograph: hyperinflated lung fields. EKG: right axis deviation, nonspecific ST-T wave changes. Oxygen saturation: room air 88%, 92% on 2 L oxygen. Echocardiogram: mildly reduced left ventricular ejection fraction, right ventricular hypertrophy, PA pressure 62 mmHg. Serial cardiac biomarkers:

Time	CK (IU/L)	CKMB (ng/ml)	Relative Index	Troponin I
Baseline	66	3	4%	< 0.5
6 hours	1864	42	2.25	3.8
12 hours	13,264	299	2.25	4.6

CK = creatine kinase, CKMB = MB isoenzyme of creatine kinase

Question: How should the cardiac biomarker results be interpreted in this clinical setting?

Diagnosis: Acute myocardial infarction.

Discussion: When patients have multiple sources of biomarker release, results may be difficult to interpret. The present patient, for instance, could have had elevated CKMB from a myocardial infarction or from damage to his thigh muscles sustained in his fall. Also note that any cause of cardiac injury can produce elevated biomarker values. Thus, acute damage to the right ventricle due to acute pulmonary emboli, for instance, could release CKMB or cardiac troponin into the circulation.

The **creatinine kinase relative index** was developed to assist the differential diagnosis of cardiac versus skeletal muscle as a source of CK release. Because more CKMB fraction is found in cardiac muscle than skeletal muscle, an elevated CK relative index supports the diagnosis of myocardial injury. For patients who have only skeletal muscle or cardiac injury—but not both—the relative index works passably well as a diagnostic aid. Unfortunately, there is substantial heterogeneity in the amount of B-chain protein and, consequently, the amount of CKMB released from different skeletal muscle groups. In addition, skeletal muscle has much more total CK per gram than does cardiac tissue. Thus, unless there is abundant CKMB in the skeletal muscle, percentages are low if there is both cardiac and skeletal muscle injury.

Patients with chronic myopathies re-express the B-chain of CK; this is the usual response of damaged tissue. During neonatal development, all CK in skeletal muscle is BBCK. Thus, B-chain protein is re-expressed after muscle injury in later life. Patients with myopathies often have elevated CKMB results and high relative indexes.

Assay of **serum cardiac troponin** is clearly much more specific for diagnosis of cardiac injury when patients have combined skeletal muscle and cardiac injury. To date, no convincing reports exist of a biologic false-positive result from cardiac troponin. In the absence of laboratory error or analytic problems, the presence of elevated cardiac troponin levels in the blood is definitive evidence that cardiac injury has occurred.

In addition to being more specific than CKMB for detecting cardiac injury, cardiac troponin assays are also more sensitive. Patients with known ischemic heart disease are more likely to have elevated cardiac troponin assays after episodes of chest pain due to myocardial ischemia than elevated CKMB levels.

Indeed, up to a third of patients with unstable angina pectoris have mild elevations of cardiac troponin with normal CKMB levels, which is associated with an adverse short- *and* long-term prognosis.

Although an elevated cardiac troponin result signifies cardiac injury, it does not indicate the underlying mechanism for injury. It is not possible for any cardiac biomarker to distinguish between an acute myocardial infarction due to coronary artery disease and right ventricular injury due to pulmonary embolism. In fact, patients with pulmonary emboli who have elevated troponin levels as compared with normal levels have a worse prognosis, which probably reflects the magnitude of the pulmonary emboli and the degree of right ventricular injury. Other conditions without overt ischemic heart disease that are associated with elevated troponin levels include:

Cardiac trauma (cardiac contusion, ablation, pacing, ICD pacing, cardioversion, cardiac surgery)
Congestive heart failure—acute and chronic
Hypertension
Hypotension, often with arrhythmias
Pulmonary embolism
Noncardiac surgery in the postoperative period
Renal failure
Critical illness
Hypothyroidism
Myocarditis
Amyloidosis
Acute neurologic disease

The present patient had an elevated troponin level, which indicated the presence of cardiac injury, and a normal CK relative index, which was considered to be a false-negative result due to the extensive thigh muscle injury sustained from the fall. Considering the patient's hypoxia, hypercapnia, and clinical evidence of pulmonary hypertension, pulmonary embolism with a right ventricular source for cardiac troponin needed to be considered. A lung scan was indeterminate, and a pulmonary angiogram was negative. The patient was found to have congestive heart failure and an acute myocardial infarction. He improved with an increase in his beta blocker and diuretic medications. Cardiac catheterization demonstrated a patent internal mammary graft and occluded right coronary and circumflex grafts, with worsening of the inferior wall dysfunction.

Clinical Pearls

1. The CK relative index is an unreliable test for myocardial ischemia in patients who have both skeletal muscle and cardiac muscle injury, because the large content of CK released by injured skeletal muscle obscures the CKMB released by the heart. When chronic skeletal muscle disease is present, false-positive relative indices occur due to re-expression of the B chain.

2. In the absence of laboratory error, an elevated cardiac troponin value indicates the presence of cardiac injury. It is both more sensitive and more specific than CKMB, but does not define the underlying mechanism by which injury has occurred.

3. Consider nonischemic causes of cardiac injury when patients present with elevated troponin levels without confirmatory evidence of myocardial ischemia. Some of these alternative diagnostic considerations include congestive heart failure, pulmonary embolism, hypertension, and hypothyroidism.

REFERENCES

1. Adams JE III, Bodor GS, Davila-Roman VG, et al: Cardiac troponin I. A marker with high specificity for cardiac injury [see comments]. Circulation 1993;118:101–106.

2. Adams JE III, Sicard GA, Allen BT, et al: Diagnosis of perioperative myocardial infarction with measurement of cardiac troponin I [see comments]. N Engl J Med 1994;330:670–674.

3. Adams JE III, Davila-Roman VG, Bessey PQ, et al: Improved detection of cardiac contusion with cardiac troponin I. Am Heart J 1996;131:308–312.

4. Apple FS, Falahati A, Paulsen PR, et al: Improved detection of minor ischemic myocardial injury with measurement of serum cardiac troponin I. Clin Chem 1997;43:2047–2051.

5. Hamm CW: Risk stratifying acute coronary syndromes: Gradient of risk and benefit. Am Heart J 1999;138:S6–11.

6. Muller-Bardoff MGE, Weidtmann B, Kurowski V, et al: Prognostic value of troponin T in patients with pulmonary embolism. Circulation 1999;100, abstract 3102.

Reshma Kewalramani, MD
Anil Chandraker, MD
Mohamed H. Sayegh, MD

PATIENT 55

A 39-year-old man with a pigmented skin lesion after
renal transplantation

A 39-year-old man complains of a small area of "rash" on his right leg during a routine office visit. He has a history of end-stage renal disease, for which he received a renal allograft from a living, related donor 18 months ago. His immunosuppression consists of prednisone, azathioprine, and cyclosporine. The patient has had no rejection episodes, and his renal function has remained stable. He feels well and has no complaints other than his rash.

Physical Examination: Temperature 97.2°; pulse 78; respirations 16; BP 120/80. General: appears well. HEENT: unremarkable. Cardiac: regular rate without murmur. Chest: good air entry, normal breath sounds. Abdomen: soft, nontender. Extremities: no edema; cluster of pigmented lesions on right calf.

Laboratory Findings: Creatinine 2 mg/dl; BUN 30 mg/dl. HIV negative. Biopsy of calf lesion: infiltration of spindle-like cells surrounding eccrine ducts, with hyaline globules and hemosiderin among slit-like vascular pores.

Question: What is the lesion?

Diagnosis: Kapsosi's sarcoma in an immunosuppressed patient.

Discussion: The risk of malignancy after transplantation is 100 times that in the general population, with approximately 6% of solid organ transplant recipients developing some form of malignancy. A wide variety of neoplasms have been described in transplanted patients, with a particular preponderance to certain forms of malignancy. These include (expressed as percentages of the overall cancer occurrence) squamous cell carcinomas of the skin and lips, non-Hodgkin's lymphomas (24% vs. 5%), Kaposi's sarcoma (1.8% vs. 0.5%), vulvar and perineal cancers (3.5% vs. 0.4%), hepatobiliary cancers (2.4% vs. 1.5%), and non-Kaposi's sarcomas (1.8% vs. 0.5%). Conversely, the rates of occurrence of some of the most common tumors in the general population, such as lung, colon, and prostate, are not increased in transplant patients, with the incidence of breast cancer actually being decreased by 25–30%. This suggests that regulation by the immune system may be responsible for tumor growth *and* tumor suppression.

Immunosuppressive agents promote cancer development in two basic ways: (**1**) immunosuppression, and (**2**) direct carcinogenesis.

Most immunosuppressive agents enhance cancer development by affecting immune surveillance. Prolonged suppression of the immune system impairs the body's ability to cope with cancers caused by carcinogens such as sunlight and oncogenic viruses. Examples of diseases linked to oncogenic viruses include B-cell lymphoproliferative disease related to Epstein-Barr virus (accounting for the majority of patients with **post-transplant lymphoproliferative disorder** [PTLD]); human papillomavirus causing carcinoma of the cervix, vulva, and other skin areas; and hepatitis B and hepatitis C–related hepatocellular carcinoma. More recently, Kaposi's sarcoma (KS) has also been touted as having a viral etiology.

Treatment with antilymphocyte agents such as OKT3 specifically predisposes to PTLD induced by Epstein-Barr virus. With this exception, there is no correlation between any specific immunosuppressant and any particular cancer, although there has been limited experience with some of the newly approved immunosuppressive drugs. The major risk factors for malignancy in transplant recipients are the dose, duration, and number of immunosuppressants used. Certain immunosuppressives such as cyclosporine, however, may themselves induce cancer progression. The mechanism of action of direct cyclosporine carcinogenesis appears to be related to the production of TFG-β.

Tumors in transplant patients tend to occur at a mean age of 41 and at a mean of approximately 5 years after transplantation. Certain cancers have been noted to occur at distinct time points after transplantation. These tumors include KS presenting at approximately 21 months, PTLD at 33 months, and carcinoma of the vulva and perineum at 67 months. Kaposi's sarcoma is classically diagnosed in transplant patients belonging to Arabic, Italian, Black, Greek, or Jewish ancestry who present with reddish-blue skin or oropharyngeal lesions. Once a diagnosis of KS is made, undertake a thorough work-up to exclude any visceral involvement, as KS with visceral involvement portends a worse prognosis with significantly increased mortality.

The term PTLD encompasses all lymphoproliferative disorders that occur post-transplant. The majority of these tumors tend to be **B-cell lymphomas** that commonly involve extranodal sites, the central nervous system, and the graft itself. The clinical picture of PTLD is highly variable and runs the gamut from no symptoms to widely disseminated disease with bulky lymphadenopathy. Presentations include an infectious mononucleosis-like syndrome and isolated organ dysfunction, including allograft dysfunction. Diagnosis is made by biopsy.

The approach to treatment of post-transplant malignancies must begin with preventive measures. Routine pelvic exams and pap smears and encouragement of barrier methods of contraception are important. Administer hepatitis B and C vaccinations when appropriate. Advise limited sun exposure, and encourage the use of sun block. In addition, repeated exposure to antilymphocyte agents should be avoided, and antiviral agents such as acyclovir or ganciclovir should be considered during periods of intense immunosuppression. Once a lesion has developed, the treatment depends on the particular neoplasm. Treatment of skin cancers includes cryosurgery, surgery, and radiation therapy. Recurrent or multiple skin cancers have also been treated with oral retinoids. These therapies are effective, and reduction in the level of immunosuppression is usually not required. Other solid tumors are treated in the standard manner, with surgery, radiation therapy, and/or chemotherapy. The withdrawal of immunosuppression in PTLD and Kaposi's sarcoma can lead to regression and even remission; therefore, it is recommended as first-line treatment for these lesions. However, since withdrawal of immunosuppression may result in allograft rejection, this approach may be precluded in certain situations.

Additional strategies used in the treatment of PTLD and Kaposi's sarcoma include treatment with antiviral agents (more efficacious and established in the treatment of PTLD than KS). Two novel therapeutic strategies that have been attempted and shown to improve outcome in PTLD are interferon-alpha and anti-B cell antibodies.

In the present patient, Kaposi's sarcoma developed as a consequence of immunosuppressive medications, and responded to withdrawal of cyclosporine. However, cyclosporine was later reintroduced because of worsening renal function, and the patient again developed Kaposi's sarcoma. Cyclosporine was once again discontinued, and azathioprine was replaced with mycophenolate. Renal function remained stable, and there has been no recurrence of the Kaposi's sarcoma.

Clinical Pearls

1. Malignancies in transplant patients have a different pattern than in the general population, with skin and lip cancers, lymphomas, and Kaposi's sarcoma having higher incidences.

2. Major risk factors for post-transplant malignancy development include the dose, duration, and number of immunosuppressive agents used.

3. Complete or partial withdrawal of immunosuppression may result in regression of PTLD and KS and has the potential to lead to remission of KS.

REFERENCES

1. Nalesnik MA, Makowka L, Starzl TE: The diagnosis and treatment of posttransplant lymphoproliferative disorders. Curr Probl Surg 1988;25:367–472.
2. Penn I: Cancers complicating organ transplantation. N Engl J Med 1990;323:1767–1769.
3. Swinnen LJ, Costanzo-Nordin MR, Fisher SG, et al: Increased incidence of lymphoproliferative disorder after immunosuppression with monoclonal antibody OKT3 in cardiac transplant patients. N Engl J Med 1990;323:1723–1728.
4. Stewart T, Tsai S-C, Grayson H, et al: Incidence of de-novo breast cancer in women chronically immunosuppressed after organ transplantation. Lancet 1995;346:796–798.
5. Gazdar AF: Tumors arising after organ transplantation: Sorting out their origins. JAMA 1997;277(2):154–155.
6. Penn I: Kaposi's sarcoma in transplant recipients. Transplantation 1997;64:669–673.
7. Hojo M, Morimoto T, Maluccio M, et al: Cyclosporine induces cancer progression by a cell-autonomous mechanism. Nature 1999;397:830–834.
8. Paya CV, Fung JJ, Nalesnik MA: Epstein-Barr virus-induced posttransplant lymphoproliferative disorders. Transplantation 1999;68(10):1517–1525.
9. Antman K, Chang Y: Kaposi's sarcoma. N Engl J Med 2000;342:1027–1038.
10. Peddi VR, First MR: Medical complications of kidney transplantation. In Owen WF, Pereira BJ, Sayegh MH (eds): Dialysis and Transplantation: A Companion to Brenner and Rector's The Kidney. Philadelphia, W.B. Saunders Co., 2000.

Richard V. Paul, MD
Arthur P. Wolinsky, MD

PATIENT 56

A 63-year-old woman with confusion and hypokalemia

A 63-year-old Hispanic-American woman presents with her third episode of confusion and somnolence. She was first admitted 6 weeks ago after being brought to the emergency department (ED) by her family because of confusion and generalized weakness of 3-day duration. She was on no medications and did not use alcohol. Her family had noted some slowing of mentation for 3 months. Urinary frequency, burning, and incontinence had been present for 1 day. She had low-grade fever and pyuria, and her urine culture was positive for 10^5 colonies/ml of *Escherichia coli*, which were sensitive to most antibiotics. The patient also had hypokalemia. Her liver function tests were abnormal (see table).

The patient was treated with trimethoprim-sulfamethoxazole and potassium chloride. Her fever resolved and mental status returned to normal within 48 hours. She was given a follow-up appointment, to recheck her elevated liver enzymes, but she did not appear for her appointment. Four weeks later, she was again admitted from the ED with disorientation and somnolence. Hypokalemia was again present, and liver function tests were still abnormal, but the pyuria had resolved. A diagnosis of hypothyroidism was made, and levothyroxine and potassium chloride were prescribed. The patient's mental status again cleared completely, and she was discharged on the second hospital day.

Her family now states that the patient has been compliant with her levothyroxine, but she does not like the taste of her potassium supplement.

Physical Examination: Temperature 36.6°C; pulse 84 and regular, respirations 22, blood pressure 142/76. HEENT: unremarkable. Chest: clear. Cardiac: grade II/VI flow murmur along left sternal border. Abdomen: no organomegaly or masses, no ascites, no flank pain. Extremities: no edema; excoriations over forearms and shins. Neurologic: recognizes family, thinks year is 1936, frequently falls asleep during exam; no focal cranial nerve or motor findings; toes downgoing, reflexes diminished but symmetrical.

Laboratory Findings: See table.

Questions: What is the likely etiology of the abnormal liver function tests? What is the connection between the hypokalemia and the patient's intermittent mental status changes?

Laboratory Summary

	First Admission	Second Admission	Third Admission
Complete blood count	Normal	Normal	Platelets 106,000/μl
Serum Na^+ (mEq/L)	141	141	140
Serum K^+ (mEq/L)	2.3	2.5	2.6
Serum total CO_2 (mEq/L)	19	19	20
BUN (mg/dl)	11	12	11
Serum creatinine (mg/dl)	1.0	0.9	0.9
AST/ALT (U/L)	75/63		69/62
Alkaline phosphatase (U/L)	402	305	361
Bilirubin (mg/dl)	2.5	1.9	2.3
Urine findings	UTI (*E. coli*)	Na+ 87 mEq/L, K^+ 24 mEq/L	K^+ 35 mEq/L
Plasma pH		7.48	7.51
Plasma pCO_2 (mmHg)		24.7	23
TSH (mU/L)		26.9 (normal 0–6)	

Diagnoses: Primary biliary cirrhosis with hepatic encephalopathy. Renal potassium wasting probably due to renal tubular acidosis.

Discussion: Hypokalemia may cause a multitude of symptoms in hospitalized patients, including muscle weakness, ileus, and cardiac arrhythmias, but it is not associated with changes in mental status. Secondary hyperaldosteronism is frequent in liver disease, but the high spot urine sodium concentration and the absence of ascites or edema in the present patient suggest that the sodium-retaining effects of hyperaldosteronism were not present. Nevertheless, the inappropriately elevated spot urine potassium values, obtained while serum potassium was very low, indicate that renal potassium wasting was the proximate cause of hypokalemia.

The exact role of **ammonia** in hepatic encephalopathy remains controversial, but ammonia almost certainly contributes to this condition even if it does not entirely account for it. Ammonia predominantly exists as the ammonium ion, NH_4^+, at physiologic pH, but the unionized fraction, which is freely diffusible across lipid membranes, is increased in alkaline conditions and decreased when pH is low. Consequently, alkalemia results in increased diffusion of unionized ammonia across the blood-brain barrier, and may precipitate hepatic encephalopathy in susceptible individuals.

Hypokalemia is a direct stimulus for the production of ammonia from glutamine by the renal tubule. Ammonium ion is secreted into the proximal tubule and is reabsorbed by substituting for the missing potassium in the Na/K/2 Cl cotransporter of the medullary thick ascending limb of the loop of Henle, resulting in high interstitial ammonia levels within the renal medulla. Ammonia can diffuse into the medullary collecting duct, where proton secretion and an acid urinary pH trap it in the ionized form within the collecting duct lumen for excretion. This process is the major reason for the almost invariant occurrence of metabolic alkalosis in hypokalemia. However, if a primary decrease in **collecting duct proton secretion** occurs, ammonia trapping in the collecting duct decreases, potentially resulting in an increased fraction of ammonia returning to the system circulation.

A complete or incomplete defect in collecting duct proton excretion is known as distal renal tubular acidosis (RTA). Distal RTA has been recognized for many years as a frequent consequence of primary biliary cirrhosis as well as other liver diseases. Its presence in liver disease is often masked by an alkaline systemic pH, which is a consequence of the primary respiratory alkalosis usually associated with liver disease. Because the inability to secrete protons into the collecting duct obligates potassium secretion for sodium reabsorption, distal RTA still results in renal potassium wasting even if systemic acidemia is not seen.

A history of pruritus was elicited from the present patient. Her serum ammonia was markedly elevated at 87 mg/dl, and CT scanning revealed a finely nodular liver. Liver biopsy and serological findings confirmed the diagnosis of primary biliary cirrhosis. The striking feature of the illness, in retrospect, was the association of episodes of encephalopathy with hypokalemia; each time, the symptoms resolved with correction of the serum potassium. Earlier recognition of the role of hypokalemia in the patient's mental status changes might have resulted in earlier diagnosis.

At a follow-up visit several months later, the patient was taking potassium citrate, spironolactone, ursodeoxycholate, and levothyroxine. Her electrolytes were normal, and she was feeling entirely well.

Clinical Pearls

1. Hypokalemia does not characteristically produce mental status changes in the absence of liver disease. However, it is a frequent precipitating factor for hepatic encephalopathy.

2. Hypokalemia may worsen hepatic encephalopathy directly by increasing renal ammoniagenesis, or indirectly by favoring alkalemia and subsequent ammonia diffusion across the blood-brain barrier.

3. Distal renal tubular acidosis is not infrequently associated with liver disease, particularly primary biliary cirrhosis, but its presence in this setting is generally obscured by coexistent respiratory alkalosis.

REFERENCES

1. Stabenau J, Warren K, Rall D: The role of pH gradient in the distribution of ammonia between blood and cerebrospinal fluid, brain, and muscle. J Clin Invest 1959;38:373–383.
2. Baertl J, Sancetta S, Gabuzda G: Relation of acute potassium depletion to renal ammonium metabolism in patients with cirrhosis. J Clin Invest 1963;42:696–706.
3. Shear L, Bonkowsky H, Gabuzda G: Renal tubular acidosis in cirrhosis: A determinant of susceptibility to recurrent hepatic precoma. N Engl J Med 1969;280:1–7.
4. Pares A, Rimola A, Bruguera M, Mas E, Rodes J: Renal tubular acidosis in primary biliary cirrhosis. Gastroenterology 1981;80:681–686.

Richard G. Wunderink, MD

PATIENT 57

A 65-year-old woman with new pulmonary infiltrates during mechanical ventilation

A 65-year-old woman, with a history of type II diabetes mellitus and hypertriglyceridemia, is admitted to the intensive care unit for increasing respiratory distress and fever in association with severe pancreatitis. She requires intubation. Chest radiograph shows diffuse alveolar infiltrates consistent with the acute respiratory distress syndrome (ARDS). A bronchoscopy is negative for pneumonia, and she is started on levofloxacin and metronidazole for suspected intra-abdominal infection. Her original ARDS pattern clears substantially, and she is weaned to 40% oxygen. Active pancreatitis resolves, but she remains on total parenteral nutrition because of a persistent ileus. After 13 days of mechanical ventilation, she develops increased endotracheal secretions.

Physical Examination: Temperature 38.5; pulse 106; respirations 22 on mechanical ventilation with a total minute ventilation of 13 L; blood pressure 126/72. General: obese, no acute distress. HEENT: oral endotracheal tube and a nasogastric tube in her right naris, no nasal purulence. Cardiac: regular tachycardia without murmur. Chest: symmetrical movement without crackles or signs of consolidation. Abdomen: protuberant, mildly tender diffusely, no bowel sounds. Extremities: left femoral triple lumen catheter with no purulence or erythema, no rash, diffuse pitting edema of all four extremities.

Laboratory Findings: WBC 16,400/μl; 76% neutrophils, 12% bands. Chest radiograph: bilateral pleural effusions, new left lower lobe infiltrate, minimal residual infiltrates throughout the rest of the lungs (see figure). Gram stain of endotracheal aspirate: many WBCs, gram-positive cocci and gram-negative bacilli. Subsequent culture grew 4+ *Proteus mirabilus*, 1+ *Staphylococcus aureus*, and 1+ *Candida albicans*.

Questions: What is the probability that this patient has ventilator-associated pneumonia? Which antibiotic therapy would you initiate?

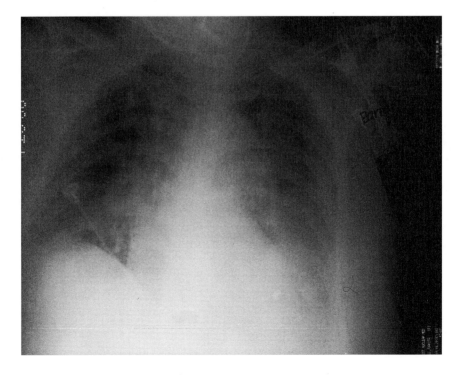

Diagnoses: Methicillin-resistant *S. aureus* pneumonia, left femoral deep venous thrombosis, and pansinusitis.

Discussion: The work-up of a febrile, ventilated patient is one of the most difficult diagnostic challenges in medicine. The number of possible causes for fever is extensive, and diagnostic testing is often compromised.

When a systematic approach to the evaluation of fever in critically ill patients is used, multiple potential causes of fever, both infectious and non-infectious, can infrequently be identified. Noninfectious etiologies can include pancreatitis, infarction of any organ, drug fever, venous thrombosis, and fibroproliferative ARDS. The range of infections is broad and varies with the underlying condition. While **ventilator-associated pneumonia** (VAP) is the greatest concern in mechanically ventilated patients, **intravascular catheter infections** and **sinusitis** are also common. Of significance, sinusitis can overlap with VAP in as many as 30% of cases. Many non-pneumonic infections in the critically ill are associated with medical devices and require some intervention, such as catheter removal or drainage procedures, in addition to antibiotics for optimal treatment.

The assumption that fever, leukocytosis, or purulent secretions and a new radiographic infiltrate represent pneumonia is frequently incorrect. An accurate clinical diagnosis of the presence or absence of VAP can be made only in about 70% of cases. However, only 33% of therapeutic plans would have represented appropriate and effective therapy.

The difficulty in accurately determining the presence or absence of VAP has led to substantial research in the use of **quantitative cultures of respiratory secretions**, usually obtained bronchoscopically, for diagnosis. Some investigators have found that approximately 50% of patients with clinical criteria for VAP do not meet a quantitative culture threshold. While the most accurate data appears to be from bronchoscopic specimens, quantitative cultures of other specimens, including non-bronchoscopic bronchoalveolar lavage, bronchial brushing, or even routine tracheal aspirates, significantly increase the accuracy of the diagnosis. The need and cost-effectiveness of routine use of quantitative cultures is still debatable, although recent studies have suggested a survival advantage to routine use of quantitative cultures. Fewer antibiotics and more narrow-spectrum antibiotic therapy with the use of quantitative cultures is a consistent pattern in comparative studies.

The choice of empiric antibiotic therapy is difficult. The probability of inappropriate therapy is greatest in those patients who have been mechanically ventilated longer than 7 days and who have received prior antibiotic therapy. One study suggests that only the combination of vancomycin, imipenem, and amikacin covers more than 80% of organisms. An empiric treatment protocol utilizing these drugs would not only still result in inappropriate therapy for a significant number of patients, but also be extremely expensive. A more practical empiric strategy is to use both patient-specific factors, such as prior antibiotic history, and local epidemiology, including common etiologies of VAP and drug sensitivity patterns, to design an appropriate empiric antibiotic strategy. The ability to stop antibiotics and narrow coverage is dependent on the accuracy of the cultures obtained.

In the present patient, an extensive diagnostic work-up was initiated. Bronchoscopy was performed of the left lower lobe. The lavage showed 95% neutrophils on the differential and gram-positive cocci in clusters on the Gram stain. Subsequent culture grew > 10^5 cfu/ml of *S. aureus*. Pleural fluid obtained by a thoracentesis showed an increased amylase level and a protein level of 3.0 mg/dl, but was sterile. A sinus CT scan showed pansinusitis, with total opacification of the right maxillary sinus and air fluid level on the left. The nasogastric tube was replaced with an oral tube, and saline nasal lavage and topical decongestants were started. An abdominal CT scan showed resolution of peripancreatic fluid and no abscess formation. Doppler ultrasound of her lower extremities showed an extensive deep venous thrombosis (DVT) of her left lower extremity. The central venous catheter was removed and replaced at an alternative site. Culture of the catheter was sterile. The patient was started on vancomycin and heparin, and other antibiotics were discontinued. The patient's fever, leukocytosis, and high-minute ventilation resolved over the next 3 days. She was extubated 6 days after the diagnosis of pneumonia and DVT and discharged home after 2 weeks.

Clinical Pearls

1. The accuracy of the clinical diagnosis of pneumonia in ventilated patients is as low as 50% and should always be taken as a tentative diagnosis.

2. A systematic search for both alternative and concomitant causes of fever in patients suspected of ventilator-associated pneumonia is required for optimal treatment.

3. Quantitative cultures, especially of bronchoscopy specimens, consistently lead to fewer antibiotic prescriptions and may be associated with lower mortality.

4. Sinusitis is common in mechanically ventilated patients and often occurs concomitantly with ventilator-associated pneumonia.

REFERENCES

1. Fagon JY, Chastre J, Hance AJ, et al: Evaluation of clinical judgement in the identification and treatment of nosocomial pneumonia in ventilated patients. Chest 1993;103:547–553.
2. Meduri GU, Mauldin GL, Wunderink RG, et al: Causes of fever and pulmonary densities in patients with clinical manifestations of ventilator-associated pneumonia. Chest 1994;106:221–235.
3. Trouillet JL, Chastre J, Vuagnat A, et al: Ventilator-associated pneumonia caused by potentially drug-resistant bacteria. Am J Respir Crit Care Med 1998;157:531–539.
4. Fagon JY, Chastre J, Wolff M, et al: Invasive and noninvasive strategies for management of suspected ventilator-associated pneumonia. A randomized trial. Ann Intern Med 2000;132:621–630.

Richard B. Berry, MD

PATIENT 58

A 55-year-old man with loud snoring

A 55-year-old man is seen for evaluation of loud snoring of many years duration. He originally contacted an ENT surgeon for surgical treatment of his snoring. The patient's wife has refused to sleep in the same bedroom for over a year. Previously, she noticed that there were pauses in his breathing followed by a loud snort and resumption of snoring. The patient gained about 50 pounds over the last 2 years. He denies being sleepy during the day, but does admit to drinking many cups of coffee to maintain alertness. At supper he typically drinks several glasses of wine.

Physical Examination: Weight 210 pounds, height 5'10", blood pressure 165/95, pulse 60. HEENT: crowded oropharynx with long uvula and dependent palate. Neck: 18-inch circumference, no thyromegaly. Chest: normal. Cardiac: normal. Extremities: no edema. Neurological: nonfocal.

Laboratory Findings: Frequent events such as the one below were noted during the first 2 hours of sleep monitoring.

Question: What treatment would you recommend?

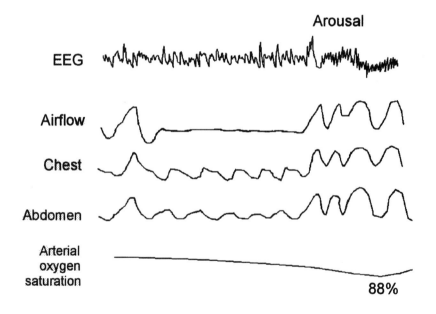

Diagnosis: Severe obstructive sleep apnea. Treatment with nasal continuous positive airway pressure is recommended.

Discussion: Obstructive sleep apnea (OSA) is a common disorder affecting about 2% of all women and 4% of all men. During sleep, the decrease in upper airway muscle activity results in either a severe narrowing or complete closure of the upper airway in susceptible individuals. Despite continued inspiratory efforts, airflow is either absent (obstructive apnea) secondary to airway closure (see figure), or reduced as a result of airway narrowing (obstructive hypopnea).

Apnea and hypopnea are associated with falls in the arterial oxygen saturation to a varying degree. Event termination is usually associated with evidence of cortical arousal (brief awakening) on electroencephalographic (EEG) monitoring and a large increase in upper airway muscle activity, restoring upper airway patency. Typically, patients with OSA fall back to sleep quickly, and apnea or hypopnea occurs again. This results in repetitive cycles of apnea/hypopnea separated by periods of ventilation.

In milder cases, apnea is present only in the supine position (positional apnea) or during REM sleep. In most patients, the longest apneas and most severe arterial oxygen desaturations occur in rapid eye movement (REM) sleep. A common practice is to compute the **apnea + hypopnea index** (AHI) by dividing the total number of apneas and hypopneas by the total sleep time in hours. Various schemes for classifying the severity of OSA exist. A simple one is AHI ≤ 5 /hr normal, < 20/hr mild, AHI 20–40/hr moderate, AHI > 40/hr severe. In assessing severity, also consider the severity of falls in the arterial oxygen saturation and the presence of apnea-associated arrhythmias.

The repetitive arousals in OSA prevent sleep from being restorative, and patients usually report varying degrees of excessive daytime sleepiness. However, the severity of sleepiness correlates poorly with the frequency of apnea. Therefore, patients with significant disease may not complain of severe daytime sleepiness. Many patients also underestimate the degree of their impairment. In one study, the best **clinical predictors** of OSA were **(1)** heavy snoring, **(2)** bedmate observed apnea/gasping, **(3)** a large neck circumference, and **(4)** hypertension. While obesity is a definite risk factor, the AHI correlates better with neck circumference. Many patients also have nasal congestion, retrognathia (overjet), and large tongues. The regular use

of ethanol also can play a contributing role, as this substance preferentially reduces upper airway muscle activity. Endocrine factors may influence the predilection for apnea. The male gender, hypothyroidism, and acromegaly all appear to predispose to apnea.

Surgical treatments of OSA include tracheostomy (bypassing the area of obstruction); uvulopalatopharyngoplasty (UPPP) which involves removal of the uvula, part of the soft palate, and redundant pharyngeal tissue; and complex maxillofacial surgery. **Medical treatments** include weight loss, the side sleep position (positional apnea), nasal continuous positive airway pressure (CPAP), and oral appliances. Nasal CPAP is the most reliably effective treatment for moderate to severe OSA and has virtually replaced tracheostomy. Nasal CPAP works by keeping the airway open with a "pneumatic splint." A pressure titration is usually required to determine a pressure effective in preventing apnea/hypopnea/snoring in all body positions and stages of sleep (higher pressures are required supine and in REM sleep). Unfortunately, an appreciable number of patients will not accept or comply with CPAP treatment. UPPP overall effectively drops the AHI by 50% or more to less than 20/hr in only about 40% of patients. Hence, it is not a reliable treatment for more severe cases. Oral appliances are effective in many cases of mild to moderate severity and in a few severe cases. Mandibular advancing devices, the most commonly used oral appliances, are believed to work by moving the tongue forward, away from the back of the throat. They may also tense the palate.

In the present patient, the AHI was 60 events/hour during the first 2 hours of the sleep study, associated with desaturations down to 80%. A typical obstructive apnea was evident (see figure), with absent airflow despite persistent inspiratory effort (chest and abdominal movement). During the second part of the study, the patient underwent a nasal CPAP titration. On 10 cm H_2O the AHI was reduced to 5 /hr. Because of the severity of the apnea, treatment with nasal CPAP (10 cm H_2O) rather than UPPP was recommended. The patient was also encouraged to lose weight and reduce his alcohol intake. On this treatment, the patient reported more energy, and his wife returned to the bedroom.

Clinical Pearls

1. Suspect obstructive sleep apnea in any patient reporting heavy snoring.
2. Not all patients with significant sleep apnea report excessive daytime sleepiness.
3. The snorer's bedmate can provide important clinical clues that OSA is present.
4. Nasal continuous positive airway pressure is considered the treatment of choice for most patients with moderate to severe obstructive sleep apnea.

REFERENCES

1. Flemons WW, Whitelaw WA, Brant R, et al: Likelihood ratios for a sleep apnea clinical prediction rule. Am J Respir Crit Care Med 1994;150:1279–1285.
2. Schmidt-Nowara W, Lowe A, Wiegand L, et al: Oral appliances for the treatment of snoring and obstructive sleep apnea. A review. Sleep 1995;18:501–510.
3. Sher AE, Schechtman KB, Piccirillo JF: The efficacy of surgical modification of the upper airway in adults with obstructive sleep apnea syndrome. Sleep 1996;19:156–177.
4. Strollo PJ, Rogers RM: Obstructive sleep apnea. N Engl J Med 1996:334:99–104.
5. Strollo PJ Jr, Sanders MH, Atwood CW: Positive Pressure therapy. Clin Chest Med 1998;19:55–68.

Timothy M. Lenardo, MD
Gary S. Hoffman, MD

PATIENT 59

A 29-year-old woman with flank pain, hypertension, and gross hematuria

A 29-year-old woman has a 4-week history of bilateral flank pain, nausea, vomiting, and intermittent hematuria. She has a prior history of "vein stripping," vaginal hysterectomy for uterine prolapse, easy bruising, and "abnormal scars." She is gravida 5 para 3, with three uncomplicated, term, vaginal deliveries. A maternal grandfather and a brother both died in their 50s with ruptured aneurysms. The patient has a 20-pack-year smoking habit, and there was a short period of marijuana and powder cocaine use 3 years ago.

Physical Examination: Temperature 37°; pulse 100; respirations 23; blood pressure 149/104. Skin: bruises, normal turgor and mobility; two hypertrophic yellow-brown scars on left shoulder. HEENT: facial narrowing with prominent eyes; oropharynx, lymph node, and carotid auscultation normal. Chest: clear. Cardiac: grade 2/6 systolic and diastolic murmurs, peripheral pulses without bruits. Abdomen: mild left flank tenderness. Extremities: "aged" appearance of hands; joint mobility normal.

Laboratory Findings: WBC 10,410/µl, creatinine 0.7 mg/dl, albumin 4.0 g/dl, AST 25 IU/L, alkaline phosphatase 37 IU/L. PT, PTT, anticardiolipin antibodies, antiglomerular basement membrane antibody, anti-neutrophil-cytoplasmic antibodies: normal or negative. ESR 31 mm/hr (normal 0–20), C-reactive protein 0.9 mg/dl (0–2.0 mg/dl). Punch biopsy of left shoulder skin lesion (light microscopy): consistent with fibromatosis. Cardiac echo: moderate aortic and tricuspid valve regurgitation. CT of the chest and abdomen (contrast): see below, *left*. Renal angiography: see below, *right*. Cardiovascular MRI with edema weighting technique: distal pulmonary artery irregularities at the right lung base and truncus anterior.

Question: What disorder best accounts for this patient's clinical presentation?

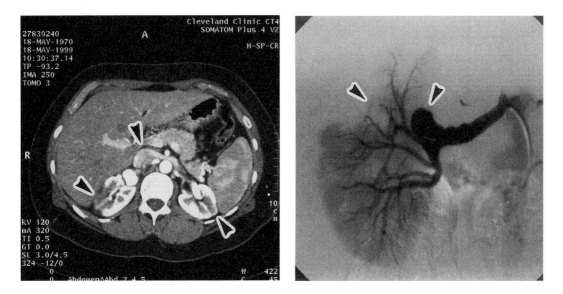

Diagnosis: An inherited abnormality of collagen synthesis.

Discussion: The most common cause of large vessel disease is atherosclerosis, which typically occurs in the elderly. When large vessel disease occurs in children or young adults, several other inherited and acquired diagnostic possibilities should be considered (see table). Often, a careful review of the patient's clinical presentation can assist the differential diagnosis of large vessel aneurysms, as occurred in the present patient.

Etiologic Classification of Arterial Aneurysms

Congenital (collagen vascular disease)
Ehlers-Danlos syndrome
Marfan syndrome

Mechanical (hemodynamic)
Post-stenotic, arteriovenous fistula-associated
Traumatic (penetrating or blunt)

Inflammatory (noninfectious)

Takayasu disease	GCA (17% elderly cases)
Behçet disease	Cogan's disease
Kawasaki disease	Sarcoidosis
Polyarteritis nodosa	Spondyloarthropathies
Periarterial inflammatory disease (e.g., pancreatitis)	Systemic lupus erythematosus (very rare)

Infectious
Bacterial, fungal, spirochetal, viral (e.g., EBV)

Degenerative
Atherosclerotic
Fibromuscular dysplasia

Surgical (anastomotic)
Postarteriotomy (post-surgical anastomotic aneurysms secondary to infections, arterial wall failure, suture failures, graft failures or unknown causes)

Adapted from Santos-Ocampo AS, Hoffman GS: Aneurysms and hypermobility in a 45-year-old woman. Cleve Clin J Med 1999;66(7):426–433.

Mechanical causes of renal and pulmonary artery aneurysms are unlikely in the absence of a history of vascular surgery or blunt trauma. A history of smoking and ingestion of a Western diet, which is cholesterol-rich, might promote premature vascular damage in a young patient. The resulting aneurysms, however, would not be expected to involve multiple vascular beds not typically involved with atherosclerosis (i.e., pulmonary) and would not explain the facial, ocular, and cutaneous findings noted in the present patient.

Infectious causes of arterial aneurysms are usually associated with fever, chills, peripheral blood leukocytosis, and elevated acute phase reactants (e.g., C-reactive protein). Inherited conditions causing large vessel disease in young patients are suggested by a family history of aneurysm. These conditions include congenital defects in connective tissue composition. A vasculitis generally is considered unlikely in the absence of constitutional symptoms and the other clinical features that define these syndromes. Note, however, that a recent clinical and histopathologic study of over 1200 patients with various causes of aortitis demonstrated that only 1 of the 52 patients with idiopathic inflammatory aortitis had systemic symptoms. MRI with "edema-weighted" images can assist the diagnosis of these patients with asymptomatic aortitis because MRI is a sensitive tool for detecting vessel wall inflammation. Inflamed vessels have increased wall thickness and enhancement with T2-weighted or STIR imaging techniques.

Ehlers-Danlos syndrome (EDS) is the most common of the inherited connective tissue disorders. It is a remarkably heterogeneous group of disorders that is comprised of at least 11 major clinical variants or types (see table next page). Classic features include: skin fragility, skin hyperextensibility, and joint hypermobility. The estimated prevalence of all types of EDS is 1:500,000 population. Types I (gravis—moderate to severe skin and joint involvement) and II (mitis—similar to Type I, but milder) account for 40% of all cases of EDS. The mode of inheritance is most commonly autosomal dominant.

EDS Type IV, also known as "vascular-type" EDS, accounts for 3–5% of all EDS cases. Men and women are equally represented among patients with this severe form of EDS. Common clinical features include joint hypermobility (usually confined to digits), minimal or no skin hyperextensibility, pale/translucent skin, easy bruising, varicosities, deeply pigmented and hypertrophic scars, and short stature. Its most severe form, the **acrogeric variant** (prematurely aged hands, prominent eyes, narrow face with beaked nose, arched palate, and lobeless ears), is associated with catastrophic vascular events (aneurysm rupture) involving one or multiple visceral beds, intestinal rupture (sigmoid), and uterine rupture or prolapse.

EDS Type IV is one among only five (I, II, IV, VI, VII) types for which a specific collagen defect has been identified. The clinical features result from an inherited disorder of Type III collagen. Type III collagen in its mature form is an integral part of elastic arteries and tissues throughout the body. A recent study of Type IV EDS patients with documented impairment of fibroblast Type III collagen synthesis identified over 87 different mutations in the COL3A1 gene coding for the alpha chains of

Clinical, Diagnostic, and Genetic Features of Ehlers-Danlos Syndrome

Type	Clinical Features	Inheritance	Molecular Defect
I: Gravis	Soft, velvety skin, cigarette paper hyperextensible skin, easy bruising, hypermobile joints, varicose veins, prematurity	AD	Unknown
II: Mitis	Similar to EDS Type I but less severe	AD	Unknown ? COL1A2 (Ar cases)
III: Familial Hypermobility	Soft skin, no scarring, marked small and large joint hypermobility	AD	Unknown
IV: Arterial	Thin, translucent skin, visible veins	AD	COL3A1 mutations with altered Type III collagen synthesis, secretion and structure
V: X-linked	Similar to EDS Type II	XLR	Unknown
VI: Ocular	Velvety, hyperextensible skin; hypermobile joints; scoliosis; ocular fragility; keratoconus	AR	Lysyl hydroxylase deficiency due to mutations in LOH gene
VII: Arthrochalasis multiplex congenita (A and B)	Congenital hip dislocation; joint hypermobility; soft skin	AD	A and B: COL1A1 exon 6 skipping mutation deleting N-proteinase cleavage site
C: Dermatospraxis	Soft, fragile, bruisable skin, hypermobile		C: Procollagen N-proteinase deficiency
VIII: Periodontal	Generalized periodontitis; skin findings as in EDS Type II	AD	Unknown
IX: X-linked Cutis laxa; Occipital	Soft, extensible, lax skin; bladder diverticuli; bladder rupture; short arms; limited pronation and supination; broad clavicles; occipital horns	XLR	Abnormal cellular copper handling with defect in lysyl oxidase (Menkes syndrome)
X: Fibronectin Defect	Similar to EDS Type II	AR	Defect in fibronectin

AD = autosomal dominant, AR = autosomal recessive, XLR = x-linked recessive
Adapted from Byers PH: Ehlers-Danlos syndrome: Recent advances and current understanding of the clinical and genetic heterogeneity. J Invest Dermatol 1994;103:47S0–52S.

Type III procollagen. These genetic alterations resulted in amino acid substitutions, deletions, and post-transcriptional splicing errors. In parallel with this vast number of genetic polymorphisms, the study population exhibited an impressive degree of phenotypic variability in disease expression. However, the investigators did not find a significant correlation between specific genotypes and phenotypes. The heterozygosity of these mutations parallels the autosomal dominant pattern of inheritance for EDS Type IV; however, parental gonadal mosaicism (individual parent's germline comprised of a mixed population of normal and mutation bearing cells) may account for interspersed disease-free generations within a family of affected individuals.

The clinical features and presentation provide important clues to the possibility of EDS Type IV.

Radiographic procedures (preferably noninvasive) serve as adjuncts in the confirmation of vascular involvement. Radiographic imaging demonstrates lesions involving medium- to large-sized arteries. They may also demonstrate distal vessel "pruning" and segmental renal artery occlusions. The etiology of these findings remains unknown, but may result from microemboli showers from the main renal artery aneurysm.

Skin biopsy demonstrates dermal thinning. Immunofluorescence staining with anti-human Type III collagen antibodies demonstrates absence or reduction in Type III collagen fibril content. Electron microscopy confirms the existence of irregular collagen fibrils and may also show distention of the rough endoplasmic reticulum with abnormal, unsecreted procollagen. Fibroblast cultures allow measurement of the quality and quantity of Type III collagen production using gel electrophoretic techniques. Messenger ribonucleic acid isolated from culture cells may be probed for specific mutations in the COL3A1 gene. This information can be used for family screening and genetic counseling.

The genetic heterogeneity of EDS Type IV precludes the development of a novel single gene therapy for the disorder. Current guidelines for management of these patients center upon the avoidance or, if necessary, judicious use of invasive procedures. Embolization and ligation techniques for surgical management are favored as substitutes for grafting or stenting of vessels. Total colectomy is recommended in cases of colonic rupture. Conservative measures include avoidance of contact sports, bracing of hypermobile joints, stool softeners (reduce the risk of colonic rupture), pregnancy counseling (25% associated risk of sudden death from uterine rupture), frequent medical surveillance by individuals who are aware of the diagnosis of EDS Type IV, genetic counseling (offspring at 50% risk of having EDS), and referral to an EDS support group. Prognosis for most forms of EDS (90% cases) is good. However, EDS Type IV, with its potential complications, is associated with a poorer prognosis: almost 50% of affected individuals die by 40 years of age.

The present patient's CT scan of the abdomen (left figure, previous page) demonstrated multiple areas of acute hypoperfusion of the renal cortices bilaterally (*arrows*). A beaded appearance of both renal arteries and a 2-cm aneurysm with associated thrombus at the right renal hilum were also noted. Her abdominal and renal angiogram (right figure, previous page) demonstrated normal-appearing mesenteric vessels and aorta. A 2-cm distal right renal aneurysm was present, with occlusion of the upper pole branch vessel and associated perfusion defects (*arrows*). Left renal images revealed perfusion defects in the mid and upper poles of the left kidney. Fibroblasts isolated from her skin biopsy grown in culture synthesized 10% of the normal amount of Type III collagen and normal amounts of Type I (skin predominant) collagen. Electrophoretic studies confirmed the retention of abnormal procollagen forms within the cells as well. These findings confirmed the diagnosis of EDS type IV.

Clinical Pearls

1. The development of acute arterial aneurysms in a previously healthy, young patient should arouse suspicion of an underlying collagen synthesis disorder.

2. Ehlers-Danlos syndrome is a genetically and phenotypically heterogeneous disorder.

3. EDS Type IV, while rare (only 3–5% of cases of EDS), poses a significant risk of catastrophic vascular events and is associated with a 50% mortality by 40 years of age.

4. Fibroblast culture demonstrating reduced quantity and quality of Type III collagen helps confirm the diagnosis of EDS Type IV.

5. Management of patients with EDS Type IV centers on avoidance of invasive techniques or surgery, unless warranted by life-threatening illness.

REFERENCES

1. Ainsworth SR, Anlicino PL: A survey of patients with Ehlers-Danlos syndrome. Clin Ortho Rel Res 1993;296:250–256.
2. Byers PH: Ehlers-Danlos syndrome: Recent advances and current understanding of the clinical and genetic heterogeneity. J Invest Dermatol 1994;103:47S–52S.
3. De Paepe A: Ehlers-Danlos syndrome type IV: Clinical and molecular aspects and guidelines for diagnosis and management. Dermatology 1994;189(suppl 12):21–25.
4. Jeannette JC, Falk RJ, Andrassy K, et al: Nomenclature of systemic vasculitides: Proposal of an international consensus conference (review). Arthr Rheum 1994;37:187–192.
5. Bergquist D: Ehlers-Danlos type IV syndrome: A review from a vascular surgical point of view. Eur J Surg 1996;162:163–170.
6. Oyen O, Clausen OP, Brekke IB, et al: Spontaneous rupture of the renal artery in a patient with Ehlers-Danlos type IV. Eur J Vasc Endovasc Surg 1997;13:509–512.
7. Witz M, Lehmann JM: Aneurysmal arterial disease in a patient with Ehlers-Danlos syndrome: Case report and literature review. J Cardiovasc Surg 1997;38:161–163.
8. Flamm SD, White RD, Hoffman GS: The clinical application of "edema-weighted" magnetic resonance imaging in the assessment of Takayasu's arteritis. Intern J Cardiol 1998;66(suppl 1):S151–S159.
9. Santos-Ocampo AS, Hoffman GS: Aneurysms and hypermobility in a 45-year-old woman. Clev Clin J Med 1999;66(7): 426–433.
10. Pepin M, Schwarze U, Superti-Furga A, Byers PH: Clinical and genetic features of Ehlers-Danlos syndrome type IV, the vascular type. New Engl J Med 2000;342(10):673–680.
11. Rojo-Leyva F, Ratliff NB, Cosgrove DM, Hoffman GS: Study of 52 patients with idiopathic aortitis from a cohort of 1204 surgical cases. Arthr Rheum 2000;43(4):901–907.

Omar A. Minai, MD
Alejandro C. Arroliga, MD

PATIENT 60

A 72-year-old man with severe COPD and progressive dyspnea

A 72-year-old man with a long smoking history presents with increasing dyspnea and a history of two hospital admissions over the previous year for "emphysema." He has never had a pneumothorax and has never been intubated. He has minimal cough with mainly clear phlegm and no history of hemoptysis. His medications include prednisone 15 mg/day, theophylline, fluticasone inhaler, nebulizers with albuterol and ipratropium bromide every 6 hours and as needed, supplemental oxygen for the last 2 years, and furosemide. The patient quit smoking 2 years ago. He enrolled in a pulmonary rehabilitation program last month, and his exercise capacity has improved.

Physical Examination: Pulse 85; respirations 20; blood pressure 138/70; afebrile. General: thinly built; in mild respiratory distress; wearing an oxygen cannula. Chest: increased anteroposterior diameter, minimal chest excursion with respiration, very poor air entry bilaterally with occasional faint wheezing and no crackles. Cardiac: distant heart sounds heard best in the epigastric area; normal S_1 and S_2; no murmurs or rubs. Abdomen: nontender without organomegaly. Extremities: no edema.

Laboratory Findings: CBC: normal. Chest radiograph: see below. ABG: pH 7.43, PCO_2 43 mmHg, PO_2 73 mmHg, HCO_3 29 mEq/L, HbO_2 93.7%, COHb 2.1%. Pulmonary function: FVC 2.07 L (74%); FEV_1 0.62 (29%); FEV_1/FVC 30%; total lung capacity (TLC; by helium) 6.17 L (128%); residual volume (RV) 3.94 L (194%); TLC (by plethysmography) 4.41 (161%); DLCO 8.5 (43%); "coving" of the flow volume loop (see graph). Echo: LVEF 55%; normal RV size and function; no pulmonary hypertension.

Question: Would this patient be a candidate for any surgical procedures to improve his dyspnea?

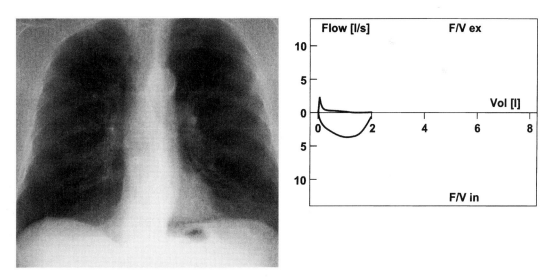

Answer: This patient is an appropriate candidate for lung volume reduction surgery (LVRS).

Discussion: Protease-induced damage to walls of air sacs causes enlargement of distal air spaces and is the major pathophysiologic mechanism in emphysema. Cigarette smoking increases the inflammatory process, tilting the protease-antiprotease balance in favor of lung damage. The main physiologic consequence is loss of lung elastic recoil, resulting in expiratory airflow limitation. The flow limitation causes a decrease in FEV_1 and in FEV_1/FVC ratio, and reduces the driving pressure for expiratory flow as well as the transmural pressure distending the airway. The dynamic compliance of the lungs is decreased, and the respiratory rate and work of breathing are increased in patients with emphysema.

Hyperinflation, characterized by an increased TLC, RV, and functional residual capacity, also occurs. It initially increases lung elastic recoil and decreases airway resistance, allowing improved expiratory airflow. Eventually these changes place the lungs at a "mechanical disadvantage" by flattening the diaphragms and decreasing the radial traction on the airways in the remaining lung producing airflow limitation.

The **rationale for LVRS** is to resect approximately 20–30% of the most diseased-appearing lung tissue from both lung apices. This decreases hyperinflation, allows better diaphragmatic excursion, and increases radial traction on the airways. Thus, expiratory resistance to airflow and residual volume are decreased. LVRS may also allow relatively less-damaged lung tissue, which was compressed by the hyperinflated and severely damaged lung tissue, to expand and take part in gas exchange.

Patients considered **candidates for LVRS** should have moderate to severe emphysema causing significant restriction of daily activities despite maximal medical therapy. Typically, patients with marked hyperinflation and heterogeneous disease have better results with LVRS. All patients should undergo a thorough history and physical examination, along with a full pulmonary function survey including spirometry, lung volumes by body plethysmography, diffusion capacity for CO, arterial blood gases, and a 6-minute walk test for assessment of exercise capacity and oxygen requirements. A chest x-ray, CT scan of the chest, and echocardiography of the heart to assess left ventricular function and rule out significant pulmonary hypertension should also be performed. Further work-up is done as needed, based on the results of these preliminary tests.

Pulmonary function tests typically show moderate to severe airflow limitation characterized by $FEV_1 \leq 40\%$, total lung capacity $\geq 100\%$ predicted, and residual volume $\geq 150\%$ predicted. Arterial blood gases typically show variable degrees of hypoxemia depending upon the extent of regional ventilation/perfusion mismatch. Hypercapnia may or may not be present and is not a contraindication to LVRS unless severe (≥ 60 mmHg).

Chest x-ray and CT scans should show heterogeneous, predominantly apical lung involvement with emphysema ("target areas") for patients to be considered good candidates for LVRS. Patients should have an acceptable nutritional status and be 70–130% of their ideal body weight. Baseline functional status is a very important consideration, and potential candidates should have the ability to participate actively in a pulmonary rehabilitation program. Patients who are current smokers or have smoked in the last 4 to 6 months prior to evaluation are not considered suitable candidates for LVRS. Other **exclusionary criteria** include active systemic disease that may cause debility or pulmonary disease, pulmonary hypertension, pleural or interstitial lung disease, untreated significant coronary artery disease, uncontrolled arrythmias, and LVEF $\leq 45\%$.

Patients should continue medical therapy for their lung disease. Systemic corticosteroids are not considered an absolute contraindication to LVRS, but they should be used in the lowest dose necessary to obtain the desired benefit. Surgery may be performed either via video-assisted thoracoscopy or median sternotomy, depending upon the expertise of the surgeon, with comparable results. Small prospective studies have shown a significant improvement in pulmonary function, PO_2, PCO_2, functional capacity, and subjective quality of life measures (e.g., Borg dyspnea index), 1, 2, and 3 years post LVRS compared with patients on medical therapy alone. The initial improvement declines with time; the need for oxygen supplementation during exercise occurs first. The reduction in RV and dyspnea is the most persistent benefit. Although positive results have been obtained, these studies suffer from a variety of limitations such as improper controls and lack of randomization. A nationwide NIH-sponsored trial—the National Emphysema Treatment Trial (NETT)—is currently underway in an effort to better define the role of LVRS in patients with emphysema.

The present patient underwent successful LVRS with improvement in quality of life indices, improvement in functional status, and decrease in hypercapnia.

Clinical Pearls

1. Resection of 20–30% of the most diseased-appearing lung tissue from both lung apices decreases hyperinflation, allows better diaphragmatic excursion, and increases radial traction on the airways. Thus, expiratory resistance to airflow decreases.

2. Patients with moderate to severe emphysema causing severe restriction of daily activities despite maximal medical therapy; marked hyperinflation; and heterogeneous disease are considered good candidates for LVRS.

3. Exclusionary criteria include recent history of smoking, active systemic disease that may cause debility or pulmonary disease, pulmonary hypertension, pleural or interstitial lung disease, untreated significant coronary artery disease, uncontrolled arrythmias, and LVEF $\leq 45\%$.

REFERENCES:

1. Rogers RM, Sciurba FC, Keenan RJ: Lung reduction surgery in chronic obstructive lung disease. Med Clinics North Am 1996;80(3):623–644.
2. Sciurba FC, Rogers RM, Keenan RJ, et al: Improvement in pulmonary function and elastic recoil after lung reduction surgery for diffuse emphysema. New Engl J Med 1996;334:1095–1099.
3. Yusen RD, Lefrak SS, and the Washington University Emphysema Surgery Group: Evaluation of patients with emphysema for lung volume reduction surgery. Sem Thoracic Cardiovasc Surg 1996;8:83–93.
4. Cooper JD, Lefrak SS. Lung reduction surgery: 5 years on. Lancet 1999;353 Suppl 1:SI26–27.

Leonard Sigal, MD

PATIENT 61

A 36-year-old woman with fatigue, impaired memory, and "total body pain"

A 36-year-old woman requests a second opinion for the management of her profound fatigue, "total body pain," and impaired concentration and memory. She was diagnosed with Lyme disease 5 years ago while living in New York City. The initial illness included fever, headache, myalgia, and fatigue. She did not experience a rash, seventh nerve palsy, brady-arrhythmias, or focal neurologic abnormalities. After 8 weeks of her illness, she went to a physician who stated he confirmed the diagnosis with serologies and gave her 6 weeks of oral antibiotics. Her symptoms, however, did not abate. She has been on a series of 6- to 12-week courses of oral antibiotics, often in combination, for the last 4.5 years. Occasionally her symptoms diminish, but she experiences remarkable worsening of her symptoms every 4 weeks. She has been told by her physician that the worsening represents "Herxheimer reactions." Her physician has not noted any abnormal physical findings during the 5 years of her disease.

Physical Examination: Vital signs: normal. General: chronically fatigued-appearing, but no acute distress. Skin: normal. Chest: clear. Cardiac: no murmurs. Extremities: joints normal. Neurologic: no abnormalities.

Laboratory Findings (from patient's previous medical records):   CBC and blood chemistries done every 4 to 6 weeks for 5 years: normal. Initial "Lyme disease serologies": IgG ELISA 1.05; ELISA IgM ELISA < 0.8 (normal < 1.00); IgG immunoblot reactive with the 41 and 66 kDa bands; IgM reactive with the 41 kDa band. Serial, monthly serologies for 5 years: same pattern. "Lyme urinary antigen test": 65 (normal < 25). Polymerase chain reaction (PCR) for the ospA gene: negative on five occasions over the last 2.5 years.

Question: What is the probable etiology of the patient's long-term complaints?

Diagnosis: Fibromyalgia.

Discussion: Lyme disease (LD) is an infection with *Borrelia burgdorferi*, spread by the tick *Ixodes scapularis* in the Northeast, Southeast, and Midwest and by *Ixodes pacificus* on the Pacific coast. In Europe and Asia, other organisms and ticks are involved. The hallmark of LD is the rash erythema migrans, which occurs 1 to 30 days (mean 7 days) after the tick bite; 90% or more of all patients with LD experience this rash.

Early localized LD includes erythema migrans and associated symptoms, usually fever, headache, myalgia, and arthralgia. **Early disseminated LD** typically occurs weeks to 6 months following the tick bite and includes cardiac and neurologic disease. Cardiac features of LD include heart block and rare examples of mild congestive cardiomyopathy; both typically begin to resolve *even before institution of antibiotic therapy*. Neurologic features can include cranial neuropathy (most commonly the facial nerve), radiculoneuritis, and lymphocytic meningitis. **Late LD** includes arthritis (migratory polyarthritis or less commonly chronic, usually monoarticular, arthritis, most often affecting the knee) and neurologic disease (mild peripheral neuropathy, mild to progressive/severe encephalopathy).

There is no defined "chronic Lyme disease" syndrome. Most patients who have long-term subjective complaints have a normal physical examination and prove to have alternative diagnoses.

The treatment of LD is antibiotic therapy. Patients with early LD can be treated with 3 to 4 weeks of oral antibiotic therapy. (Note that there is no proof that 3 to 4 weeks is superior to 2 weeks.) Doxycycline, tetracycline, or amoxicillin are primary therapy for adults with early disease. Intravenous antibiotics are reserved for patients with central nervous system infection, arthritis refractory to oral therapy, and severe instances of heart disease. There is no role for long-term oral antibiotics after the initial 3- to 4-week course of therapy. Approximately 10% of patients with LD experience a Jarisch-Herxheimer reaction following their initial antibiotic treatment. This is a short-term immunologic reaction manifested by fever, chills, headache, myalgias, and exacerbation of cutaneous lesions. No evidence exists that Herxheimer reactions re-occur after an initial course of treatment.

Confusion exists among clinicians about the appropriate diagnostic evaluation of patients with suspected Lyme disease. On the basis of explicit historical evidence and objective findings on examination that suggest LD, a physician can make a clinical diagnosis of LD. Nonspecific symptoms without evidence explicitly suggesting the diagnosis remain nonspecific. *A clinical diagnosis of LD cannot rest on nonspecific symptoms alone.*

Use serologic testing only to confirm the diagnosis of LD for patients with clinical signs of the disease. Screening patients with these tests yields a very high proportion of false-positive results. The available serologic tests only detect anti-*B. burgdorferi* antibodies, and cannot in themselves diagnose LD. IgM serologic tests should be positive within 6 weeks of the tick bite. The onset of signs of clinical infection follow shortly thereafter, along with IgG seroconversion. Any positive or equivocal ELISA result should be corroborated by immunoblot. In the instance of the present patient, the initial weakly positive IgG ELISA should have been confirmed by an immunoblot. In the setting of nonspecific clinical findings, a weakly positive IgG ELISA is most likely a false-positive result. The "Lyme urinary antigen test" is of no proven value in the diagnosis or management of LD and should not be used. Likewise, PCR and culture techniques should not be routinely used in the evaluation of possible LD.

The present patient demonstrated no historical findings that explicitly suggested the diagnosis of LD. Her absence of abnormalities on the physical examination was not compatible with a diagnosis of active *B. burgdorferi* infection, which is *always* accompanied by abnormal findings. The initial laboratory tests were done at a time after onset of her symptoms when they would have been positive had she had LD. Also, the lack of response to what amounted to 60 or 80 times the necessary antibiotics for true LD excluded LD as the cause of her symptoms. Upon further evaluation, it became clear that the patient had fibromyalgia, which is a common misdiagnosis in patients who are referred for evaluation at LD centers.

Clinical Pearls

1. Carefully review the medical records of patients referred for evaluation of "chronic Lyme disease." The most common cause of a lack of response to antibiotic therapy is an initial misdiagnosis.

2. A clinical diagnosis of Lyme disease can be made in a patient with history and physical findings that explicitly suggest the disease. Nonspecific and vague complaints are never sufficient to make a diagnosis of Lyme disease.

3. Active Lyme disease is accompanied by objective physical findings; the absence of these findings strongly decreases the likelihood of active disease.

4. Use serologic tests to confirm a clinical diagnosis of Lyme disease, but *never* use these tests as screening tools for patients with nonspecific complaints.

5. Specific serologic tests used in patients with possible Lyme disease are *not* "Lyme disease tests"; they are merely anti-*Borrelia burgdorferi* antibody assays.

REFERENCES

1. Hsu V, Patella S, Sigal L: "Chronic Lyme disease" as the incorrect diagnosis in patients with fibromyalgia. Arthritis Rheum 1993;36:1493–1500.
2. Steere A, Taylor E, McHugh G, Logigian E: The overdiagnosis of Lyme disease. JAMA 1993;269:1812–1816.
3. Rahn D, Malawista S: Treatment of Lyme disease. In Mandell GL, Bone RC, Cline MJ, et al (eds): Year Book of Medicine. St. Louis, MO, Mosby-Year Book, Inc., 1994.
4. Sigal L: Persisting complaints of Lyme disease: A conceptual review. Am J Med 1994;96:365–374.
5. Sigal LH: National Clinical Conference on Lyme disease. Am J Med 1995;98:1S–92S.
6. Sigal L: Lyme disease: A review of aspects of its immunology and immunopathogenesis. Ann Rev Immunol 1997;15:63–92.
7. Sigal LH: Pitfalls in the diagnosis and management of Lyme disease. Arthritis Rheum 1998;41:195–204.
8. Sigal LH, Zahradnik JM, Lavin P, et al: A vaccine consisting of recombinant *Borrelia burgdorferi* outer-surface protein A to prevent Lyme disease. N Engl J Med 1998;339:216–222.
9. Steere AC, Sikand WK, Meurics F, et al: Vaccination against Lyme disease with recombinant *Borrelia burgdorferi* out-surface lipoprotein A with adjuvant. N Engl J Med 1998;339:209–215.

Lewis Blevins, Jr., MD
Shubhada Jagasia, MD

PATIENT 62

A 44-year-old woman with weight loss, nausea, and vomiting

A 44-year-old woman with no significant past medical history presents with a 2-month history of feeling extremely unwell. During this time, she lost 40 pounds and experienced anorexia, nausea, and daily vomiting. She complains of diffuse myalgias and arthralgias, decreased libido, hair thinning, and occasional dyspnea on exertion. Over the last few months, she became so weak that she needed assistance with her activities of daily living. Another physician ascribed her problems to depression secondary to her mother's recent demise.

Physical Examination: Temperature 97.6; pulse 116; respirations 18; blood pressure 70/30 with orthostasis. General: very tanned; appears cachectic. HEENT: dry mucous membranes with some hyperpigmented patches on buccal mucosa. Cardiac: normal rhythm with tachycardia. Chest: normal. Abdomen: soft, no tenderness. Neurologic: normal. Extremities: hyperpigmented knuckles and palmar creases.

Laboratory Findings: WBC 6600/μl (50% neutrophils, 48% lymphocytes, 2% eosinophils), PCV 33%, platelets 207,000/μl. Na^+ 131 mEq/L, K^+ 5.8 mEq/L, Cl^- 95 mEq/L, HCO_3^- 25 mEq/L, BUN 33 mg/dl, Cr 2 mg/dl, glucose 92 mg/dl, Ca^{2+} 11 mg/dl, phosphate 2.5 mg/dl, albumin 3.8 g/dl, Mg 1.5 mg/dl and total bilirubin 0.5 mg/dl.

Question: What disorder explains this patient's clinical presentation?

Diagnosis: Primary adrenal insufficiency.

Discussion: Adrenal insufficiency can be caused by diseases of the adrenal glands (primary) or by interference with corticotropin (ACTH) secretion by the pituitary (secondary) or corticotropin-releasing hormone (CRH) by the hypothalamus (tertiary). Primary adrenal insufficiency (**Addison's disease**) has an incidence of 6 per million adults per year.

The most common cause of Addison's disease is **autoimmune adrenalitis** (isolated adrenal insufficiency or polyglandular autoimmune syndrome types 1 and 2). The various postulated mechanisms include defective CD4+ activity, "molecular mimicry" with infectious agents, anticytoplasmic adrenal antibodies, certain HLA sub-types (HLA-DR3, HLA-DR4, HLA-B8), or circulating IgGs that block ACTH action. Enzymes such as CYP 21, CYP 17, and CYP 11 mediate steroidogenesis within the adrenal gland. Antibodies are produced against these enzymes if the underlying etiology of the adrenal insufficiency is autoimmune in nature. Patients with positive antibodies but normal adrenal function at the outset have a yearly adrenal function detriment of 19%.

Addison's disease can also be caused by infectious adrenalitis (TB, histoplasmosis, HIV), metastatic cancer (lung, breast, stomach, and colon), adrenal hemorrhage or infarction, drugs (ketoconazole, rifampin, phenytoin, megestrol acetate) and inherited disorders (adrenomyeloneuropathy and adrenoleukodystrophy). Panhypopituitarism, isolated ACTH deficiency, or drugs such as megestrol acetate may cause secondary adrenal insufficiency. Tertiary adrenal insufficiency occurs due to chronic high-dose glucocorticoid therapy or after successful treatment of Cushing's disease, due to suppression of the hypothalamic-pituitary-adrenal axis.

Symptoms and clinical manifestations of primary adrenal insufficiency include weakness, fatigue, and anorexia (100% of patients), weight loss (100%), **hyperpigmentation** (94%), systolic BP < 110 mmHg (88%), nausea (92%), vomiting (86%), constipation (33%), diarrhea (16%), abdominal pain (31%) salt craving (16%), postural dizziness (12%), muscle or joint pains (13%), vitiligo (20%), and auricular calcification (5%). Laboratory anomalies include hyponatremia (88%), hyperkalemia (64%), hypercalcemia (6%), azotemia (55%), anemia (40%), and eosinophilia (17%).

In secondary or tertiary adrenal insufficiency, hyperpigmentation is not seen because ACTH levels are low. Hypoglycemia sometimes occurs secondary to chronic glucocorticoid deficiency and concomitant growth hormone deficiency. Manifestations of mineralocorticoid deficiency, such as hypotension, hyponatremia, or hyperkalemia, are not seen since aldosterone secretion is under regulation of the renin-angiotensin axis. Pituitary involvement might produce other trophic hormone deficiencies, headache, or visual field deficits.

Primary adrenal insufficiency is characterized by the presence of low cortisol values in the face of very elevated ACTH values. The definitive diagnosis is made when a **cortrosyn (ACTH) stimulation test** is unable to stimulate a cortisol response above 18 µg/dl. Adrenal imaging and antibody testing is indicated in patients with an abnormal cortrosyn stimulation test. Secondary or tertiary adrenal insufficiency produces both low cortisol and ACTH values. The low-dose (1 µg) ACTH stimulation test may be superior in assessment of secondary adrenal insufficiency as compared to the high-dose (250 µg) ACTH stimulation test. The insulin-induced hypoglycemia test remains the gold standard to test integrated function of the hypothalamic-pituitary-adrenal axis.

Treatment of Addison's disease involves maintenance therapy with **hydrocortisone** 20–30 mg daily in 2–3 divided doses, **dexamethasone** 0.5 mg daily, or **prednisone** 5 mg daily. Occasionally, patients require variations in the doses and timing of the doses based on clinical effects. Dexamethasone and prednisone may be given in a single daily dose at night to suppress morning ACTH levels more effectively and also provide adequate glucocorticoid activity when the patients awakens. Take care to avoid glucocorticoid excess, which may result in osteopenia, osteoporosis, impaired glucose tolerance, and hypertension. ACTH levels are not reliable parameters to judge adequacy of replacement, since approximately one-third of patients with Addison's disease have elevated levels despite adequate glucocorticoid replacement. This is in contrast to TSH levels, which are reliable markers of thyroid hormone replacement in primary hypothyroidism.

Mineralocorticoid replacement with fludrocortisone 0.5–0.2 mg daily is required in patients with primary adrenal insufficiency. Liberal salt intake is encouraged to maintain adequate intravascular volume. Doses may have to be increased in the summer. Salt intake needs to be increased when exercising. Lower doses might be required if there is concomitant treatment with a glucocorticoid such as hydrocortisone, which has some mineralocorticoid activity. Treat essential hypertension in patients with adrenal insufficiency by reducing the salt intake and lowering doses of fludrocortisone. Recent reports have suggested that dehydroepiandrosterone replacement therapy might improve the sense of well being and sexuality in women.

Treatment of acute adrenal crisis or treatment in response to acute physiologic stress (infection, surgery, and injury) requires intravenous hydrocortisone in doses of 50–100 mg every 8 hours. This is rapidly tapered to maintenance therapy based on the clinical condition of the patient. Patients undergoing surgery should receive higher doses of steroids starting at the time of induction of anesthesia.

Explain to the patient, in detail, the nature of the hormonal deficit and rationale for replacement. All such patients should wear medic alert tags. Adequacy of replacement is judged on the basis of overall sense of well being, weight gain, and disappearance of hyperpigmentation and associated symptoms. Mineralocorticoid replacement is followed by observing resolution of electrolyte abnormalities, improvement of blood pressure, and absence of peripheral edema. Overall prognosis is excellent, with normal life expectancy resulting from standard management.

The present patient presented with classic signs and symptoms of Addison's disease. Her laboratory results revealed a random cortisol < 1 μg/dl and an aldosterone < 2.5 ng/dl. Cortrosyn (ACTH) stimulation resulted in a cortisol of 1.2 μg/dl. Her adrenal antibody titer was positive at 1:8. CT scan of the adrenals revealed no distinct pathology. She was treated with oral hydrocortisone 30 mg in divided doses and Florinef (fludrocortisone) 0.1 mg daily. She continues to do well at this time.

Clinical Pearls

1. Mineralocorticoid deficiency leading to hyponatremia and hyperkalemia is seen only in primary adrenal insufficiency.

2. Individualize treatment of Addison's disease, based on clinical and biochemical parameters.

3. A high index of clinical suspicion is required for the diagnosis since symptomatology may be quite nonspecific.

4. Hyperpigmentation occurs in patients with primary insufficiency due to the elevated ACTH levels, which stimulate melanocyte receptors.

REFERENCES

1. Betterle C, Scalici F, Presotto F, et al: The natural history of adrenal function in autoimmune patients with adrenal antibodies. J Endocr 1988;117:467–475.
2. Thaler LM, Blevins LS Jr: The low-dose (1-mcg) adrenocorticotropin stimulation test in the evaluation of patients with suspected central adrenal insufficiency. Clin Endocrinol Metab 1998;83(8):2726–2729.
3. Arlt W, Callies F, Allolio B, et al: Dehydroepiandrosterone replacement in women with adrenal insufficiency. N Engl J Med 1999;341:1013–1020.

Liza C. O'Dowd, MD

PATIENT 63

**A 25-year-old woman with drug allergies, cystic fibrosis, fever,
and worsening cough**

A 25-year-old woman with cystic fibrosis presents with worsening cough productive of copious greenish sputum, fevers, and increasing shortness of breath with wheezing. Frequent exacerbations of her cystic fibrosis over the past several years have required treatment with multiple courses of parentally administered antibiotics. During an exacerbation 4 weeks ago, piperacillin was discontinued because she developed urticaria, angioedema of the tongue, and worsening wheeze immediately after infusion of the drug. She has had a similar reaction to ceftriaxone in the past.

Physical Examination: Temperature 38.6°; pulse 120; blood pressure 110/70; pulse oximetry 88% on room air. General: thin, audibly wheezing and using accessory muscles. HEENT: nasal polyps bilaterally. Cardiac: tachycardic without murmer. Chest: diffuse rhonchi and wheezes. Abdomen: soft, nontender; normal-active bowel sounds. Extremities: clubbing; no rash or edema.

Laboratory Findings: WBC 22,000/µl with 70% neutrophils, 15% bands. Chest radiograph: new right lower lobe infiltrate; hyperinflation, diffuse bronchiectasis. Pulmonary function tests: FEV_1 1.25 L (45% of predicted), FEV_1/FVC 35%. Sputum cultures: *Burkholderia cepacia*, sensitive *only* to imipenem and tobramycin.

Question: How would you manage this patient with a history of a beta-lactam allergy?

Answer: Desensitize the patient to imipenem in a monitored setting.

Discussion: Five to ten percent of adverse drug reactions are allergic or IgE-mediated. Clinical features of these immediate hypersensitivity reactions include urticaria (hives), bronchospasm, angioedema, and in the most severe cases, anaphylaxis. Beta-lactam antibiotics are among the most frequent and clinically important causes of IgE-mediated reactions.

Appropriate management of patients who require therapy with a beta-lactam antibiotic, but who have a history an allergic reaction to this drug class, begins with assessment of risk for a recurrent reaction. Historical features that place the patients at **high risk** for a potentially life-threatening reaction upon re-challenge include: immediate reaction (occurring within 30 minutes of drug administration), history of a systemic reaction, and recent reaction (occurring within the last year.) The patient is at **low risk** if the reaction occurred more than 2 hours after drug administration, was limited to the skin, or if occurred in the remote past (more than 10 years ago). The patient is at **intermediate risk** if there is a history of severe reaction (anaphylaxis) that occurred more than 10 years ago.

Skin testing to penicillin is the preferred method to determine if the patient with a prior history of a beta-lactam allergy is truly at risk for an IgE-mediated reaction to penicillin. Sensitivity to either the major or minor antigenic determinants of penicillin results in a positive skin test. The negative predictive value of a negative test to both major and minor determinants (i.e., percentage of patients who will tolerate penicillin without an immediate allergic reaction) is 97%. If such a patient does have an immediate allergic reaction, it tends to be mild. In contrast, the positive predictive value of the test (i.e., percentage of patients with a positive test who will experience a life-threatening reaction on receiving a beta-lactam) is 40–73%. The results of the penicillin skin test *cannot* be used to assess the risk of non-IgE-mediated reactions such as hemolytic anemia, interstitial nephritis, serum sickness, Stevens-Johnson syndrome, drug fever, or maculopapular rashes.

Skin tests should be considered if a patient with a beta-lactam allergy requires a beta-lactam to treat a serious infection, and no other alternative antibiotic is appropriate. However, they should be **avoided** if a patient has been found to be at high risk for an anaphylactic reaction as determined by history. They are also contraindicated if the patient has used an antihistamine in the last 5 days or doxepin within the 6 weeks prior to the skin test, has no suitable site to perform the test (e.g., diffuse skin disease), or lacks a positive reaction to skin test controls. Patients with any of these characteristics should be desensitized to penicillin if the drug must be given. Importantly, a history of penicillin-induced Stevens-Johnson syndrome or toxic epidermal necrolysis is an **absolute contraindication** to both skin testing as well as desensitization to a beta-lactam antibiotic.

Patients with Ig-E mediated sensitivity to penicillin, as determined by a positive penicillin skin test, are at a fourfold increased risk of an allergic reaction to cephalosporins compared to those patients who are skin test negative, particular if the drug is a first- or second-generation agent. If a patient with a history of an allergic reaction to a cephalosporin has a negative penicillin skin test, a penicillin can be safely administered, but cephalosporins should be avoided. Similarly, a patient who has a history of a life-threatening reaction to a semi-synthetic penicillin (such as nafacillin), but a negative skin test to penicillin, may safely be given penicillin. However, avoid the semi-synthetic agent that caused the reaction.

Carbapenems, such as imipenem, cross-react with penicillin and should be avoided in penicillin-allergic patients unless they are first desensitized (see figures). While the monolactam aztreonam does not cross-react with penicillin, it does cross-react with ceftazidime. A patient with a history of an allergic reaction to ceftazidime or aztreonam should avoid both.

Desensitization is a method to **induce immunologic tolerance and reduce the risk of anaphylaxis** to a drug. Consider desensitization if your

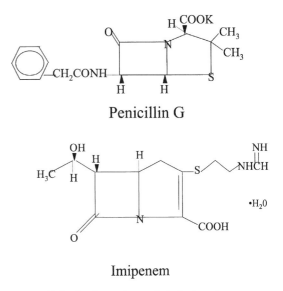

Penicillin G

Imipenem

Both structures share a beta-lactam ring.

patient is at high risk for an anaphylaxis to a drug, as determined either by history or positive penicillin skin test, and no other alternative antibiotic is available. Also consider it if history is uncertain, and the skin test cannot be performed. Note that desensitization does not protect a patient from developing a non-IgE-mediated reaction to the drug, such as serum sickness or maculopapular rashes.

Both oral and parenteral desensitization can be performed, although in critically ill patients the parenteral method is preferred, because it can generally be completed within 3 hours. Dilutions of the antibiotic are prepared, starting at one millionth of the full-strength final dose. Each subsequent dilution is slowly given, and the patient is carefully observed before the next higher-strength dilution is administered. Perform parenteral desensitization in a monitored setting; 30% of patients have an allergic reaction during the procedure. These reactions may be severe and require aggressive therapy.

After desensitization is complete, tolerance to the antibiotic persists only as long as the patient continues to receive the drug. Once the drug is discontinued for more than 24 hours, the patient is again at risk for an immediate hypersensitivity reaction if exposed to the drug. Repeat desensitization is required if the antibiotic is again needed.

The present patient required therapy with a class of antibiotics that are known to cross-react with penicillin. Penicillin skin testing was contraindicated because she had a recent life-threatening reaction to a beta-lactam agent. Because no alternative antibiotic was available, she was desensitized to imipenem in the intensive care unit without incident. With the initiation of the antibiotic, steroids, and aggressive pulmonary toilet, her pulmonary status slowly improved over the next 2 weeks.

Clinical Pearls

1. Penicillin skin testing, coupled with a careful drug allergy history, is the most reliable way to accurately assess a patient's risk of an immediate hypersensitivity reaction to penicillin.

2. In addition to cephalosporins, carbepenems such as imipenem can cross-react with penicillin. Aztreonam and ceftazidime cross-react with each other, but not with penicillin.

3. If an antibiotic is required to treat a life-threatening condition and no appropriate alternative agent exists, desensitization can safely induce temporary immunologic tolerance to the drug.

4. A history of a penicillin- induced exfoliative dermatitis is an absolute contraindication to both skin testing with and desensitization to a beta-lactam.

REFERENCES

1. Borish AL, Tamit R, Rosenwasser LJ: Intravenous desensitization to beta-lactam antibiotics. J Allergy Clin Immunol 1987; 80:314.
2. Weiss ME, Adkinson NF: Immediate hypersensitivity reactions to penicillin and related antibiotics. Clin Allergy 1988;18:515.
3. Lin RY: A perspective on penicillin allergy. Arch Intern Med 1992;152:930.
4. Bates DW, Cullen DJ, Laird N, et al: Incidence of adverse drug events and potential adverse drug events. Implications for prevention. JAMA 1995;274:29.
5. Torres MJ, Mayorga C, Pamles R, et al: Immunologic response to different determinants of benzylpenicillin, amoxicillin, and ampicillin. Comparison between urticaria and anaphylactic shock. Allergy 1999;54:936.

Jon T. Mader, MD
Saul G. Trevino, MD
James W. Galbraith Jr., BS
Mark E. Shirtliff, PhD

PATIENT 64

A 41-year-old man with pain and fever related to an old wound

A 41-year-old man with a history of an open right tibia/fibula fracture secondary to a motor vehicle accident 8 months ago complains of drainage from the original wound. The patient is status-post open reduction internal fixation (ORIF). He has fever, tenderness, and erythema over the right anterior tibial region, with off and on drainage. The patient also has a social history of tobacco use and intravenous drug abuse.

Physical Examination: Temperature 38.3°. Chest: clear to auscultation. Cardiac: regular rhythm with no murmurs. Abdomen: nontender with normal bowel sounds. Extremities: two 0.5×0.5 cm, draining sinus tracts, one with yellow purulent drainage, on the anterior aspect of the right leg below the knee; erythema surrounds both sinus tracts.

Laboratory Findings: WBC 17,000/µl with 70% neutrophils. Sinus drainage: *Staphylococcus aureus* susceptible to methicillin. Leg radiograph (see below): three screws at the proximal tibia; lytic changes around the distal screw.

Question: What is the primary diagnostic concern?

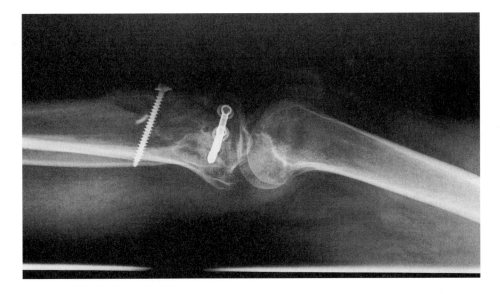

Answer: The primary diagnostic concern is to make sure the bone is stable (x-ray). Hardware cannot be removed unless there is union at the fracture site.

Discussion: Osteomyelitis is characterized by infection of the bone, commonly the cortical and/or medullary portions. This infectious disease is progressive and results in inflammatory destruction of bone, bone necrosis, and new bone formation. While there are many causative micro-organisms, osteomyelitis is predominately bacterial in origin.

Osteomyelitis can be classified by duration, pathogenesis, location, extent, and host status. It is currently classified by either the Waldvogel or Cierny-Mader classification systems. The Waldvogel staging system (see table) describes three categories of osteomyelitis based on the etiology of the infection. These categories are (1) hematogenous and contiguous focus, (2) with or, (3) without vascular insufficiency. These etiologies are further described as acute or chronic processes. Although the Waldvogel classification system remains the most popular, it is limited to the etiology and does not lend itself well to the classification of different clinical aspects for diagnosis and treatment.

Osteomyelitis: Waldvogel Classification

- Hematogenous osteomyelitis
- Osteomyelitis secondary to a contiguous focus of infection
    No generalized vascular disease
    Generalized vascular disease
- Chronic osteomyelitis (necrotic bone)

The Cierny-Mader system (see table, right) classifies osteomyelitis in 12 stages based on a combination of anatomical disease types and physiological host categories. The present patient has Stage 3Bs osteomyelitis, or **localized osteomyelitis**. Because this patient has a history of noninsulin-dependent diabetes mellitus, the "Bs" represents a patient with compromised systemic, physiologic, metabolic, and immunologic capabilities. The terms acute and chronic osteomyelitis are not used in this staging system, since areas of macronecrosis and/or infected hardware must be removed regardless of the acuity or chronicity of the infection.

Contiguous focus osteomyelitis results when bacteria are introduced into the bone by direct trauma or by extension of an adjacent soft tissue infection. **Open fractures**, **chronic soft tissue infections**, **hardware implantation**, and **surgical procedures** are common causes. Most infections of hardware occur by endogenous or exogenous contamination during surgery. Unlike hematogenous osteomyelitis, multiple bacterial species are usually isolated from the infected bone. *Staphylococcus aureus*, coagulase-negative *Staphylococcus* sp., and *Streptococcus* sp. represent the most frequently isolated species. In addition, Gram-negative bacilli and anaerobic organisms are commonly isolated. Hardware is less commonly infected by a hematogenous route.

The clinical features of contiguous focus osteomyelitis include local pain, draining sinus, tenderness, and erythema over the involved bone. The patient is often afebrile. Patients with peripheral vascular disease usually display more subtle symptoms and have foot ulcers. Infection of hardware may become evident shortly after surgery, especially if the organism is virulent. Erythema and drainage at the operative site are common. The onset of infection is often delayed, with erythema, sinus tracts, persistent pain, and hardware loosening noted 3 to 12 months after surgery.

Bacterial osteomyelitis is confirmed by identification of the causative organism(s) via bone culture or histology. Bone cultures are usually obtained at the time of surgical debridement. Optimal antibiotic treatment is selected by isolation of causative organisms and determination of their antibiotic susceptibilities.

Cierny-Mader Staging System

- Anatomic Type
    Stage 1—Medullary osteomyelitis
    Stage 2—Superficial osteomyelitis
    Stage 3—Localized osteomyelitis
    Stage 4—Diffuse osteomyelitis
- Physiologic Class
    A Host—Normal host
    B Host—Systemic compromise (Bs)
        Local compromise (B1)
        Systemic and local compromise (B1s)
    C Host—Treatment worse than the disease
- Systemic and local factors that affect immune surveillance, metabolism, and local vascularity

Systemic (Bs)	Local (B1)
Malnutrition	Chronic lymphedema
Renal, hepatic failure	Venous stasis
Diabetes mellitus	Major vessel compromise
Chronic hypoxia	Arteritis
Immune disease	Extensive scarring
Malignancy	Radiation fibrosis
Extremes of age	Small vessel disease
Immunosuppression or immune deficiency	Neuropathy
	Tobacco abuse

Although radiographic evidence of osteomyelitis lags behind the bone infection by at least 2 weeks, x-ray findings include soft tissue swelling, periosteal thickening or elevation, local osteopenia, lytic changes, and new bone formation. Radiographic changes in contiguous focus osteomyelitis may be vague and in association with other non-specific radiographic findings. In hardware infections, there may be evidence of lytic changes around the hardware and/or hardware loosening.

Radionuclide scans such as technetium-99m bisphosphonate, gallium-67 citrate, or indium-111 chloride–labeled leukocyte scans may be obtained when the diagnosis of osteomyelitis is ambiguous or to help gauge the extent of bone and soft tissue inflammation. In general, it is not usually necessary to obtain these scans for the diagnosis of long bone osteomyelitis.

Computed axial tomography (CT) may play a role in the diagnosis of osteomyelitis. Increased marrow density occurs early in the infection, and intramedullary gas has been reported in patients with hematogenous osteomyelitis. The CT scan can also help to identify areas of necrotic bone and to assess the involvement of the surrounding soft tissues. In a recalcitrant infection, the CT scan may assist in identifying the surgical approach and augment debridement. One disadvantage of this study is the scatter phenomenon, which occurs when metal is present in or near the area of bone infection. This scatter results in a significant loss of image resolution.

Magnetic resonance imaging (MRI) has become the most useful diagnostic tool for determining the presence and extent of musculoskeletal sepsis. The spatial resolution of MRI makes it useful in differentiating between bone and soft tissue infections. However, metallic implants in the region of interest may produce focal artifacts, thereby decreasing the utility of the image. MRI displays greater anatomical detail than radionucleotide scans, and greater specificity for abnormalities than CT scans or radiographs. Furthermore, patients do not have to be exposed to ionizing radiation.

The components of osteomyelitis treatment include patient evaluation, staging assessment, identification of micro-organism(s) and their sensitivity, administration of antibiotics, debridement surgery, dead space management, and, if necessary, stabilization. Reconstruction is considered at the first surgery. Antibiotics that cover the clinically suspected pathogens should be administered until sensitivities can be determined from cultures (see table, next page).

Surgical exposure should be direct and designed to avoid unnecessary devitalization of bone and soft tissue. The cortical and cancellous bone remaining in the wound after debridement surgery must bleed uniformly to ensure antibiotic perfusion and avoid sequestration. Appropriate **management of the dead space created by surgery** is mandatory to arrest the disease and maintain the integrity of the bone involved. The goal of dead space management is to replace dead bone and scar with durable, vascularized tissue. Local tissue flaps, free tissue flaps, vascularized bone grafts, bone transfers, and antibiotic beads can be used to fill dead space. Cancellous bone grafts can be placed beneath local or transferred tissues when surgical augmentation is necessary. If motion is present before or after surgery, stability of the bone must be achieved. Stabilization of the bone is usually managed with internal or external fixation. An Ilizarov external fixator allows segmental resection and bone lengthening or shortening.

Since the soft tissue envelope enclosing the debrided bone requires 3 to 4 weeks in a normal host and up to 6 weeks in a compromised host to become revascularized after debridement surgery, antibiotics are used to treat live infected bone and to safeguard soft tissue and bone undergoing revascularization. Traditionally, parenteral antibiotics are administered for 4 to 6 weeks following the last major debridement surgery. We treat osteomyelitis with 2 weeks of parenteral antibiotics followed by 4 weeks of oral antibiotics.

Hospitalization times with traditional antibiotic therapy have decreased in recent years due to the development of outpatient catheters and oral antibiotic therapy. Outpatient intravenous therapy using long-term intravenous access catheters, such as Hickman or Groshong catheters, has allowed patients to administer intravenous antibiotics without the need for hospitalization. For treatment of methicillin-sensitive *S. aureus*, nafcillin or oxacillin is the antibiotic of choice. Clindamycin, which provides excellent bone penetration, can be administered every 8 hours. The quinolones or the 3rd- or 4th-generation cephalosporins are used to treat gram-negative organisms.

In addition to outpatient IV-therapy, long-term oral therapy with the quinolone class of antibiotics has been shown to arrest osteomyelitis caused by gram-negative organisms. Normally, the quinolones are given parenterally for 1 to 3 days, and then switched to oral therapy. Coverage of aerobic gram-positive organisms should be obtained with other antibiotics such as nafcillin, clindamycin, or ampicillin and a β-lactamase inhibitor. Before changing to an oral regimen with these agents, it is recommended that the patient initially receive at least 2 weeks of parenteral antibiotic therapy. For all outpatient treatments, the patient must be compliant and agree to close outpatient follow-up.

Initial Choice of Antibiotics for Therapy of Infectious Arthritis and Osteomyelitis (Adult Doses)

Organism	Antibiotics of First Choice	Alternative Antibiotics
Staphylococcus aureus	Nafcillin 2 gm every 6h or clindamycin 900 mg every 8h	Vancomycin, cefazolin
Methicillin-resistant *S. aureus*	Vancomycin 1 gm every 12 h	SXT + rifampin, minocycline + rifampin
Staphylococcus epidermidis	Vancomycin 1 gm every 12 h or nafcillin 2 gm every 6 h	Cefazolin, clindamycin
Group A streptococcus	Penicillin G 2 million every 4 h*	Clindamycin, cefazolin
Group B streptococcus	Penicillin G 2 million every 4 h*	Clindamycin, cefazolin
Enterococcus sp.	Ampicillin 2 gm every 6 h ± gentamicin 5 mg/kg/day every 8 h	Vancomycin, ampicillin-sulbactam
Escherichia coli	Ampicillin 2 gm every 6 h or Levofloxacin 500 mg qd	Cefazolin, tobramycin
Proteus mirabilis	Ampicillin 2 gm every 6 h or Levofloxacin 500 mg qd	Cefazolin, gentamicin
Proteus vulgaris *Proteus rettgeri* *Morganella morganii*	Cefotaxime 2 gm every 6 h ± gentamicin 5mg/kg/day every 8 h	Mezlocillin + gentamicin, levofloxacin
Serratia marcescens	Cefotaxime 2 gm every 6 h ± gentamicin 5 mg/kg/day every 8 h Levofloxacin 500 mg qd	Ciprofloxacin, Mezlocillin + gentamicin
Pseudomonas aeruginosa	Piperacillin 3 gm every 4 h or Ceftazidime 2 gm every 8 h + tobramycin 5 mg/kg/day every 8 h	Ciprofloxacin, amikacin, cefepime
Bacteroides fragilis group	Clindamycin 900 mg every 8 h	Metronidazole, ampicillin-sulbactam
Peptostreptococcus sp.	Clindamycin 900 mg every 8 h	Penicillin, metronidazole, ampicillin-sulbactam

SXT = sulfamethoxazole-trimethoprim, ± = with or without, + = with
* There is a national shortage of penicillin G.

Antibiotic-impregnated acrylic beads can be used to sterilize and temporarily maintain dead space. Although this method is limited by the rate and duration of antibiotic elution from the implant, it has many advantages. With local delivery, high concentrations of antibiotics can be administered to the site of infection without increasing the systemic antibiotic concentrations that can lead to high toxicity. The most common antibiotics used in beads are tobramycin and vancomycin. The beads are usually removed within 2 to 4 weeks and replaced with a cancellous bone graft.

For patients with stable bone and hardware infections, treatment requires removal of the hardware, thorough debridement, and antibiotic therapy. If bone is unstable, rigid and strong bony union must be established. Debridement of infected material is essential to permit strong bony union to occur. The patient is maintained on suppressive oral antibiotics. Once stability is re-established, the hardware can be removed, the bone debrided, and another course of antibiotics administered.

The present patient was taken to surgery, and the screws were removed. He had bony continuity and stability after the surgical procedure. The cultures taken at surgery were positive for methicillin-sensitive *S. aureus*. The patient was treated with 2 weeks of parenteral clindamycin (900 mg every 8 hours). Following the parenteral antibiotic therapy, he received 4 weeks of oral clindamycin 300 mg QID. The patient was protected with a cast and then a brace for 6 months after surgery. At follow-up 1 year later, the osteomyelitis was arrested.

Clinical Pearls

1. Due to the late presentation of osteomyelitis on plain films, bacterial osteomyelitis can only be confirmed by identification of the causative organism via deep bone biopsy.

2. Adequate drainage thorough debridement, dead space management, removal of hardware, bone stability, wound coverage with viable soft tissue, and specific antimicrobial coverage are essential to the treatment of contiguous focus osteomyelitis due to hardware infections.

3. Close patient follow-up is necessary to prevent osteomyelitis from becoming a chronic infection.

REFERENCES:

1. Waldvogel FA, Medoff G, Swatz MM: Osteomyelitis: a review of clinical features, therapeutic considerations, and unusual aspects. N Engl J Med 1970;282:198–206, 260–266, 316–322.
2. Gold RH, Hawkins RA, Katz RD: Bacterial osteomyelitis: Findings on plain radiography, CT, MR, and scintigraphy. Am J Roentgenol 1990;157:365–370.
3. Lew DP, Waldvogel FA: Quinolones and osteomyelitis: State-of-the-Art. Drugs 1995;49(suppl. 2): 100–111.
4. Calhoun J, Mader JT: Treatment of osteomyelitis with a biodegradable antibiotic implant. Clin Orthop 1997;341:206–214.
5. Lew DP, Waldvogel FA: Current concepts: Osteomyelitis. N Engl J Med 1997;336:999–1007.
6. Mader JT, Mohan D, Calhoun J: Staging and staging application in osteomyelitis. Clin Infect Dis 1997;25:1303.
7. Rissing JP: Antimicrobial therapy for chronic osteomyelitis in adults: Role of the quinolones. Clin Infect Dis 1997;25: 1327–1333.
8. Gugenheim JJ: The Ilizarov method. Orthopedic and soft tissue applications. Clin Plast Surg 1998;25(4):567–578.
9. McAndrew PT, Clark C: MRI is best technique for imaging acute osteomyelitis. BMJ 1998;316:147.
10. Schutz M, Sudkamp N, Frigg R, et al: Pinless external fixation. Indications and preliminary results in tibial shaft fractures. Clin Orthop 1998;347:35–42.
11. Tice AD: Outpatient parenteral antimicrobial therapy for osteomyelitis. Infect Dis Clin North Am 1998;12:903–917.
12. Mader JT, Shirtliff ME, Bergquist SC, Calhoun J: Antimicrobial treatment of chronic osteomyelitis. Clin Orthop 1999;360:47–65.

Marie-Florence Shadlen, MD
Kathryn Dobmeyer, MD

PATIENT 65

A 74-year-old woman with urinary incontinence

A 74-year-old woman with a history of hypertension and breast cancer treatment 10 years previously comes to the primary care clinic with symptoms of urinary incontinence exacerbated by a recent upper respiratory infection. She has had numerous urinary tract infections, and a past evaluation included a normal cystoscopy and unremarkable CT scan of her upper urinary tract. She complains of urgency, frequency, and leakage of small volumes of urine with cough and sneezes. The leakage requires use of four pads a day. She has no enuresis and no spontaneous incontinence. She denies constipation, hematuria, or vaginal bleeding. Water intake is six cups per day, with two cups of coffee daily. Her medications are Tamoxifen and Amlodipine.

Physical Examination: Vital Signs: normal. Abdomen: nondistended and nontender. Extremities: no edema. Pelvic examination: smooth vaginal mucosa with moderate atrophy, no vaginal prolapse, mild hypermobility of the anterior vaginal wall with cough and valsalva; apex of the vaginal vault is supported, uterus surgically absent, no enterocele or cystocele; pelvic floor muscle localization fair, with good strength of contraction. Normal perineal sensation, anal wink, and rectal examination. Post-void residual urine volume: 20 ml.

Laboratory Findings: Normal WBC count, hematocrit, electrolytes, and urine dipstick.

Question: What is the role of behavioral management of this patient's urinary incontinence?

Diagnosis: Urinary incontinence.

Discussion: Most cases of urge, stress, or mixed stress and urge incontinence can be initially managed in the primary care setting (see figure next page). In the present patient, diagnosis of mixed urinary incontinence depended on the constellation of symptoms of urgency, frequency, and leakage of small volumes of urine with coughs and sneezes. Other reversible causes (see **DIAPPERS mnemonic** in the algorithm) of urinary incontinence—including urinary tract infection—were ruled out. The pelvic exam and postvoid residual ruled out bladder outlet obstruction and neurogenic bladder.

The involuntary leakage of urine is a common and disruptive condition that can be managed effectively for the majority of patients. Approximately 15–30% of community dwelling elderly, one-third of hospitalized patients, and up to half of residents of nursing homes have urinary incontinence. Many patients assume that urinary incontinence is a normal consequence of aging and do not report their symptoms to their care providers. Moreover, many primary care physicians are not comfortable with their ability to evaluate and treat urinary incontinence. The focus of medical management of urinary incontinence has involved the use of anticholinergic agents to increase bladder contractility; however, behavioral techniques may be more effective and have no potential side effects.

The cerebral cortex coordinates micturition through inhibition, and the brainstem facilitates urination. Bladder filling occurs when sympathetic tone from T11-L2 causes detrusor muscle relaxation and sphincter contraction, and inhibits parasympathetic tone from S2-S4. Somatic nerves from the sacral plexus contribute to continence by increasing pelvic floor muscle contraction. When parasympathetic innervation overcomes sympathetic tone, detrusor muscle contracts, and the bladder empties. The physiological changes of aging predispose to symptoms of urinary incontinence. Older persons have decreased bladder capacity, increased residual urine, and more frequent bladder contractions. Older women are susceptible to laxity of pelvic musculature following childbirth and the decreased influence of estrogen on bladder outlet and urethral resistance pressures. These physiological changes contribute to the three types of incontinence most commonly seen in women: **stress incontinence**, **urge incontinence**, and **mixed stress and urge urinary incontinence**.

Stress urinary incontinence is suspected clinically when a patient gives symptoms of involuntary leakage of urine with coughing, sneezing, and laughing. Women with stress urinary incontinence often give a history of being postmenopausal, having multiple childbirths, and/or prior hysterectomy. Bladder cystometrics reveal that a cough causes intra-abdominal pressures that exceed urethral pressures, leading to urinary leakage. Patients who report symptoms of urinary frequency, urgency, nocturia and voiding of variable volumes of urine have urge urinary incontinence. Both local genitourinary factors (e.g., urinary tract infection, bladder irradiation) and central nervous system conditions (e.g., dementia, stroke, multiple sclerosis) contribute to urge incontinence. In the case of urge urinary incontinence, bladder cystometrics reveal uninhibited bladder contractions and small voiding volumes.

The targeted history and physical exam is focused on identifying potentially reversible causes of urinary incontinence and detecting gynecologic or urologic problems for which referrals would be needed. At this point in the evaluation, a **voiding diary** and **bedside cystometrics** may provide additional information when the diagnosis and type of incontinence is still unclear. The management of stress and urge incontinence requires lifestyle and behavioral techniques that may be more effective than any pharmacologic treatment. Instruct the patient to avoid caffeine, bladder irritants, and alcohol, and not to consume any liquids after 8:00 PM. She should record the timing, frequency, and setting of incontinence episodes in a voiding diary to establish a baseline. This patient is having 4–8 incontinence episodes daily.

Most interventions do not cure the incontinence, but may significantly reduce the frequency of episodes. Instruct the patient to void every 2 or 3 hours during the day. Verify that the patient can localize her pelvic floor muscles and contract them during the pelvic exam. The patient should perform 15 **pelvic muscle exercises** three times a day, gradually increasing the contractile period to 10 seconds. A recent study found pelvic muscle exercises, delayed voiding, and caffeine restriction to be the most effective in reducing incontinence severity. Subjects were taught with biofeedback to respond to the urge to void by sitting down, relaxing their body, and contracting pelvic muscles selectively while keeping their abdominal muscles relaxed.

Estrogen treatment for atrophic vaginitis was the next most beneficial management strategy for urinary incontinence. In contrast, systemic pharmacological treatment of urinary incontinence in older women is often unhelpful. A randomized trial found that a biofeedback-based behavioral approach (81%) was significantly more effective than oxybutynin (68.5%) or placebo (39%). Only 14%

of women given behavioral therapy wished to change their treatment, compared with 75% in the drug and placebo groups. Selection of systemic urinary incontinence drugs such as imipramine, oxybutinin, and hyoscyamine is made on the basis of minimizing side effects or cost rather than differences in efficacy.

The present patient was treated with daily estrogen vaginal cream, daily voiding control, and pelvic muscle exercises. She was given a prescription of hyoscyamine to use as needed on days of vigorous exercise or for air travel or long car rides, when access to the toilet could be restricted. The patient's symptoms improved, and her incontinence episodes decreased to once or twice per week. This case underscores that in older women atrophic vaginitis can be a contributing factor, and that stress and urge incontinence often coexist.

Algorithm for Management of Female Urinary Incontinence

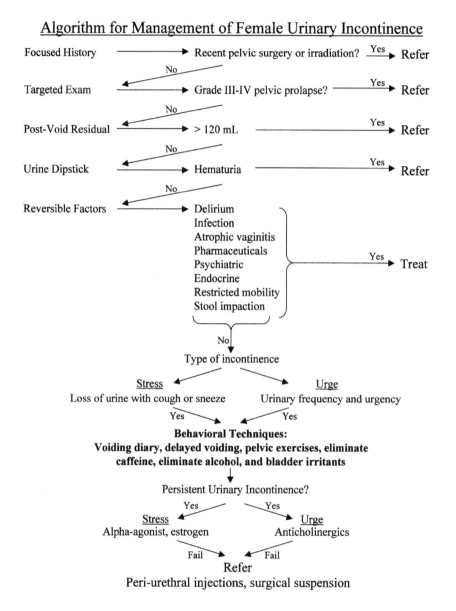

Clinical Pearls

1. Most cases of urge, stress, or mixed incontinence can be initially managed in the primary care setting.

2. Compared with pharmacological treatment, behavioral techniques are more effective in reducing urinary incontinence severity.

3. Selection of systemic urinary incontinence drugs is made on the basis of minimizing side effects or cost rather than differences in efficacy.

REFERENCES

1. Resnick NM, Ouslander JG, eds: National Institutes of Health Consensus Development Conference on Urinary Incontinence. J Am Geriatr Soc 1990;38:263–286.
2. Bergio KL, Locer JL, Goode PS, et al: Behavioral vs. drug treatment for urge urinary incontinence in older women: a randomized controlled trial. JAMA 1998;280:1995–2000.
3. Anderson RU, Mobley D, Blank B, et al: Once daily controlled versus immediate release of oxybutynin chloride for urge urinary incontinence. OROS Oxybutynin Study Group. J Urol 1999;161(6):1809–1812.
4. Johnson TM, Ouslander JG: Urinary incontinence in the older man. Med Clin North Am 1999;83(5):1247–1266.
5. Weinberger MW, Goodman BM, Carnes M: Long-term efficacy of nonsurgical urinary incontinence treatment in elderly women. J Gerontol: Med Sci 1999;54A:M117–M121.

Spencer V.B. Wilking, MBBS
Daniel Berlowitz, MD

PATIENT 66

A 78-year-old woman with a pressure ulcer and knee pain

A 78-year-old, obese woman is admitted to a nursing home following a 15-day hospitalization for a cerebrovascular accident. She had been in good health, except for type 2 diabetes, hypertension, and mild degenerative joint disease of the knees, until the day of acute hospitalization when she was found lying on the floor of her apartment for an undefined period. She had a dense right hemiparesis, and a left middle cerebral artery infarction was diagnosed. Hospital course was complicated by the development of a pressure ulcer over the right greater trochanter; no improvement in her neurological status was noted. The patient has been transferred to the nursing home for long-term placement.

Physical Examination: Vital signs: temperature 99.8°. General: obese, appeared comfortable. Skin: 6 cm × 4 cm stage 4 pressure ulcer on right hip; ulcer base discolored at center, but otherwise clean and with evidence of granulation; small amount of serosanguinous exudate noted on dressing. Chest: normal. Extremities: mild crepitation in both knees with no erythema or effusion. Neurologic: right hemiparesis with dysarthric speech; mini-mental status score 25.

Nursing Home Course: Shortly following admission, the patient began to complain of a new, aching pain in the right knee. Acetaminophen every 6 hours provided partial relief. The examination was unchanged, and a radiograph of the knee revealed moderate degenerative changes. The patient had a low-grade fever of 37.3°–38.1°. WBC 10,400/μl, hemoglobin 11.3 g/dl, total protein 7.5 g/dl, albumin 3.1 g/dl. Care for the pressure ulcer consisted of wet-to-dry dressings every shift. The patient was placed on a mattress overlay and turned every 2 hours. Nutritional supplements were provided, and her intake appeared good. Despite this care, the pressure ulcer increased in size to 8 × 4 cm. The wound appeared clean with good granulation tissue, except for the central area. There was only a minimal exudate. Hip radiograph: see below.

Question: What diagnostic procedures were performed?

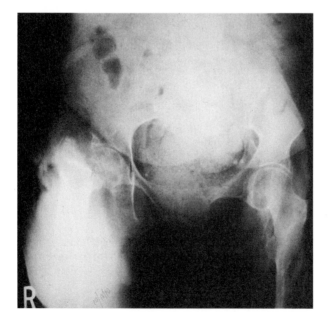

Answer: Evaluation for osteomyelitis.

Discussion: Pressure ulcers are defined as localized areas of tissue necrosis that tend to develop when soft tissue is compressed between a bony prominence and an external surface for a prolonged period of time. The appearance of pressure-induced skin injury may range from non-blanchable erythema of intact skin (**stage 1**) to ulcers that extend through the skin and fascia into muscle and other supporting tissues (**stage 4**). Pressure ulcers can be associated with numerous complications. Deep ulcers may extend down to bone, resulting in osteomyelitis, or joints, causing septic arthritis. Infected pressure ulcers may also be the source of bacteremia, meningitis, and endocarditis. Sinus tracts may occur even in pressure ulcers that appear superficial. These may communicate with internal organs, including the rectum and bladder. Other rare complications include development of squamous cell carcinoma, amyloidosis, and pseudoaneurysm.

Diagnosing osteomyelitis complicating a stage 4 pressure ulcer is frequently difficult. A high degree of suspicion for this complication is required—particularly, as in this case, when the wound does not heal despite aggressive wound care. Routine radiographs of the underlying bone are indicated if osteomyelitis is a concern. However, these are often normal, and early osteomyelitis may be difficult to differentiate from changes in the bone due to pressure and an overlying ulcer. Among the changes that may be seen on radiography are periosteal elevation, defacement and/or thickening of cortical margins, osteonecrosis, or marked radiolucency. Technetium Tc 99m bone scans have a high sensitivity for detecting osteomyelitis, but specificity is low. MRI, either alone or with gladolinium contrast to increase specificity, may be a valuable alternative. Recently, the **probe-to-bone test** has been promoted as a simple bedside technique for the detection of osteomyelitis in infected diabetic foot ulcers. Palpating bone on probing had a sensitivity of 66% and a specificity of 85% for the presence of osteomyelitis. This compares favorably to the other, more expensive tests. The use of the probe-to-bone test has been expanded beyond diabetic foot ulcers and should be included as part of the evaluation of a deep pressure ulcer. The gold standard for detecting osteomyelitis, though, remains a **bone biopsy**.

Despite extensive damage to the hip secondary to osteomyelitis, the patient complained only of knee pain. Knee pain can occur as a result of hip pathology. The obturator and femoral nerves, which arise from the anterior and posterior divisions of the lumbar plexus (L2, L3, L4), send branches to both the hip and knee. Thus, *referred pain in the knee can arise from diseases of the hip.*

A surgical consultant re-examined the present patient's pressure ulcer. Probing the center of the wound with a sterile, blunt probe, palpable bone was easily detected. A positive probe-to-bone sign is highly suggestive of the presence of osteomyelitis. A subsequent radiograph revealed extensive destruction of the hip joint presumed secondary to osteomyelitis (see figure). The knee pain was now recognized as being referred pain from the hip.

Treatment of the patient's osteomyelitis was complicated by her poor prognosis for functional recovery. A decision was made not to proceed with surgical debridement of the hip, and she was treated with a prolonged course of intravenous antibiotics. Some improvement in the pressure ulcer was evident 3 months later, when the patient was transferred to another nursing home.

Clinical Pearls

1. Consider osteomyelitis when a pressure ulcer does not improve or heal despite good wound care.
2. Probing to bone is a useful bedside test for the detection of osteomyelitis.
3. Hip pathology should always be considered when confronted with unexplained knee pain.

REFERENCES:
1. Bergstrom N, Bennett MA, Carlson CE, et al: Treatment of Pressure Ulcers. Clinical Practice Guideline, No. 15. Rockville, MD, U.S. Department of Health and Human Services. Public Health Service, Agency for Health care Policy and Research. AHCPR Publication No. 95-0652. December 1994.
2. Grayson ML, Gibbons GW, Balogh K, Levin E, Karchmer AW: Probing to bone in infected pedal ulcers: A clinical sign of underlying osteomyelitis in diabetic patients. JAMA 1995;273:721–723.
3. Smith DM: Pressure ulcers in the nursing home. Ann Intern Med 1995;123:433–442.

S. J. Bickston, MD

PATIENT 67

A 61-year-old man with epigastric pain

A 61-year-old professor comes to the clinic for a yearly visit. He complains of burning epigastric pain. It occurs almost daily, particularly at night and after certain foods. The pain lasts for several minutes to half an hour. It seems to be aggravated by job-related stress. He wonders if it could be an ulcer, and asks specifically if he could be infected with *Helicobacter pylori*. His only medicines are over-the-counter ranitidine and antacids that he takes on a prn basis with some relief. He had an appendectomy in childhood and is scrupulous about his colorectal cancer screening with fecal occult blood tests and flexible sigmoidoscopy.

Physical Examination: Vital signs: normal. Oropharynx: clear. Sclerae: anicteric. Chest: clear. Abdomen: flat with well-healed surgical scar; soft, with mild epigastric tenderness to deep palpation; no palpable organomegaly.

Laboratory Findings: Hemogram: normal. Electrolytes and urine indices: normal. Upper GI series: see below.

Question: What clinical condition best explains this man's symptoms?

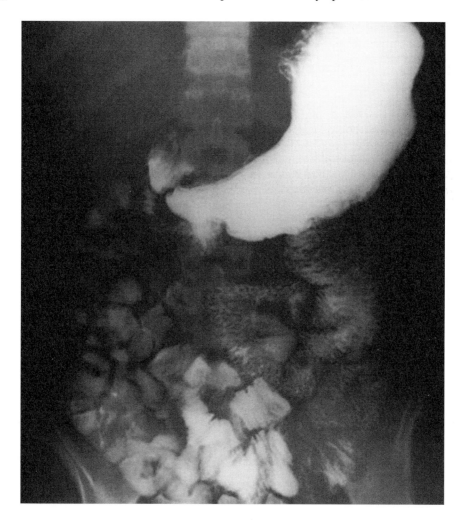

Answer: Gastroesophageal reflux disease (GERD).

Discussion: GERD is far more common than peptic ulcer disease (PUD). More than 60 million American adults experience heartburn at least once a month, and about 25 million adults suffer daily from heartburn. The rows of antacids on the shelves of every mini-mart are testimony to the widespread impact of this condition. Educational campaigns have promoted an emerging lay interest in *H. pylori* infection, but its role in GERD is not entirely understood.

H. pylori has been recognized in gastric biopsy specimens for nearly a century. It was thought to be a contaminant or colonizing organism until Marshall's pivotal investigation (and self-infection). The mode of infection is generally thought to be fecal-oral or oral-oral. Recognition of *H. pylori*'s important role in PUD has encouraged physicians to look for the organism and to eradicate it in a variety of non-ulcer conditions. The popularity of this approach now brings information that has caused the the pendulum to swing back— sometimes it is best not to test or treat at all.

Individuals who have never been infected with *H. pylori* appear to be at greater risk for developing GERD than those infected. To date there is **no conclusive evidence** that *H. pylori* eradication helps (or harms) patients with GERD. The infection itself does not appear to directly contribute to the pathogenesis of GERD, since its prevalence in those with reflux is no greater than in control populations. Data do suggest that infection with the organism may actually have a *protective* role: some duodenal ulcer patients develop GERD symptoms following bacterial eradication. In addition, GERD appears to be less severe in infected individuals. *H. pylori* infection appears to augment the antisecretory properties of both H2 receptor antagonists and proton pump inhibitors, suggesting that eradication may not always be beneficial if prolonged acid suppressive treatment is planned.

Since most experts feel that anyone who tests positive for the bacteria should be treated, it may be wise not to test in the first place in patients with GERD. Noninvasive testing is preferred in the initial diagnosis of this infection; this is *not* a question to be answered with an endoscope. When testing is appropriate, **serologic testing for IgG** is preferred as the most cost-effective approach. With the introduction of stool assays, the test of choice may change. Established indications for *H. pylori* testing and treatment include active or past duodenal and gastric ulcer, complicated ulcer, and low-grade gastric MALT lymphoma. Controversial indications include dyspepsia, severe endoscopic gastritis (especially hypertrophic), and patients taking NSAIDs. Currently, there is no reason to test asymptomatic individuals hoping to prevent ulcer disease or subsequent cancer.

Treatment of *H. pylori* infection is cumbersome, requiring combinations of several drugs. Currently approved FDA regimens successfully cure infection in 70–90% of patients. Combinations of two antibiotics (clarithromycin and amoxicillin or metronidazole) and a proton pump inhibitor (lansoprazole or omeprazole) or ranitidine bismuth citrate appear to be the most effective regimens. Additionally, they delay development of antibiotic resistance. Most experts now favor a 14-day course.

The present patient had a normal upper GI series and chose to be tested for *H. pylori* infection. Serology was negative. He is asymptomatic on once-a-day treatment with omeprazole.

Clinical Pearls

1. GERD is far more common than peptic ulcer disease.
2. Eradication of *H. pylori* can provoke GERD.
3. Serology is the most cost-effective way to diagnose *H. pylori*.

REFERENCES

1. Labenz J, Blum AL, Bayerdörffer E, et al: Curing *Helicobacter pylori* infection in patients with duodenal ulcer may provoke reflux esophagitis. Gastroenterol 1997;112:1442–1447.
2. Holtmann G, Cain C, Malfertheiner P: Gastric *Helicobacter pylori* infection accelerates healing of reflux esophagitis during treatment with the proton pump inhibitor pantoprazole. Gastroenterol: 1999;117:11–16.

Ayalew Tefferi, MD

PATIENT 68

A 40-year-old man with erythrocytosis

A 40-year-old Caucasian man, a nonsmoker, was incidentally discovered to have an increased hemoglobin (Hb) level (20.2 g/dl) in July 1998. He was asymptomatic at the time, and diagnostic work-up elsewhere suggested an increased red blood cell mass and a normal arterial oxygen saturation. The patient experienced headaches in December 1998 and was treated with phlebotomy. His symptoms did not improve, and he is now (8 months later) seeking a second opinion. The patient's mother had a history of requiring phlebotomies for a similar illness.

Physical Examination: Vital signs: normal. General examination: unremarkable. HEENT: facial plethora. Funduscopic examination: normal. Cardiac: normal. Chest: normal. Abdomen: no palpable organomegaly. Extremities: palmar erythema.

Laboratory Findings: Hb 18.9 g/dl, mean corpuscular volume 88 fL, WBC 5100/μl, platelet count 167,000/μl, leukocyte alkaline phosphatase score 53, vitamin B_{12} 319 ng/L, ferritin 47 μg/L. Abdominal ultrasound examination: normal. Hb-oxygen dissociation curve: left shifted (see figure).

Question: What is the differential diagnosis and the most likely diagnosis?

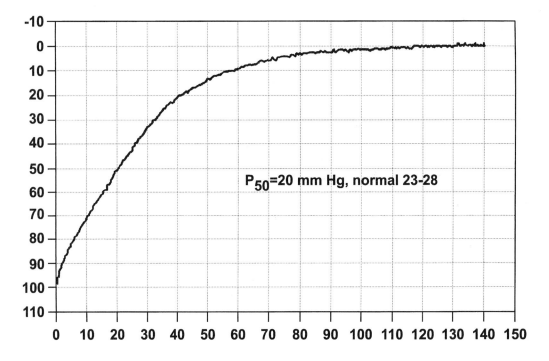

P_{50}=20 mm Hg, normal 23-28

Diagnosis: High-oxygen-affinity hemoglobinopathy (Hb Heathrow), as suggested by Hb electrophoresis and confirmed by DNA sequence analysis.

Discussion: An increased Hb concentration (or hematocrit) may represent the upper tail end distribution among normal persons, a relative polycythemia (normal red cell mass associated with decreased plasma volume), or an absolute erythrocytosis. Erythrocytosis may result from an autonomous (usually clonal) proliferation of erythrocytes (polycythemia vera [PV]), a growth factor (erythropoietin)-mediated increase in erythrocytes (secondary erythrocytosis), or a defective erythropoietin (EPO) receptor resulting from a congenital mutation.

In order to distinguish PV from both relative polycythemia and secondary erythrocytosis, the PV study group established widely used diagnostic criteria more than 30 years ago (see table). Although these criteria remain useful for the uniform selection of patients for clinical studies, they lack both specificity and sensitivity. Furthermore, with the current availability of biologic assays, red cell mass measurement may not always be required to diagnose PV.

Investigation of "erythrocytosis" is indicated in the following circumstances:
- Hb > 18 g/dL in a male Caucasian or the corresponding value in female patients and in those of different ethnic origin.
- A documented and persistent increase in Hb of > 2 g/dL.
- Presence of a high-normal Hb (16-18 g/dl) that is associated with a PV-associated clinical feature (thrombosis, aquagenic pruritus, increased leukocytosis or thrombocytosis, microcytosis, splenomegaly, or erythromelalgia).

Diagnostic work-up may start with a determination of the serum EPO level (sEPO). In PV, sEPO is usually low, but can be normal. Therefore, the diagnosis of PV is considered only if the sEPO is low or normal. If a repeat sEPO confirms a low value, a bone marrow biopsy is indicated to look for morphologic and immunohistochemical evidence of PV. The characteristic histologic features include bone marrow hypercellularity, atypical megakaryocytic hyperplasia and clustering, and decreased bone marrow iron stores. In addition, the demonstration, by standard immunoperoxidase methods, of reduced megakaryocyte expression of the thrombopoietin receptor, is consistent with a diagnosis of PV and complements the morphologic findings.

Another relatively specific diagnostic test for PV is the in vitro demonstration of EPO-independent erythroid colony formation. However, the particular assay is not widely available, and it requires a high level of expertise in test performance and interpretation of results.

A bone marrow biopsy is also indicated if a "normal" sEPO level is accompanied by a PV-associated feature. Otherwise, careful follow-up with a 3-month repeat of Hb and sEPO is reasonable. In the presence of an increased sEPO or a normal sEPO not associated with any clear evidence of PV, a diagnostic work-up for congenital or acquired SE may be started with the determination of P_{50} (oxygen pressure at 50% Hb-oxygen saturation). A low P_{50} suggests either a high-oxygen-affinity hemoglobinopathy (as in the current case report) or 2,3-diphosphoglycerate deficiency. In the presence of a normal P_{50}, the diagnostic possibilities include autosomal dominant or recessive familial erythrocytosis and acquired EPO-mediated processes. The latter may be self-limited (central hypoxia) or feedback insensitive (EPO-producing tumors, renal artery stenosis). In most instances, the correct diagnosis is suggested by the history and physical findings. Useful laboratory tests include arterial blood gas measurement and computed tomography of the abdomen.

The Polycythemia Vera Study Group Diagnostic Criteria for Polycythemia Vera*

Major Criteria	Minor Criteria
Increased red cell mass	Platelets > 400,000/μl
Males ≥ 36 ml/kg	Leukocytes > 12,000/μl
Females ≥ 32 ml/kg	Leukocyte alkaline phosphatase > 100
Normal arterial oxygen saturation, ≥ 92%	Vitamin B_{12} > 900 pg/ml *or* unbound vitamin B_{12} binding
Splenomegaly	capacity > 2200 pg/ml

* Diagnosis requires the presence of all three major criteria *or* the presence of the first two major criteria and any two minor criteria.
From Tefferi A, Silverstein MN: Myeloproliferative diseases. In Goldman L, Bennett JC (eds): Cecil Textbook of Medicine. 21st ed. Philadelphia, WB Saunders Company, 2000, pp 935–941; with permission.

Clinical Pearls

1. Bone marrow immunoperoxidase staining for the thrombopoietin receptor (c-Mpl) may be helpful for complementing the morphologic distinction between SE and PV.

2. Investigation of "erythrocytosis" is indicated if a patient has Hg > 18 g/dl, a documented and persistent increase in Hb of > 2 g/dl, or Hb that ranges from 16 to 18 g/dl in a patient with a PV-associated clinical feature.

3. The diagnostic evaluation of erythrocytosis begins with determination of a serum erythropoietin level.

REFERENCES

1. Berlin NI: Diagnosis and classification of the polycythemias. Semin Hematol 1975;12:339–351.
2. Cotes PM, Dore CJ, Yin JA, et al: Determination of serum immunoreactive erythropoietin in the investigation of erythrocytosis. N Engl J Med 1986; 315:283–287.
3. Valla D, Casadevall N, Huisse MG, et al: Etiology of portal vein thrombosis in adults. A prospective evaluation of primary myeloproliferative disorders. Gastroenterology 1988;94:1063–1069.
4. Prchal JT, Sokol L: "Benign erythrocytosis" and other familial and congenital polycythemias. Eur J Haematol 1996;57:263–268.
5. Wajcman H, Galacteros F: Abnormal hemoglobins with high oxygen affinity and erythrocytosis. Hematol Cell Ther 1996;38:305–312.
6. Arcasoy MO, Degar BA, Harris KW, et al: Familial erythrocytosis associated with a short deletion in the erythropoietin receptor gene. Blood 1997;89:4628–4635.
7. Weinberg RS: In vitro erythropoiesis in polycythemia vera and other myeloproliferative disorders. Semin Hematol 1997; 34:64–69.
8. Moliterno AR, Hankins WD, Spivak JL: Impaired expression of the thrombopoietin receptor by platelets from patients with polycythemia vera. N Engl J Med 1998;338:572–580.
9. Tefferi A: Diagnosing polycythemia vera: A paradigm shift. Mayo Clin Proc 1999;74:159–162.
10. Tefferi A, Yoon S-Y, Li C-Y: Immunohistochemical staining for megakaryocyte c-mpl may complement morphologic distinction between polycythemia vera and secondary erythrocytosis. Blood 2000;96:771–772..

Nicholas Hill, MD

PATIENT 69

A 69-year-old woman with COPD and increasing cough and dyspnea

A 69-year-old woman with a history of severe chronic obstructive pulmonary disease (baseline FEV_1 0.620 L) and chronic hypercapnia (baseline pCO_2 54 mmHg) presents to the emergency department with a 3-day history of increasing cough and dypsnea. She has been expectorating moderate amounts of yellow sputum without difficulty. The patient is an ex-smoker, but her past medical history is otherwise unremarkable.

Physical Examination: Respirations 28, pulse 132, blood pressure 168/70. General: moderate respiratory distress, with use of accessory respiratory muscles. Chest: bilateral expiratory wheezes, prolonged expiration. Cardiac: distant heart sounds, irregular pulse, no jugular venous distension. Extremities: no edema. Neurologic: alert, anxious but not agitated.

Laboratory Findings: ABG (NC 2 L/min): pH 7.27, pCO_2 66, pO_2 86. Chest radiograph: hyperinflated lung fields without infiltrates. EKG: multifocal atrial tachycardia (MAT).

Questions: Should this patient receive ventilatory support? What methods of assisted ventilation should be used?

Diagnosis: Moderate exacerbation of chronic obstructive pulmonary disease (COPD).

Discussion: Several randomized controlled trials have demonstrated that **noninvasive positive-pressure ventilation** (NPPV) used in the initial therapy of selected patients with COPD exacerbations avoids the need for intubation in the majority of patients. In addition, NPPV decreases the incidence of complications, mortality, and the length of ICU and hospital stay as compared to conventional management with intubation in this patient population. On the basis of these observations, consensus groups have considered NPPV as the ventilatory modality of first choice in selected COPD patients with acute respiratory insufficiency. Note that appropriate patient selection is a critical factor in obtaining benefit from this form of ventilatory support.

Randomized trials demonstrate that *mildly ill* patients with COPD exacerbations are unlikely to receive benefit from NPPV. Patients sufficiently ill to benefit from NPPV usually have *moderate to severe* respiratory distress with tachypnea (respiratory rate > 24) and use their accessory respiratory muscles, or abdominal paradox is present. They should also have evidence of an acute or acute on chronic deterioration of gas exchange (PCO_2 > 45 mmHg with a pH < 7.35).

Patients with some causes of respiratory failure other than COPD are also potential candidates for NPPV. Although patients with cardiogenic pulmonary edema appear to benefit from NPPV, evidence of benefit in terms of clinical outcomes is not as well established as compared with acute exacerbations of COPD. Continuous positive airway pressure (CPAP), however, remains the treatment of first choice for patients with pulmonary edema. Recent controlled studies show that patients with hypoxemic respiratory failure (PaO_2/FiO_2 < 200) and underlying immunocompromised states have lower complication rates and shorter lengths of ICU stay if treated with NPPV as compared with intubation and mechanical ventilation. Successfully treated, immunocompromised patients usually have isolated respiratory failure without evidence of other organ dysfunction, and improvement is likely within a few days.

Anecdotal evidence suggests that NPPV may be beneficial for other forms of respiratory failure, such as acute asthma, exacerbations of cystic fibrosis, and upper airway obstruction.

It is also important to appropriately exclude patients with *severe* respiratory failure who are unlikely to benefit from NPPV. A trial of face mask ventilation in a patient who needs prompt intubation may cause harm by delaying effective ventilatory support. Patients suffering respiratory arrests should be promptly intubated because insufficient time exists for mask placement and patient adaptation to NPPV breathing. Some patients may not tolerate a face mask or present anatomic impediments for a tight face mask fitting. Patients with recent head and neck surgery usually do not tolerate placement of a face mask and NPPV. Patients with nonrespiratory organ instability, as demonstrated by hypotension, uncontrolled cardiac ischemia or arrhythmias, or unremitting upper gastrointestinal bleeding, are poor candidates for NPPV because of the potential for sudden clinical deterioration.

Excessive airway secretions and poor airway control due to impaired coughing or swallowing, excessive agitation, or a limited ability to cooperate represent relative contraindications for NPPV. Clinical judgment is required in evaluating these patients because of the absence of objective criteria for patient selection. Some agitated patients may be appropriate candidates for NPPV when calmed with the judicious use of benzodiazepines.

In evaluating patients with exacerbations of COPD, recognize that only a third of patients prove to be appropriate candidates for NPPV. Also, favorable results from NPPV (70–90% success in appropriately selected patients) have been reported from centers that are highly experienced with this technique; NPPV is less effective in facilities with limited clinical experience with noninvasive forms of assisted ventilation. In establishing the use of NPPV in a healthcare setting, **extensive training of respiratory therapists** in fitting patients for appropriately sized masks and adjusting ventilatory equipment is requisite to ensure good clinical outcomes. Appropriate application of NPPV has the additional benefit of decreasing resource utilization and the cost of care.

The present patient appeared to be an ideal candidate for NPPV. She had moderate respiratory distress; her blood gas results indicated the presence of acute on chronic hypercapnia; and she was using her accessory muscles. These findings indicated that the patient was at increased risk of further deterioration if assisted ventilation was not used. Moreover, she was cooperative and had sufficient reserve to allow fitting of a mask and adaptation to NPPV. The presence of MAT is not considered a contraindication to NPPV because it is not a life-threatening arrhythmia. The patient's increased sputum production was concerning, but she was able to expectorate during brief removals of her mask. The patient was treated for 24 hours with intermittent NPPV. She subsequently improved, and was discharged on the fourth hospital day.

Clinical Pearls

1. NPPV is the ventilatory modality of first choice in selected patients with COPD exacerbations because it has been shown to reduce morbidity, mortality, and length of hospital stay.

2. Appropriate recipients for NPPV have a demonstrable need for ventilatory assistance, but are not so severely ill as to render the use of NPPV unsafe.

REFERENCES

1. Barbe F, Quera-Salva MA, de Lattre J, et al: Long-term effects of nasal intermittent positive pressure ventilation on pulmonary function and sleep architecture in patients with neuromuscular diseases. Chest 1996;110:1179–1183.
2. Meduri GU, Cook TR, Turner RE, et al: Noninvasive positive pressure ventilation in status asthmaticus. Chest 1996;110:767–774.
3. Meduri GU, Turner RE, Abou-Shala N, et al: Noninvasive positive pressure ventilation via face mask. Chest 1996;109:179–193.
4. Antonelli M, Conti G, Rocco M, et al: A comparison of noninvasive positive-pressure ventilation and conventional mechanical ventilation in patients with acute respiratory failure. N Engl J Med 1998;339:429–435.
5. Celikel T, Sungur M, Ceyhan B, Karakurt S: Comparison of noninvasive positive pressure ventilation with standard medical therapy in hypercapnic acute respiratory failure. Chest 1998; 114:1636–1642.
6. Pang D, Keenan SP, Cook DJ, Sibbald WJ: The effect of positive pressure airway support on mortality and the need for intubation in cardiogenic pulmonary edema. Chest 1998;114:1185–1192.
7. Wood KA, Lewis L, Von Harz B, Kollef MH: The use of noninvasive positive pressure ventilation in the emergency department. Chest 1998;113:1339–1346.
8. Confalonieri M, Potena A, Carbone G, et al: Acute respiratory failure in patients with severe community-acquired pneumonia. Am J Respir Crit Care Med 1999;160:1585–1591.
9. Antonelli M, Conti C, Bufi M, et al: Noninvasive ventilation for treatment of acute respiratory failure in patients undergoing solid organ transplantation. JAMA 2000;283:235–241.

Anne B. Whitehurst, MD
Stanley W. Chapman, MD

PATIENT 70

A 19-year-old HIV-infected man with fever, cough, and shortness of breath

A 19-year-old HIV-infected man from rural Mississippi is hospitalized with a 1-month history of general malaise, fever, weight loss, and cough productive of green sputum with occasional mild hemoptysis. One week ago, right-sided pleuritic chest pain developed. He was hospitalized elsewhere with pneumonia 2 to 3 weeks earlier, but did not improve after a course of antibiotics. He is not currently followed for his HIV infection and has never been on antiretroviral therapy.

Physical Examination: Temperature 39°, respirations 20, pulse 90, blood pressure 120/70. General: mild distress secondary to chest pain. HEENT: unremarkable. Skin: no lesions or nodules. Adenopathy: none palpated. Cardiac: unremarkable. Chest: poor inspiratory effort. Abdomen: mild right upper quadrant pain; positive bowel sounds; no rebound tenderness. Extremities: unremarkable. Neurologic: unremarkable.

Laboratory Findings: WBC 8800/μl with normal differential. Blood cultures (two sets): negative. Expectorated sputum: many PMNs; normal flora; all stains for fungi and mycobacterium negative. Chest radiograph: see figure. CT head scan: negative.

Hospital Course: The patient is treated for community-acquired pneumonia with levofloxacin and clindamycin. He remains febrile and undergoes fiberoptic bronchoscopy on the fifth hospital day. Bronchoscopy washings show budding yeast.

Question: Which fungal pathogen would best fit this clinical presentation?

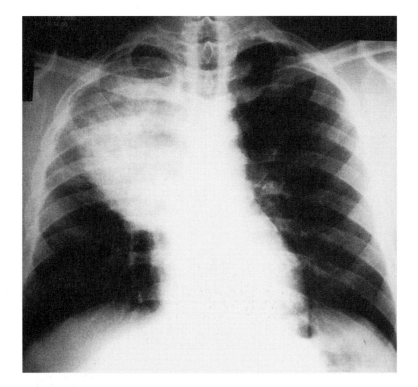

Diagnosis: Chronic pulmonary blastomycosis.

Discussion: Chronic pulmonary blastomycosis is one of several clinical conditions caused by infection with the endemic fungus *Blastomyces dermatitidis*. Blastomycosis is endemic in North America, especially in those states bordering the Mississippi and Ohio Rivers; most cases are reported from Mississippi, Arkansas, Kentucky, Tennessee, and Wisconsin. Pulmonary infection is the most common clinical manifestation because the conidia gain entry by inhalation. Isolated skin infection has been noted in cases of direct inoculation from a laboratory accident and from the bite of an infected dog.

Pulmonary manifestations are seen in approximately 80% of patients and include asymptomatic infection, an acute pneumonitis with typical features of bacterial pneumonia, and an indolent chronic pneumonia. Rarely, primary pulmonary infection may rapidly progress to adult respiratory distress syndrome (ARDS), which is associated with a high mortality. Most patients exhibit the **chronic form** of pulmonary disease and typically present with weight loss, fever, night sweats, cough with or without hemoptysis, and pleuritic chest pain.

The most common associated radiographic presentations of chronic pulmonary blastomycosis are **alveolar infiltrates** or **mass-like lesions** that tend to involve the upper lobes. It is not unusual for a patient with the nonspecific symptoms mentioned above and a pulmonary mass lesion to be presumed initially to have lung cancer. Other pathogens that can present in the same manner as chronic pulmonary blastomycosis are tuberculosis and other fungal infections. Disseminated (extrapulmonary) disease occurs in approximately 25–50% of patients and involves the skin, bone, and the male genitourinary system in order of frequency; however, virtually any organ system can be involved.

Although blastomycosis is most often associated with infections in normal hosts, there has been an increase in the incidence of infections in immunocompromised patients. The largest number of reported cases are in HIV-infected patients who have advanced immunodeficiency (e.g., counts less than 200/μl). Other populations with defective T-cell function have been reported and include patients with prolonged glucocorticoid use, pregnant women, solid organ transplant recipients, and patients with hematologic malignancies. **Immunocompromised patients** tend to present with more severe disease, and they have disseminated disease at the time of presentation more often than do patients with normal immune status. In particular, **CNS involvement** is noted to be as high as 40% in immunocompromised patients as compared to 5% or less in immunocompetent patients. ARDS with respiratory failure, though rarely associated with primary pulmonary disease in normal hosts with blastomycosis, is seen in 20–30% of patients with an altered immune status.

A presumptive diagnosis of blastomycosis can be made in an appropriate clinical setting by visualizing the characteristic broad-based yeast form, which warrants early antifungal therapy. A definitive diagnosis requires growth of the organism from clinical specimens and may require several weeks. Currently available serologic tests are of limited value, owing to their inadequate sensitivity and specificity, and are not used in diagnosis.

Although resolution without therapy has been documented in immunocompetent patients with acute pulmonary infection, the majority of patients with blastomycosis require therapy. It is important to thoroughly evaluate patients for extrapulmonary disease before a decision is made to monitor without therapy. Follow patients carefully to document either resolution or progression of disease. Although there have been no comparative trials that definitely establish the optimal therapy, it is generally agreed that all patients with life-threatening disease, those with immunosuppression, patients with CNS disease, and pregnant females should be treated with **amphotericin B**. A total dose of 1.5 g has been associated with the highest cure rate and fewest relapses.

In immunocompromised patients with mild to moderate non-CNS disease who have an initial response with amphotericin, oral therapy with an azole can be considered. In patients with CNS disease and in pregnant females, the entire course should be given as amphotericin B. In immunocompromised patients, particularly advanced HIV disease, indefinite suppressive therapy with itraconazole is considered to be prudent. Lipid formulations of amphotericin have not been studied in depth in clinical trials; however, they are generally believed to be acceptable alternatives for patients who require amphotericin B but who are intolerant of the side effects.

Immunocompetent patients with non-CNS and mild to moderate disease can be treated safely and effectively with an azole. Ketoconazole was the first azole to be proven effective in these patients. However, **itraconazole** is now the azole of choice—despite the increased cost—owing to its greater efficacy, better absorption, and lower toxicity. The recommended initial dose of itraconazole is 200 mg/day, which can be increased in 100 mg increments depending on clinical response. Limited data support the use of fluconazole in blastomycosis. In general, fluconazole appears equal in efficacy to ketoconazole, but has less drug interactions and side effects. There may be a role for fluconazole in the treatment of CNS blastomycosis owing to its excellent CNS penetration, but clinical trials are lacking.

In the present patient, a classic mass-like infiltrate was demonstrated on the chest radiograph. It is important to note in this patient the lack of CNS involvement. Despite significant pulmonary disease, a diagnosis was not made until invasive means were used to collect bronchial washings. He was treated initially with approximately 600 mg of amphotericin B, to which he had a rapid clinical response with resolution of fever, night sweats, chest pain, and cough. He was discharged on itraconazole 200 mg a day to be continued indefinitely.

Clinical Pearls

1. Immunocompromised patients with blastomycosis often have disseminated disease and have a significantly higher incidence of CNS involvement than do immunocompetent hosts.

2. The azoles, particularly itraconazole, provide a safe and effective alternative to amphotericin B in selected patients with mild to moderate disease that does not involve the CNS.

3. In a patient with suspected pulmonary blastomycosis and nondiagnostic expectorated sputum, invasive procedures are required to obtain diagnostic samples.

REFERENCES

1. Pappas PG, Threlkeld MG, Bedsole GD, et al: Blastomycosis in immunocompromised patients. Medicine 1993;72:311.
2. Bradsher RW: Clinical features of blastomycosis. Sem Respir Infect 1997;12:229.
3. Chapman SW, Lin AC, Hendricks KA, et al: Endemic blastomycosis in Mississippi: Epidemiology and clinical studies. Sem Respir Infect 1997;12:219.
4. Chapman SW, Bradsher RW, Campbell GD, et al: Practice guidelines for the management of patients with blastomycosis. Clin Infect Dis 2000;30:679.

Robert A. Kyle, MD

PATIENT 71

A 50-year-old woman with anemia and fatigue

A 50-year-old woman was found to have a hemoglobin level of 11.1 g/dl. She was given oral iron for 2 months without benefit. Eighteen months later a routine examination reveals a total protein of 8.7 g/dl. This leads to the discovery of a monoclonal gammopathy and an increased number of plasma cells in the bone marrow. The patient had noticed that she did not have as much energy as in the previous year, but attributed her fatigue to age and her children. She denies bone pain, recurrent infections, and bleeding. She gives no history of light-headedness, change in her tongue or voice, weight loss, edema, or paresthesias.

Physical Examination: Temperature, pulse, respirations, and blood pressure: normal. HEENT: unremarkable. Cardiac: normal sinus rhythm; no murmurs. Chest: no crackles. Abdomen: no organomegaly or tenderness.

Laboratory Findings: Hemoglobin 12.9 g/dl; leukocytes 4000/µl, platelets 238,000/µl. Calcium 8.2 mg/dl, creatinine 1.0 mg/dl. Serum protein electrophoresis: a gamma spike of 4.38 g/dl. Immunofixation: IgG κ monoclonal protein. Quantitative immunoglobulins: IgG 5520 mg/dl; IgA 9.3 mg/dl; IgM 14.8 mg/dl. Bone marrow: 30% plasma cells. Metastatic bone survey: no lytic lesions.

Questions: What is the likely diagnosis? Should this patient be treated now?

Diagnosis: Smoldering multiple myeloma.

Discussion: Smoldering multiple myeloma is characterized by the presence of an M-protein > 3 g/dl and more than 10% plasma cells in the bone marrow, but no anemia, hypercalcemia, renal insufficiency, or lytic bone lesions. The plasma cell labeling index (plasma cell proliferative rate) is low. Biologically these patients have monoclonal gammopathy of undetermined significance (MGUS) and should not be treated because they may remain stable and asymptomatic for several years.

When evidence of progression occurs, treatment becomes a consideration. If the patient is younger than 70 years, the physician should discuss the possibility of an autologous peripheral blood stem cell transplant. If the patient is older than 70 years, treatment with alkylating agents such as melphalan and prednisone is recommended. There is no evidence that the combination of alkylating agents is more effective than oral melphalan and prednisone. Administer chemotherapy until the patient is in a plateau state, which is defined as stable serum and urine M-protein levels and no other evidence of progression. Discontinue chemotherapy when the plateau state occurs, because continued therapy may lead to the development of a myelodysplastic syndrome or acute leukemia.

For an autologous transplant, chemotherapy is usually initiated with vincristine and Adriamycin by continuous intravenous infusion for 96 hours, plus dexamethasone 40 mg/daily on days 1–4, 9–12, and 17–20 (VAD). The dexamethasone may need to be reduced to one or two 4-day periods during the even numbered cycles because of undesirable side effects. Most patients are given three or four 1-month cycles. Dexamethasone as a single agent may also be used for induction therapy. Stem cells can be collected following high-dose cyclophosphamide and granulocyte-stimulating factor (G-CSF). The transplant can then proceed. The patient is given high-dose chemotherapy (melphalan 200 mg/m^2, *or* melphalan 140 mg/m^2 plus total body radiation [8Gy]) followed by infusion of the peripheral stem cells. Most physicians now prefer melphalan 200 mg/m^2 because the side effects, particularly mucositis, are much less. Additionally, the autologous stem cell transplant can be performed on an outpatient basis in many instances. The other choice is to treat the patient with alkylating agents after stem cell collection until a plateau is reached, and then delay high-dose therapy and infusion of the previously collected peripheral blood stem cells.

The current mortality of **autologous stem cell transplant** is about 1%. Stem cell transplantation is not curative, and most patients will relapse. The use of dendritic cells and vaccines may be of benefit in prolonging the plateau phase following autologous transplantation. The two major shortcomings of autologous stem cell transplantation are: (1) an inability to eradicate multiple myeloma from the patient, and (2) autologous peripheral blood stem cells are contaminated by myeloma cells or their precursors.

Allogeneic bone marrow transplantation is advantageous because the graft contains no tumor cells that can lead to a relapse. Unfortunately, the mortality rate is approximately 25%, and there is no evidence that a cure is possible. At present, allogeneic transplantation is not recommended. Efforts to reduce mortality by using a preparative regimen such as fludarabine and melphalan (mini-allo) as well as T cell depletion are being explored.

In the present patient, progressive disease developed 2 years later. She underwent chemotherapy with vincristine, Adriamycin, and dexamethasone. She then underwent a successful stem cell transplant.

Clinical Pearls

1. An elevation of total protein may be the first clue of a large monoclonal protein.
2. Do not treat multiple myeloma unless the patient is symptomatic or has laboratory or x-ray abnormalities that will soon progress to a symptomatic state.
3. The three most important prognostic factors are β_2-microglobulin level, plasma cell labeling index (proliferative rate), and cytogenetic abnormalities.
4. Neither autologous nor allogeneic transplantation is a curative procedure.
5. Treat patients with lytic lesions with an intravenous bisphosphonate such as pamidronate.

REFERENCES

1. Kyle RA, Greipp PR: Smoldering multiple myeloma. N Engl J Med 302:1347, 1980.
2. Attal M, Harousseau JL, Stoppa AM, et al: A prospective, randomized trial of autologous bone marrow transplantation and chemotherapy in multiple myeloma. Intergroupe Francais du Myélome. N Engl J Med 335:91, 1996.
3. Berenson JR, Lichtenstein A, Porter L, et al: Long-term pamidronate treatment of advanced multiple myeloma patients reduces skeletal events. Myeloma Aredia Study Group. J Clin Oncol 16:593, 1998.
4. Fermand JP, Ravaud P, Chevret S, et al: High-dose therapy and autologous peripheral blood stem cell transplantation in multiple myeloma: Up-front or rescue treatment? Results of a multicenter sequential randomized trial. Blood 92:3131, 1998.
5. The Myeloma Trialists' Collaborative Group: Combination chemotherapy versus melphalan plus prednisone as treatment for multiple myeloma: An overview of 6633 patients from 27 randomized trials. J Clin Oncol 16:3832, 1998.
6. Marlogie B, Jagannath S, Desikan KR, Mattox S, et al: Total therapy with tandem transplants for newly-diagnosed multiple myeloma. Blood 93:55–65, 1999.
7. Singhal S, Mehta J, Desikan R, et al: Antitumor activity of thalidomide in refractory multiple myeloma. N Engl J Med 341:1565, 1999.
8. Sirohi B, Powles R, Mehta J, et al: Complete remission rate and outcome after intensive treatment of 177 patients under 75 years of age with IgG myeloma defining a circumscribed disease entity with a new staging system. Br J Haem 107:656, 1999.
9. Desikan R, Barlogie B, Sawyer J, et al: Results of a high-dose therapy for 1000 patients with multiple myeloma: Durable complete remissions and superior survival in the absence of chromosome 13 abnormalities. Blood 95:4008–4010, 2000.
10. Kyle RA: The role of bisphosphonates in multiple myeloma. Ann Intern Med 132:734–736, 2000.

Stephanie Marglin, MD
Alan L. Rothman, MD

PATIENT 72

A 54-year-old man with fever and rash after travel to the Caribbean

A 54-year-old man presents following a trip to St. Lucia. During the 4th day of his vacation, he noted vague abdominal pain and nausea. On the 8th day, while returning home, fever and chills developed. During the next 2 days, his temperature occasionally exceeded 38.3°, and he experienced severe myalgia, for which he took acetaminophen. He continued to have nausea, without anorexia or vomiting. A retro-orbital headache developed, and he had loose stools that were dark in color. On the third day after returning home, he noted an erythematous rash on his trunk and back, which spread to his arms and legs and eventually his hands.

The patient has a history of coronary artery disease and a heart murmur. He has traveled several times previously to the Caribbean without illnesses.

Physical Examination: Temperature 37.4°, blood pressure 140/78, pulse 68, respiratory rate 18. General: thin, no distress. HEENT: eyes anicteric; throat moist, no petechiae. Cardiac: regular rate with grade II/VI systolic murmur at the left sternal border. Abdomen: normal bowel sounds, soft, slightly tender to palpation in the lower quadrants, fecal occult blood test negative. Skin: warm, blanching, erythematous rash on face, trunk, and back; maculopapular rash on arms and legs, confluent erythema on palms and between fingers; petechiae on lower extremities.

Laboratory Data: WBC 3400/μl with 62% neutrophils, 23% lymphocytes, 13% monocytes; hct 37%; platelet count 200,000/μl. Liver function tests: normal.

Question: What illness would ruin a perfect vacation in paradise?

Diagnosis: Dengue fever.

Discussion: Dengue virus is a member of the family Flaviviridae, which is comprised of small, enveloped RNA viruses. Dengue virus is transmitted to humans by mosquitoes, predominantly *Aedes aegypti*, and is widely distributed in tropical and subtropical climates, including Southeast Asia, the Pacific Islands, Central and South America, and the Caribbean.

There are two syndromes associated with dengue virus infection: **dengue fever**, which is a relatively benign, self-limited illness, and **dengue hemorrhagic fever**, which can be life threatening. The incubation period is 3 to 14 days. The characteristic features of dengue fever include fever, headache, retro-orbital pain, rash, and marked muscle and joint pains. The fever typically lasts 5 to 7 days. Many patients have nausea, vomiting, or diarrhea. Some patients also develop respiratory symptoms.

All of the above symptoms may be present in patients with dengue hemorrhagic fever, but what distinguishes it from dengue fever is the development of **plasma leakage** and a **bleeding diathesis**. Plasma leakage causes hemoconcentration, pleural effusions, and ascites; the bleeding disorder manifests as marked thrombocytopenia (< 100,000/μl), petechiae, and sometimes spontaneous bleeding. Plasma leakage typically develops suddenly, over a few hours, after several days of fever. If treatment is delayed, shock may ensue (dengue shock syndrome); the case-fatality rate in this setting may be as high as 12%.

There are four serotypes of dengue virus. Infection with one serotype provides lifelong immunity to that serotype, but does not protect against infection with other serotypes. In fact, dengue hemorrhagic fever is much more common during a second dengue virus infection than during the first infection. This observation has led many to hypothesize that the plasma leakage is caused by an immunopathologic response.

The diagnosis of dengue relies on maintaining a high index of suspicion in any febrile patient who has been in an endemic area within 14 days of the onset of illness. Leukopenia, mild thrombocytopenia, and mildly elevated hepatic transaminases are supportive findings. In endemic areas, the tourniquet test is also used to support the diagnosis—a blood pressure cuff is inflated and the lower arm observed for the development of petechiae.

The differential diagnosis of dengue is broad. Malaria, leptospirosis, and typhoid fever must be considered in the setting of travel to appropriate areas. Influenza, measles, and enteroviral infection may also present similarly to dengue fever.

Serologic testing is the mainstay for laboratory diagnosis of dengue virus infection. A four-fold or greater rise in antibody titer by hemagglutination inhibition assay or IgG ELISA between acute phase and convalescent serum samples is definitive evidence of infection. A positive IgM ELISA assay on a single acute serum sample is highly suggestive; however, a negative result does not exclude this diagnosis if serum was obtained in the first week after onset of illness. Isolation of dengue virus or detection of viral RNA in serum provides a definitive diagnosis, but neither test is widely available.

Treatment for dengue fever and dengue hemorrhagic fever is supportive, as there is currently no specific antiviral treatment for dengue. Avoid aspirin and nonsteroidal anti-inflammatory drugs because of the risk of bleeding. Corticosteroids are ineffective for the treatment of established shock. Give priority to early recognition of dengue hemorrhagic fever; marked thrombocytopenia or hemoconcentration are indications for hospitalization. Administer intravenous fluids to reverse hemoconcentration.

There is currently no vaccine against dengue. To avoid dengue, travelers are advised to wear pants and long-sleeved shirts and use insect repellent.

In the present patient, the diagnosis of dengue fever was confirmed by the finding of a positive IgM ELISA. The patient recovered completely without specific therapy.

Clinical Pearls

1. Consider dengue fever as a cause of fever in any patient who traveled to the tropics within 14 days of the onset of illness.

2. The diagnosis of dengue can be confirmed by IgM ELISA on a single acute phase serum sample or hemagglutination inhibition or IgG ELISA testing on paired (acute and convalescent) sera.

3. Dengue hemorrhagic fever, a potentially life-threatening form of dengue characterized by plasma leakage, thrombocytopenia, and a bleeding tendency, is more common during second dengue virus infections.

4. Therapy for dengue fever and dengue hemorrhagic fever is supportive, and should focus on early recognition of plasma leakage and appropriate fluid resuscitation.

REFERENCES

1. Chin CK, Kang BH, Liew BK, et al: Protocol for out-patient management of dengue illness in young adults. J Trop Med Hyg 1993;96:259–263.
2. Cobra C, Rigau-Perez JG, Kuno G, Vorndam V: Symptoms of dengue fever in relation to host immunologic response and virus serotype, Puerto Rico, 1990–1991. Am J Epidemiol 1995;142:1204–1211.
3. Gubler DJ, Clark GG: Dengue/dengue hemorrhagic fever: The emergence of a global health problem. Emerg Infect Dis 1995;1:55.
4. Schwartz E, Mendelson E, Sidi Y: Dengue fever among travelers. Am J Med 1996;101:516–520.
5. Kalayanarooj S, et al: Early clinical and laboratory indicators of acute dengue illness. J Infect Dis 1997;176:313–321.
6. Pinheiro FP, Corber SJ: Global situation of dengue and dengue haemorrhagic fever, and its emergence in the Americas. World Health Stat Q 1997;50:161–169.
7. Shirtcliffe P, et al: Don't forget dengue! Clinical features of dengue fever in returning travellers. J R Coll Physicians Lond 1998;32:235–237.
8. Rothman AL, Ennis FA: Immunopathogenesis of dengue hemorrhagic fever. Virology 1999;257:1–6.

Idelle M. Weisman, MD
R. Jorge Zeballos, MD

PATIENT 73

A 24-year-old woman with unexplained exertional dyspnea

A 24-year-old soldier is referred for evaluation of exertional shortness of breath and increasing difficulty in performing her usual required exercise routine of running two to three times per week. The dyspnea started 12 months ago. Lightheadedness and weakness while running also have been noted. She is a lifelong nonsmoker with an unremarkable past medical history.

Physical Examination: Normal.

Laboratory Findings: Hemogram, hematocrit, urinalysis, thyroid function tests, chest x-ray, ECG: all normal. Pulmonary function tests: see table. Methacholine bronchoprovocation test: negative. Incremental cardiopulmonary exercise test (CPET) to volitional exhaustion: see table and figure.

Question: Based on CPET results, what is the cause of this patient's exertional dyspnea?

Pulmonary Function and Cardiopulmonary Exercise Tests

FVC: 3.72 (103%)   FEV1: 3.37 (108%)   FEV1/FVC: 91%   Dco: 24 (87%)
Maximal Incremental CPET. Cycle ergometry 15 W/min. Stop: dyspnea 8/10

Variables	Peak	% Pred	ABGs	Rest	Peak
$\dot{V}O_2$, L/min	1.84	89	SaO_2, %	94	95
A.T., % $\dot{V}O_2$pred	53%	Nor	PaO_2	86	93
HR, beats/min	167	86	$PaCO_2$	34	28
O_2 pulse, mL/beat	11	103	pH	7.39	7.38
V_E, L/min	94	71	PAO_2–PaO_2	6	12
f, breaths/min	69	High	VD/VT	0.25	0.14
V_E/VCO_2, at A.T.	41	High	Lactate	1.6	8.4

Location: 1270 m, P_B: 655 mmHg.
FVC: forced vital capacity. FEV_1: forced expiratory volume in 1 second. Dco: diffusing capacity.

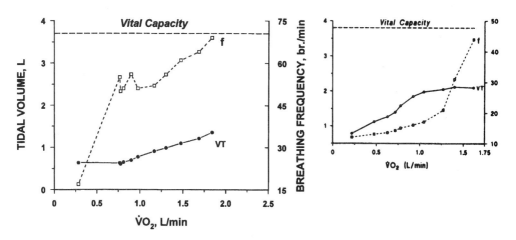

Left: The patient's breathing pattern during maximal incremental cardiopulmonary exercise test (CPET). Tidal volume (V_T) and breathing frequency (f) versus $\dot{V}O_2$. *Right:* A normal breathing pattern response during progressive CPET. Note the gradual increase in respiratory frequency and plateauing of tidal volume.

Diagnosis: Psychogenic hyperventilation.

Discussion: Exertional dyspnea is a frequent clinical problem for which a cause can be established in most cases. Several studies have noted that the most common causes include pulmonary disorders, especially reactive airways dysfunction, cardiovascular disease, psychogenic disorders including hyperventilation syndrome, deconditioning, obesity, and gastroesophageal reflux disease. An initial evaluation of the patient with exertional dyspnea includes a comprehensive medical history, detailed physical examination, and screening tests to include ECG, chest x-ray, spirometry, and appropriate laboratory tests. If the cause of exertional dyspnea remains unclear, a methacholine bronchoprovocation test is recommended to exclude hyperreactive airways disease. If a diagnosis remains elusive, a CPET is recommended.

CPET measures oxygen uptake (VO_2), carbon dioxide output (VCO_2), minute ventilation (V_E), and other variables, as well as monitors 12-lead electrocardiogram, blood pressure, and pulse oximetry or arterial blood gases during a maximal, symptom-limited exercise test. CPET provides a global assessment of functional capacity and pathophysiologic insight into the integrative exercise response (heart, lungs, and peripheral factors—muscles) that is not provided by resting cardiac and pulmonary function testing. Furthermore, CPET permits an evaluation of exercise limitation, detection of early (occult) disease, and documentation of exercise-induced hypoxemia. Increasingly, CPET is being used in the diagnostic evaluation of exertional dyspnea and is especially useful in the more challenging scenario of unexplained dyspnea, as in the present case.

The results of the CPET in this case reveal maximal/near maximal effort as demonstrated by a lactate 8.4 mmol/L and a heart rate > 85% predicted at peak exercise. VO_2 peak or aerobic (functional) capacity was normal (> 84%, 95% CI) with normal cardiovascular and ECG responses. There was significant ventilatory or breathing reserve manifested by the use of only 72% of her ventilatory capacity at peak exercise (normal $\approx$ < 80%). However, despite a normal VO_2 peak, an impressively abnormal breathing pattern is noted throughout exercise (see figure), with the respiratory frequency abruptly increasing from 16 to 50 breaths/minute during unloaded exercise, and then continuing to increase to 69 at peak exercise (normal < 60)! Tidal volume increased, but in a flattened fashion.

An abnormally (increased) ventilatory equivalent for CO_2 (V_E/VCO_2) at the anaerobic threshold and throughout exercise, but with normal V_D/V_T responses (i.e., no abnormal dead space problems) and no hypoxemia, reinforces that hyperventilation disproportionate to metabolic acidosis was responsible for the inefficient ventilation. The increase in PaO_2 with exercise is most probably due to hyperventilation. The minimal change in pH despite an impressive increase in lactate is best explained by hyperventilation due to an excessive breathing frequency and manifested by a reduced $PaCO_2$. The "turned-on" onset of rapid, shallow breathing disproportionate to the metabolic stress of exercise is highly suspicious and almost diagnostic for a psychogenic cause of unexplained exertional dyspnea.

The patient in the present case was reassured that there were no functional abnormalities responsible for her unexplained dyspnea and that some other cause was likely. At that point, she revealed some major childhood abuse problems. She was referred for psychiatric counseling. Fortunately, the patient responded to counseling and psychogenic medication. Within a year, she had resumed her regular exercise routine without problems.

Subjects with psychogenic disorders (i.e., anxiety reactions, hysteria, panic disorders, obsessional behavior, hyperventilation syndrome) may complain of several symptoms, including exertional dyspnea, chest pain, and lightheadedness. These symptoms may represent unrecognized hyperventilation due to anxiety and stress. Often, however, as in the present patient, there may be no immediately apparent psychopathology. Psychogenic disorders constitute in some series $\approx$ 30% of unexplained dyspnea cases. As such, it is important to consider these disorders in the differential diagnosis of unexplained dyspnea. Identification of hyperventilation syndrome is important since appropriate treatment is usually successful. In the present patient, early use of CPET was cost effective in avoiding additional, unnecessary testing and in facilitating therapeutic outcome.

Clinical Pearls

1. For patients with exertional dyspnea not explained by an initial evaluation consisting of a comprehensive history, physical examination, CXR, ECG, and appropriate laboratory blood testing, a bronchoprovocation challenge is warranted. Hyperreactive airways dysfunction is responsible for ≈ 30% of unexplained dyspnea and is most definitively diagnosed by a bronchoprovocation test.

2. If the bronchoprovocation challenge is nondiagnostic, a CPET is recommended.

3. Both peak and submaximal CPET response patterns, especially breathing patterns, as well as acid-base changes are helpful in establishing the diagnosis of psychogenic hyperventilation.

REFERENCES

1. Magarian GJ: Hyperventilation syndromes: infrequently recognized common expressions of anxiety and stress. Medicine 1982;61:219–236.
2. Pratter MR, Curley FJ, Dubois J, Irwin RS: Cause and evaluation of chronic dyspnea in pulmonary disease clinic. Arch Intern Med 1989;149:2277–2282.
3. DePaso WJ, Winterbauer RG, Lusk JA, et al: Chronic dyspnea unexplained by history, physical examination, chest roentgenogram, and spirometry: Analysis of a 7-year experience. Chest 1991;100:1293–1299.
4. Martinez FJ, Stanopoulos I, Acero R, et al: Graded comprehensive cardiopulmonary exercise testing in the evaluation of dyspnea unexplained by routine evaluation. Chest 1994;105:168–174.
5. Weisman IM, Zeballos RJ: An integrated approach to the interpretation of cardiopulmonary exercise testing. Clin Chest Med 1994;15:421–445.
6. Zeballos RJ, Weisman IM: Behind the scenes of cardiopulmonary exercise testing. Clin Chest Med 1994;15:193–213.
7. Gardner WN: The pathophysiology of hyperventilation disorders. Chest 1996;109:516–534.
8. Weisman IM, Zeballos RJ: Clinical evaluation of unexplained dyspnea. Cardiologia 1996;41:621–634.
9. Weisman IM, Zeballos RJ: Exercise testing. In Parsons PE, Heffner JE, (eds): Pulmonary/Respiratory Therapy Secrets. Philadelphia, Hanley & Belfus, Inc., 1997.
10. Weisman IM, Zeballos RJ: A step approach to the evaluation of unexplained dyspnea: The role of cardiopulmonary exercise testing. Pulmonary Perspectives 1998;15:8–11.

Chaim Putterman, MD
Peter Barland, MD

PATIENT 74

A 64-year-old woman with rheumatoid arthritis, facial rash, and pleuritic chest pain

A 64-year-old woman with a history of severe rheumatoid arthritis presents with a 2-week history of facial rash and left-sided pleuritic chest pain. She was diagnosed with rheumatoid arthritis 20 years ago, when she presented with fatigue, low-grade fever, morning stiffness, and symmetrical polyarthritis involving her knees, ankles, wrists, and small joints of her hands. Rheumatoid factor was strongly positive, antinuclear antibody test was negative, and the ESR was elevated at 88 mm/hr. Over the years, she has been treated with low-dose prednisone, multiple nonsteroidal anti-inflammatory drugs, and injectable gold salts with minimal relief. For the last 4 years, she has been treated with a combination regimen of maximal doses of methotrexate, sulfasalazine, and hydroxychloroquine, with good control of her symptoms. However, during the last 12 months there was a recrudescence of disease activity, with the appearance of new erosions on x-ray. Sulfasalazine was discontinued, and the patient was started on TNF-blockade therapy, with dramatic improvement.

Physical Examination: Temperature 38°, pulse 88, respirations 16, blood pressure 130/70. HEENT: erythematous malar rash. Cardiac: regular rate without murmurs or rubs. Chest: pleuritic rub at the left base, with some decreased breath sounds over the left lower lobe. Abdomen: soft without palpable organomegaly. Extremities: ulnar deviation and volar subluxation and tenderness of both wrists; no other signs of active synovitis; subcutaneous nodules palpated over both elbows.

Laboratory Findings: WBC 10,400/μl with 80% neutrophils, 1% bands, 19% lymphocytes. Electrolytes and renal indices: normal. Urinalysis: protein 30 mg/dl, 3–4 RBC/hpf, 1–2 WBC/hpf, with no casts seen. Arterial blood gas: normal. ECG: normal sinus rhythm, with no signs of pericarditis. ESR: 100 mm/hr, rheumatoid factor 200 IU/ml (normal < 20), antinuclear antibodies positive, titer 1:640, homogeneous staining pattern (normal < 1:40). Anti-double stranded DNA antibody titer elevated at 210 IU/ml (normal < 70), anti-Ro(SS-A) antibody titer elevated at 84 IU/ml (normal < 25), anti-histone antibody titer elevated at 21 IU/ml. Tests for anti-La, anti-Sm, anti-RNP, anti-cardolipin IgG and IgM antibodies: normal. C3 and C4 levels: normal. Chest radiograph: small amount of fluid at left base, lung fields clear; heart size normal.

Question: What explains the new onset of facial rash and pleuritis in this patient?

Diagnosis: Drug-induced lupus secondary to TNF-α inhibition.

Discussion: When patients with seropositive erosive rheumatoid arthritis (RA) develop a fever, malar rash, and pleuritis accompanied by a high titer antinuclear antibody (ANA) test and elevated titers of anti-DNA antibodies, several possibilities should be considered.

One possibility is a vasculitis and pleural effusion as an extra-articular feature of her RA. A vasculitis predominantly involving the skin is seen in approximately 5% of patients with seropositive RA, usually in patients with other extra-articular manifestations of RA such as subcutaneous nodules, a sensory neuropathy, and episcleritis. The rash is often papular and occurs over the extensor surfaces of the peripheral joints. Periungual infarcts are often seen. A malar rash, like that in our patient, is *not* seen. While patients with rheumatoid vasculitis often have a positive ANA test, they do not have elevated titers of anti-DNA antibodies.

Another possibility is SLE as the basic connective tissue disease with the new symptoms representing a flare of this disease. While polyarthritis and polyarthralgias are frequently the presenting symptoms of SLE, the presence of erosions and fixed deformities are extremely unusual in SLE. Also, a negative ANA test, as in the present patient, virtually excludes a diagnosis of SLE. The occurrence of both erosive RA and SLE in the same patient or clustering in the same family is also quite unusual, and the HLA-DR associations differ as well.

The most likely possibility in patients with this presentation is the development of drug-induced lupus syndrome secondary to TNF-blockade treatment. In the classic form of drug-induced lupus syndrome the most common findings are **fever, pleuropericarditis, arthralgias, pneumonitis, and rash**. Renal and CNS involvement are unusual. The most common drugs to induce this syndrome are procainamide, phenytoin, and hydralazine. More recently, carbamazepine and captopril have accounted for many reported cases of this syndrome. The clinical reactions to these drugs usually occur after prolonged exposure to the medication and are always accompanied by a strongly positive ANA test. The autoantibodies responsible for the positive ANA test are directed at the H2A-H2B histone antigens or, in the case of hydralazine, to H4 histone. Anti-n-DNA antibodies are not ordinarily found with these drugs.

The requirement for a positive ANA test as part of this syndrome may not be absolute. Recently, a clinical picture of reversible symmetrical inflammatory arthritis secondary to minocycline and quinidine has been described with negative tests for ANA and anti-histone antibodies.

More recently, TNF-α blockade with either humanized monoclonal antibodies to TNF-α (infliximab, Remicade) or soluble recombinant TNF-α receptor dimerized through linkage to human Fc chains (etanercept, Enbrel), which have been approved for the treatment of RA, have been found to elicit a lupus-like syndrome. In contrast to other drug-induced lupus syndromes, these drugs have elicited the production of anti-n-DNA antibodies. Approximately 4–15% of patients treated with TNF-α inhibition develop anti-dsDNA antibodies, albeit generally at low titers. In one large study, 3 of 770 treated patients experienced a drug-induced lupus like syndrome, which resolved after discontinuation of the medication and medical therapy. This phenomenon may be similar to the experimental observations in mouse models of SLE: TNF-α deficiency is accompanied by worsening lupus serologies and exacerbation of disease severity. The drug-induced lupus syndrome elicited by TNF-α inhibition appears to be a direct effect of the biologic activity of the drugs. This notion is supported by the observation that both etanercept and infliximab cause the same type of autoimmune response, though they are pharmacologically very different compounds. Causation by TNF-α inhibition contrasts with most other forms of drug-induced lupus, in which the syndrone appears to be mediated by pharmacologically inactive drug metabolite. Another drug used in the treatment of RA, D-penicillamine, can also cause a lupus-like syndrome accompanied by anti-n-DNA antibodies.

Our patient has also been on sulfasalazine. The number of anecdotal reports describing a drug-induced lupus syndrome in patients with RA treated with sulfasalazine has been increasing. Preliminary studies suggest an increased risk in patients with the slow-acetylator phenotype. Although sulfasalazine is a possible offender in our patient, development of drug-induced lupus after the medication had already been stopped and the presence of anti-DNA antibodies would be most unusual.

Although at the present time drug-induced autoantibodies and lupus-like manifestations do not seem like a critical problem given the effectiveness of anti-TNF-α drugs in RA and the low incidence of these reactions, recognition of these side effects by physicians may save unnecessary time and effort in diagnosis and treatment.

The present patient proved to have drug-induced lupus secondary to TNF-α inhibition. She improved with discontinuation of this agent.

Clinical Pearls

1. TNF-α inhibition therapy can cause a drug-induced lupus syndrome.
2. TNF-α inhibition therapy can induce anti-n-DNA antibodies.
3. The drug-induced lupus syndrome from TNF-α inhibition includes anti-n-DNA antibodies and malar rash—findings not present in the autoimmune syndromes induced by most other drugs.
4. Minocycline can induce a lupus-like reaction without anti-nuclear antibodies.

REFERENCES

1. Jorizzo JL, Daniels JC: Dermatologic conditions reported in patients with rheumatoid arthritis. J Am Acad Derm 1983; 8:439–457.
2. Bray VJ, West SG, Scjultz KT, Boumpas DT, Rubin RL: Antihistone antibody profile in sulfasalazine-induced lupus. J Rheum 1994; 21:2157–2158.
3. Bacon PA, Carruthers D: Vasculitis associated with connective tissue disorders. Rheum Dis Clin NA 1995; 21:1077–1096.
4. Laversuch CJ, Collins DA, Charles PJ, Bourke BE: Sulfasalazine-induced autoimmune abnormalities in patients with rheumatic disease. Brit J Rheum 1995;34:435–439.
5. Gunnarsson I, Kanerud L, Pettersson E, Lundberg I: Predisposing factors in sulfasalazine-induced systemic lupus erythematosus. Brit J Rheum 1997; 36:1089–1094.
6. Maini R, St Clair EW, Breedveld F, et al: Infliximab (chimeric anti-tumor necrosis alpha monoclonal antibody) versus placebo in rheumatoid arthritis receiving concomitant methotrexate: a randomized phase III trial. Lancet 1999; 354:1932–1939.
7. Weinblatt ME, Kramer JM, Bankhurst AD, et al: A trial of etanercept, a recombinant tumor necrosis factor: Fc fusion protein in patients with rheumatoid arthritis receiving methotrexate. N Engl J Med 1999; 340–253–259.
8. Watts RA: Musculoskeletal and systemic reactions to biological therapeutic agents. Curr Opin Rheumatol 2000; 12:49–52.

C. W. Legerton III, M.D.

PATIENT 75

A 35-year-old woman with chest pain 4 days after labor and delivery

A 35-year-old woman presents to the emergency department 4 days after delivery of her first child. She complains of pleuritic chest pain, which developed a few hours earlier. She has a history of a left lower extremity deep venous thrombosis (DVT) 5 years ago which was treated for 6 months, initially with intravenous heparin and subsequently with warfarin. At that time, she remembers that her platelet count was low, believed due to heparin-induced thrombocytopenia. Her only other history is a prior pregnancy that resulted in a fetal loss early in the second trimester.

Physical Examination: Vital signs: normal, except for respiratory rate 18. General: healthy appearing. Skin: livedo reticularis on legs (see figure). HEENT: unremarkable. Chest: clear. Cardiac: decrescendo diastolic murmur best heard in aortic area with patient sitting upright. Abdomen: normal. Musculoskeletal: normal. Neurologic: normal.

Laboratory Findings: Hct 38%, MCV 89, platelet count 80,000/μl. Chemistry: normal. Urinalysis: normal. ABG (room air): pH 7.44, PCO_2 32 mmHg, PO_2 80 mmHg. Chest radiograph: normal. Ventilation perfusion scan: high probability for pulmonary embolism.

Questions: What is the most likely cause of this patient's pulmonary embolus (PE)? What diagnostic laboratory tests should be obtained?

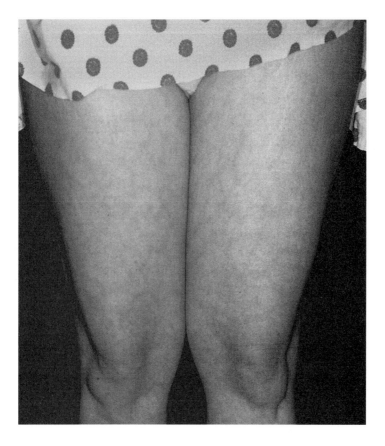

Diagnosis: Antiphospholipid syndrome.

Discussion: The antiphospholipid (aPL) syndrome is a hypercoagulable state comprised of clinical events combined with a positive test for antibodies to phospholipids or a "lupus anticoagulant" or both. The syndrome may occur in a primary form without associated disease, or may occur secondarily to another disease, such as systemic lupus erythematosis.

The classic triad of clinical features of this disease includes thrombosis, recurrent fetal demise, and thrombocytopenia. The thrombosis is severe and may include either arterial or venous thrombotic events. Fetal demise may occur in the first or second trimester and is felt to occur due to thrombosis of the placental vasculature with resultant placental insufficiency. Other clinical features may include livedo reticularis, cardiac valvular disease, or ischemic leg ulcers. Less common manifestations may result from the thrombotic occlusion of other vascular beds, including renal, adrenal, central nervous system, or even an acute, widespread, multi-organ involvement often called the "catastrophic" aPL syndrome. Features of this case that should raise concern about the aPL syndrome include the two thromboembolic events (DVT and PE), thrombocytopenia, fetal demise, livedo reticularis, and murmur of aortic insufficiency.

Much confusion surrounds the appropriate laboratory testing for this disorder. Any one of several tests or a multiple of these tests can be positive. The test for aPL (or anticardiolipin) antibodies most likely detects antibodies to any one of a number of phospholipids. Cardiolipin is most commonly employed, and hence the name, but these antibodies may recognize other antigens as well. Strong evidence implicates a phospholipid-binding protein, B_2 glycoprotein I, as the actual antigen recognized by these so-called antiphospholipid antibodies. Tests for antibodies to B_2 glycoprotein I can also be ordered, and evidence suggests that this test may be more sensitive and specific for the clinical syndrome than aPL antibodies. The IgG isotype of aPL antibody is associated more commonly with the clinical syndrome, but an isolated IgM or IgA antibody may be associated with disease. Since this test is an enzyme-linked immunosorbent assay (ELISA), patients may be anticoagulated when this test is drawn.

Tests for a lupus anticoagulant are functional clotting tests, and are believed to be more specific for the clinical syndrome than tests for aPL antibodies, but less sensitive. Any of a number of tests may be performed in a given laboratory. Commonly performed assays include an activated partial thromboplastin time, or a dilute Russell vipor venom assay. The common underlying principle to any of these tests for a lupus anticoagulant is that the patient's antibodies bind available phospholipid in the coagulation assay and increase the time to clot formation. Thus, the ratio of the patient's clotting time compared to control is increased. A mixing study will not correct, distinguishing the presence of an inhibitor from a deficiency of a clotting factor. As this is a functional test, patients may not be anticoagulated when this test is drawn unless special measures are taken to account for the anticoagulation.

Treatment involves full anticoagulation, which has been shown to reduce the incidence of recurrent thrombotic events. Warfarin is typically prescribed to attain an INR of 2.5–3.0. As warfarin is contraindicated in pregnancy, most of these women are treated with heparin plus low-dose aspirin. Increasingly, low-molecular-weight (LMW) heparin is being used in pregnancy, again in concert with low-dose aspirin. Due to pregnancy-induced fluctuations in clotting times, use of LMW heparin plus aspirin simplifies monitoring of the patient's anticoagulation.

In the present case, both activated partial thromboplastin time and dilute Russell viper venom time tests were prolonged. An ELISA test was positive for the presence of an antibody to cardiolipin. The patient was anticoagulated with heparin and subsequently converted to warfarin to maintain an INR of 3.0.

Clinical Pearls

1. The antiphospholipid syndrome is characterized by a wide variety of clinical features related to hypercoagulability. Chief among these are venous and arterial thromboses, recurrent pregnancy loss, and thrombocytopenia.

2. Diagnostic testing for the aPL syndrome requires the performance of both an ELISA test for antibodies to phospholipid and a battery of functional tests to define an inhibitor to coagulation.

3. Diagnosis of the aPL syndrome is made in the presence of both clinical events and at least one positive diagnostic test.

4. Treatment is centered around the maintenance of full anticoagulation.

REFERENCES

1. Brewer PMC, Roseove MH: Antiphospholipid thrombosis: Clinical course after the first thrombotic event in 70 patients. Ann Intern Med 1992;117:303–308.
2. Harris EN, et al: A retrospective review of 61 patients with antiphospholipid syndrome. Analysis of factors influencing recurrent thrombosis. Arch Intern Med 1997;157(18):2101–2108.
3. Petri M: Pathogenesis and treatment of the antiphospholipid antibody syndrome. Med Clin North Am 1997;81(1):151–177.
4. Asherson RA, et al: Catastrophic antiphospholipid syndrome. Clinical and laboratory features of 50 patients. Medicine 1998;77(3):195–207.
5. Anonymous: Case records of Massachusetts General Hospital. Weekly clinicopathological exercises. Case 18-1999. A 54-year-old woman with acute renal failure and thrombocytopenia [clinical conference]. New Engl J Med 1999;340(24):1900–1908.
6. Branch DW, et al: International consensus statement on preliminary classification criteria for definite antiphospholipid syndrome. Arthritis Rheum 1999;42:1309–1311.
7. Roubey RA: Immunology of the antiphospholipid syndrome: Antibodies, antigens, and autoimmune response (Review). Thrombosis Haemostasis 1999;82(2):656–661.

Katherine P. Hendra, MD
Harrison W. Farber, MD

PATIENT 76

A 40-year-old man with dyspnea on exertion and productive cough

A 40-year-old man presents with progressive dyspnea on exertion, which has worsened over the last 2 years. He reports a cough productive of white sputum, but denies wheezing, fever, chills, night sweats, dyspnea at rest, or previous pulmonary disease. He smokes two packs of cigarettes per day and also reports a history of intravenous drug use.

Physical Examination: Temperature 37°, pulse 80, respirations 16. Oxygen saturation (room air): 96%. HEENT: unremarkable. Cardiac: regular rate, without murmur. Chest: bilateral, fine inspiratory crackles. Abdomen: unremarkable, with positive bowel sounds. Extremities: no cyanosis, clubbing, edema, or rash.

Laboratory Findings: CBC: normal. Chest radiograph: bilateral, tiny, mid-lung nodules. Pulmonary function tests: FEV_1 65%, FEV_1/FVC ratio 70%, DLCO 60% of predicted. Arterial blood gas (room air, *at rest*): pH 7.44, pCO_2 38 mmHg, pO_2 78 mmHg. Cardiopulmonary exercise testing: maximum VO_2, maximum O_2 pulse and delta VO_2/delta decreased, maximum heart rate 100% predicted, breathing reserve 30 L/min. Arterial blood gas (room air, *during exercise*): pO_2 65 mmHg. High-resolution chest CT: diffuse 2- to 3-mm nodules and diffuse ground-glass pattern throughout both lung fields; small areas of peripheral emphysema at lung bases (see figure).

Question: What might explain this patient's dyspnea?

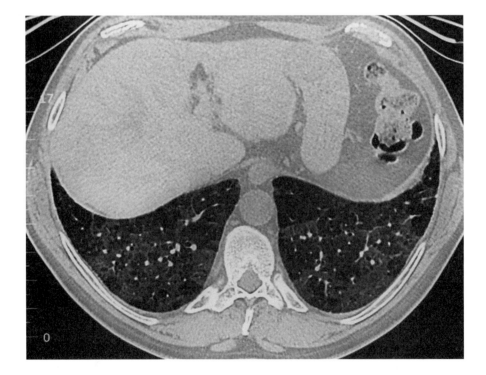

Diagnosis: Foreign body granulomatosis.

Discussion: Tablets intended for oral use contain **insoluble binding agents** such as talc, microcrystalline cellulose, potato starch, and cornstarch; when abused, they are pulverized, dissolved in water, and injected. Medications abused in this manner include methylphenidate hydrochloride (Ritalin), oral opiates, amphetamines, and antihistamines. Cellulose and talc, the most widely used fillers, can cause significant pulmonary damage. Moreover, after the tablets are pulverized, they are often heated and filtered through materials such as cotton wool; embolized cottonwool fragments may lead to additional pulmonary damage such as granuloma formation. In heroin addicts, this does not usually occur because heroin is mixed with soluble fillers such as quinine, lactose, or maltose. However, in cocaine users, particulate or foreign body embolization can occur. Thus, depending on the type of addiction, the incidence of foreign body granulomatosis in autopsy series of addicts ranges from 15–80%; yet, foreign body granulomatosis is a clinical issue in less than 5% of pulmonary complications of drug abuse.

The pathophysiology of foreign body granulomatosis varies with the responsible agent. **Talc** contains an insoluble agent that causes an initial arteritis associated with a rapid influx of neutrophils. Foreign body granulomas are formed as talc particles migrate into the perivascular and pulmonary interstitial tissue. Eventually, coalescence of small discrete nodules may occur, predominantly in a periphilar and upper lobe distribution. Emphysema, due to alveolar wall necrosis, can develop in the lower lobes. Nodules, diffuse interstitial fibrosis, and massive fibrosis have been described. Autopsy series of intravenous drug abusers have also demonstrated talc in other organs, including the spleen, liver, bone marrow, heart, and kidney. **Cellulose** can cause a process similar pathologically to talc. **Potato starch** and **cornstarch** appear to be removed rapidly from the lung and are associated with fewer pulmonary complications. Because cellulose and starch particles are much larger than talc, these agents are less likely to embolize to other organs.

Most patients with foreign body granulomatosis due to injected agents present with nonspecific complaints, such as cough, dyspnea, and an increase in sputum production. Abusers of intravenous drugs containing talc or a similar substance may experience a rapid decline in pulmonary function in comparison to individuals injecting unadulterated agents such as heroin. Patients may also present with acute pulmonary hypertension, spontaneous pneumothorax, acute respiratory distress

syndrome, progressive massive fibrosis, and panlobular emphysema. Physical exam is often unremarkable, although bibasilar end-inspiratory crackles and ophthalmological abnormalities such as birefringent particles in retinal vessels have been described. Laboratory testing is also unremarkable, except that an elevated angiotensin converting enzyme level is common. Pulmonary function testing usually reveals a decreased DLCO and either an obstructive or restrictive pattern on spirometry. Exercise testing in patients with foreign body granulomatosis may reveal a decreased arterial oxygen tension, an increase in dead space ventilation, and findings consistent with pulmonary vascular disease. Radiographic abnormalities include widespread, small, well-defined nodules often in the mid lung zones. As the disease progresses these nodules can coalesce, and massive fibrosis may be seen. High-resolution CT of the chest may demonstrate small nodules, a diffuse ground-glass appearance, confluent perihilar masses containing areas of high attenuation consistent with talc deposits, adenopathy, and severe peripheral emphysema. Lower-lobe panacinar emphysema appears more common in methylphenidate abusers than in nonmethylphenidate drug abusers.

Although the clinical history and radiographic findings may be highly suggestive of foreign body granulomatosis, further diagnostic evaluation such as bronchoscopy and/or lung biopsy are often necessary. **Lung biopsy** typically reveals fibrosis and aggregates of multinucleated foreign body giant cells containing birefringent, plate-like talc crystals. The size, shape, and color of the particles with polarizing light and PAS staining may distinguish the type of injected substance. Vascular changes include mild medial muscular hypertrophy in small- and medium-sized arteries. **Bronchoalveolar lavage** (BAL) demonstrates a marked lymphocytosis with a predominance of CD8+ lymphocytes. Inspection of BAL fluid with polarized light may reveal crystalline material. Though transbronchial or fine needle biopsy specimens of pulmonary masses may be diagnostic, the yield is less than with open lung biopsy.

The differential diagnosis of foreign body granulomatosis includes other causes of emphysema, interstitial lung disease, and granulomatosis lung disease. Alpha-1 antitrypsin deficiency should be excluded. Consider sarcoidosis, beryllium exposure, and other causes of granulomatosis lung disease. Although immunosuppressive agents have been successful in limiting lymphocyte activation and decreasing granuloma size in animal models of foreign body granulomatosis, experience in humans is extremely limited. For example, corticosteroids appear to have a limited role in patients with talc-induced granulomas. Although selected patients—particularly those with less vascular pathology—may have an initial improvement, little information exists regarding dosage duration, tapering, and durability of response. Pulmonary hypertension associated with foreign body granulomatosis may be responsive to vasodilator therapy. Lung transplantation has been successful in some patients with severe pulmonary hypertension secondary to foreign body granulomatosis. Most patients injecting pills containing talc or cellulose have poor outcomes secondary to severe emphysema, pulmonary hypertension, hypoxemia, and progressive interstitial lung disease. Patients who have injected fewer pills and discontinue injection drug and tobacco abuse may have a better prognosis.

In the present patient the diagnosis was strongly suspected due to the history, radiographic findings, and physiologic testing that demonstrated pulmonary vascular disease with exercise-induced hypoxemia. The patient subsequently underwent an open lung biopsy, which demonstrated extensive foreign body granulomatosis and material consistent with talc. Vasodilator therapy resulted in decreased pulmonary vascular resistance; however, the patient was unable to tolerate the systemic effects of the medication. Despite discontinuation of intravenous injection and cigarettes, the patient ultimately died of progressive hypoxemia and cor pulmonale.

Clinical Pearls

1. Patients with foreign body granulomatosis may present with rapidly progressive pulmonary pathology.

2. Exercise testing in these patients often reveals evidence of pulmonary vascular disease.

3. Vasodilator therapy may benefit patients with foreign body granulomatosis and associated pulmonary hypertension.

REFERENCES

1. Itkonen J, Schnoll S, Daghestani A, et al: Accelerated development of pulmonary complications due to illicit intravenous use of pentazocine and tripelennamine. Am J Med 1984;76:617–612.
2. Kringsholm B, Christoffersen P: The nature and occurrence of birefringent material in different organs in fatal drug addiction. Forensic Sci Int 1987;34:53–62.
3. Farber HW, Fairman RP, Millen JE, et al: Pulmonary response to foreign body microemboli in dogs: Release of neutrophil chemoatractant activity by vascular endothelial cells. Am J Respir Cell Mol Biol 1989;1:27–35.
4. Pare JP, Cote G, Fraser RS: Long term follow-up of abusers with intravenous talcosis. Am Rev Respir Dis 1989; 139:233–241.
5. Rhodes RE, Chiles C, Vick WW: Talc granulomatosis presenting as spontaneous pneumothorax. South Med J 1991;84:929–930.
6. Schmidt RA, Glenny RW, Goodwin JD, et al: Panlobular emphysema in young intravenous Ritalin abusers. Am Rev Respir Dis 1991;143:649–656.
7. Hashimoto M, Kobayashi K, Yamagata N, et al: Suppression of pulmonary granulomatous inflammation by immunosuppressive agents. Agents Actions 1992:37:99–106.
8. Ward S, Heyneman LE, Reittner P, et al: Talcosis associated with IV abuse of oral medications: CT findings. AJR Am J Roentgenol 2000;174:789–793.

John E. Heffner, MD

PATIENT 77

A 43-year-old man with pneumonia and severe hypotension

A 43-year-old man presents with a 3-day history of shortness of breath and diffuse chest pain accompanied by fever, purulent sputum, and nausea. He also notes sharp, left-sided chest pain when he takes a deep breath. The patient smokes cigarettes and occasionally injects himself with intravenous illicit drugs. Four days before admission, he injected heroin into a "neck vein."

Physical Examination: Temperature 36.4°, pulse 78, respirations 22, blood pressure 105/55 mmHg. General: moderate discomfort with breathing. Skin: decreased turgor. Neck: no venous distension at 30° upright. Chest: crackles, tubular breath sounds, and decreased fremitus at the left lung base. Cardiac: no murmurs, rubs, or gallops. Abdomen: benign. Rectal: negative for occult blood. Extremities: no edema.

Laboratory Findings: Hct 39%, WBC 11,400/μl with 76% neutrophils and 9% bands, Na⁺ 141 mEq/L, K⁺ 3.5 mEq/L, Cl⁻ 101 mEq/L, HCO₃⁻ 26 mEq/L, BUN 30 mg/dl, creatinine 1.5 mg/dl. Sputum: patient could not produce. Chest radiograph (see below, *left*): left lower lobe alveolar opacification, increased cardiac silhouette. ECG: borderline low voltage in frontal leads.

Hospital Course: The patient was started on intravenous nafcillin and ticarcillin disodium-clavulanic acid for a presumed pneumonia. A chest CT scan (see below, *right*) was obtained to evaluate mediastinal structures and the pleural space. On return from radiology, rigors, hypotension with a blood pressure of 90/40, tachycardia with a heart rate of 125, and severe dyspnea developed.

Question: What is the most likely cause of the patient's sudden deterioration?

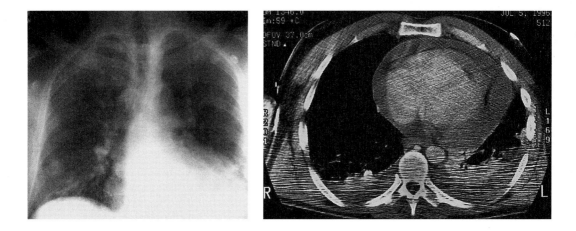

Diagnosis: Sepsis with intrapleural empyema and cardiac tamponade from purulent pericarditis.

Discussion: Purulent pericarditis was a common condition in the pre-antibiotic era and accounted for 40% of all etiologies for pericarditis in general. As many as 0.8% of autopsies detected postmortem evidence of purulent pericarditis. Since the advent of antibiotics, pericardial infections are much less common and are found in only 0.006% of autopsies. Although a relatively rare disorder, it remains an acute and potentially catastrophic condition that is, in most instances, difficult to diagnose. The diagnosis is first suspected in most patients only after the onset of cardiac tamponade and severe hemodynamic instability, when the infection has already progressed to a severe degree.

Four primary mechanisms exist for the development of purulent pericarditis: (1) spread of infection from contiguous sites within the chest, (2) spread from a cardiac source of infection, such as endocarditis, (3) hematogenous spread from a distant site, and (4) direct inoculation of the pericardium as a result of cardiothoracic surgery or penetrating trauma. Underlying conditions that cause pericardial abnormalities, such as uremia, postoperative pericarditis, and collagen vascular diseases, predispose patients for purulent pericarditis. Pneumonia with contiguous spread of infection is the most commonly found underlying disease. Up to 50% of patients with purulent pericarditis have an associated **intrapleural empyema**. The second most common underlying condition is a distant site f infection with hematogenous spread. Rarely, there is no identifiable primary source of infection.

Patients with purulent pericarditis most often present in an acute and fulminant manner, with obvious signs and symptoms of a severe infectious disease. Patients may complain of cough, shortness of breath, fever, and shaking chills. Various forms of chest pain due to pericardial inflammation and associated conditions, such as empyema, are common occurrences. Characteristic patterns of pain associated with pericarditis, however, occur in less than a third of patients. Cardiac tamponade produces signs and symptoms of hemodynamic instability. Other manifestations of purulent pericarditis vary depending on the existence and nature of a primary site of infection. The prehospital course of symptoms is usually < 3 days in duration. Typically, the presenting clinical features are ascribed to a more apparent site of infection, such as pneumonia or endocarditis, which can obscure the presence of the pericardial infection. For this reason, < 50% of patients in most series who die with purulent pericarditis have an antemortem diagnosis.

Cardiac tamponade is the most serious complication of purulent pericarditis. Rapid development of pericardial fluid compromises cardiac filling and decreases cardiac output. In order to maintain blood pressure, patients initiate compensatory mechanisms, which include increased blood volume, elevated diastolic intracardiac pressures, tachycardia, and vasoconstriction. When the degree of tamponade supercedes these compensatory mechanisms or when vasodilation due to sepsis or intravascular volume depletion intervenes, sudden and life-threatening drops in blood pressure occur.

A diverse array of microbiologic pathogens have been described associated with purulent pericarditis. In most clinical series, however, *Staphylococcus aureus* is the most commonly isolated agent, accounting for 30% of all instances of the disease. Other common bacteria include *Streptococcus pneumoniae*, other *Streptococcal* species, *Haemophilus pneumoniae*, and aerobic gram-negative rods. Anaerobic pathogens are frequently isolated in up to 40% of patients with purulent pericarditis in institutions that have specialized laboratory skills and resources for anaerobic microbiology. Various fungal pathogens, such as *Actinomycetes* and *Nocardia* species, have the capacity to cause purulent pericarditis.

The diagnosis requires a high clinical suspicion because of the underlying infectious conditions that can obscure the pericardial site of infection. Moreover, the presence of cardiac tamponade may be difficult to recognize in patients who present with signs and symptoms of generalized sepsis. Only a small minority of patients with cardiac tamponade present with the classic triad of hypotension, elevated neck veins, and a quiet precordium. Although elevated neck veins are the most sensitive of these findings, establishing their presence is difficult in critically ill patients. More common manifestations of tamponade, such as dyspnea, abdominal discomfort, and sinus tachycardia are nonspecific and usually ascribed to other more clinically obvious conditions. Pulsus paradoxus occurs in only three-quarters of patients. Friction rubs are frequently absent; their presence in purulent pericarditis portends a poor prognosis.

Routine laboratory and imaging studies have a similarly low diagnostic value for identifying the presence of purulent pericarditis or cardiac tamponade. Standard chest radiographic findings of an enlarged cardiac silhouette have little diagnostic value because a rapidly developing, small pericardial effusion can produce tamponade without enlarging the silhouette. The ECG findings of low voltage, electrical alternans, and P-R segment depression are classic manifestations of pericardial tamponade, but recent case series indicate that they have

232

an extremely poor sensitivity. **Cardiac catheterization** and **echocardiography** remain the diagnostic procedures of choice to establish the presence of cardiac tamponade. Echocardiography is preferred because it is noninvasive and can detect the presence of pericardial fluid before tamponade occurs. Some patients may be first suspected as having purulent pericarditis when an incidental chest CT demonstrates pericardial fluid with thick pericardial membranes. CT may be more sensitive than ultrasound for identifying pericardial fluid and may suggest the infectious nature of pericarditis by providing information on fluid density and the thickness of the pericardium.

Pericardiocentesis remains the diagnostic procedure of choice for confirming the presence of purulent pericarditis. Detection of purulent fluid or a positive pleural fluid Gram stain or culture are diagnostic. Suggestive findings in the appropriate clinical setting include a pleural fluid leukocyte count > 50,000/μl, protein > 3 g/dl, glucose < 40 mg/dl, and lactate dehydrogenase > 4000 U/L.

Management of purulent pericarditis requires the *prompt* initiation of **antibiotic therapy** and effective **drainage of the pericardial space**. Medical therapy alone has an unacceptably high mortality rate that approaches 100%. Empiric antibiotic therapy is directed at pathogens previously isolated from primary sites of infection or the common etiologic agents of purulent pericarditis. Identification of pathogens in pericardial fluid and their drug susceptibility patterns guide subsequent therapy. Although consensus exists regarding the need to establish drainage, the selection of the specific drainage procedure is controversial and benefits from individualization of care. Some patients with early infection and free-flowing pericardial fluid may respond to pericardiocentesis alone or percutaneous catheter drainage. Patients with more established infections with intrapericardial loculations or viscous pericardial fluid require surgical drainage. Subxiphoid pericardiotomy is effective in most patients, although some may require a partial or complete pericardiectomy to prevent an early recurrence of tamponade. A few reports exist of intrapericardial instillation of fibrinolytic agents to promote adequate drainage of pericardial fluid.

Despite adequate therapy, the mortality of purulent pericarditis remains as high as 40–80%. Most patients, however, die of the underlying disease or site of infection rather than the hemodynamic instability of cardiac tamponade. Pericardial constriction due to thickened pericardial membranes may occur during the early phase of recovery, but chronic constriction is rare in long-term survivors of purulent pericarditis.

The present patient had CT evidence of a left pleural effusion, left lower lobe infiltrate, and pericardial fluid. He stabilized with aggressive fluid resuscitation; an echocardiogram demonstrated cardiac tamponade. Pericardiocentesis with placement of an intrapericardial catheter resulted in hemodynamic stabilization. A left chest tube was required for drainage of an empyema. Both the pericardial and pleura fluid grew *S. aureus*. He gradually improved and was discharged 2 weeks later with good cardiopulmonary function. From the history and clinical course, it was conjectured that the patient developed a cervical infection from his drug injections that resulted in descending mediastinitis, which progressed to empyema and purulent pericarditis.

Clinical Pearls

1. Although pneumonia with contiguous spread of infection is the most common cause of purulent pericarditis, it can also occur from a cardiac or extrathoracic site of infection or from direct inoculation by trauma or surgery.

2. Patients with pre-existing pericardial abnormalities, as caused by collagen vascular disorders, uremia, or post-operative pericarditis, are at increased risk for purulent pericarditis.

3. Physical findings, 12-lead electrocardiograms, and standard chest radiographs have a low sensitivity and specificity for cardiac tamponade.

4. *S. aureus* is the most common etiologic agent for purulent pericarditis; pericardial infections can also occur from *S. pneumoniae*, other *Streptococcal* species, *H. pneumoniae*, aerobic gram-negative rods, and anaerobic pathogens.

REFERENCES

1. Isner JM, Carter BL, Bankoff ME, et al: Computed tomography in the diagnosis of pericardial heart disease. Ann Intern Med 1982;97:473–479.
2. Sagristà-Sauleda J, Barrabés JA, Permanyer-Miralda G, Soler-Soler J: Purulent pericarditis: Review of a 20-year experience in a general hospital. J Am Coll Cardiol 1993;22:1661–1665.
3. Winkler W-B, Karni R, Slany J: Treatment of exudative fibrinous pericarditis with intrapericardial urokinase. Lancet 1994;344:1541–1542.
4. Brook I, Frazier E: Microbiology of acute purulent pericarditis. A 12-year experience in a military hospital. Arch Intern Med 1996;156:1857–1860.
5. Eisenberg MJ, Munoz de Romeral L, Heidenreich PA, et al: The diagnosis of pericardial effusion and cardiac tamponade by 12-lead ECG. A technology assessment. Chest 1996;110:318–324.

Acknowledgement: This case has been modified from Heffner JE: What caused severe hypotension in this 43-year-old man with pneumonia? J Crit Illness 1998;13:37–40.

Robert A. Larson, MD
Ronald M. Fairman, MD

PATIENT 78

A 35-year-old man with sudden onset of left flank pain, fever, and hypertension

A 35-year-old man, normally in good health, experienced sudden left flank pain that radiated to the front. The pain was constant and tearing. He denies nausea, vomiting, diarrhea, dysuria, or hematuria. He also denies a history of kidney stones, hernias, or previous abdominal surgery. His only past history is for a head injury 15 years ago that required a craniotomy.

Physical Examination: Temperature 38°, pulse 100, blood pressure 210/100. General: uncomfortable, but not in distress. HEENT: unremarkable. Cardiac: tachycardic, regular rate with no murmurs. Chest: lungs clear bilaterally, moderate left costovertebral angle tenderness. Abdomen: soft, non-distended, non-tender, normal bowel sounds, no masses, no bruits. Extremities: no rashes; no edema; palpable femoral pulses bilaterally, but posterior tibial and dorsalis pedis pulses palpable only on the right leg.

Laboratory Findings: WBC 5700/µL, HCT 39%, creatinine 1.2 mg/dl. Urinalysis: trace occult blood. Electrocardiogram: normal. Chest radiograph: normal. Intravenous urogram: delayed excretion by left kidney, but no ureteral dilatation or stones. Abdominal CT scan: see figure below. Aortogram: see figures, next page.

Question: What is the cause of this patient's constellation of symptoms?

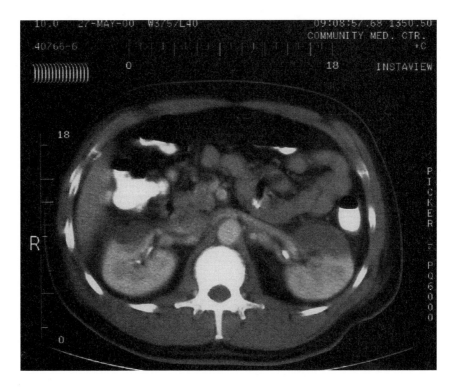

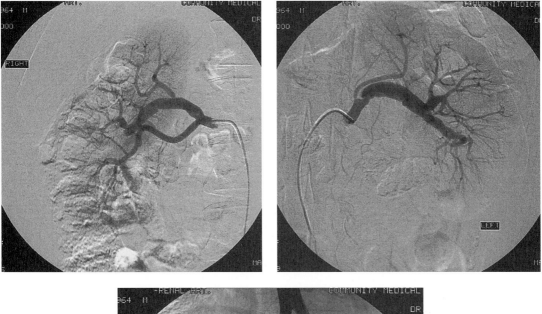

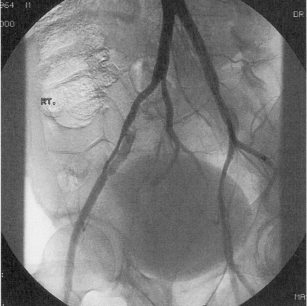

Diagnosis: Spontaneous renal artery dissection secondary to fibromuscular dysplasia with bilateral renal parenchymal infarcts.

Discussion: Fibromuscular dysplasia (FMD) is a heterogeneous group of mostly fibrotic arteriopathies that typically present as thickening in the arterial media. FMD most commonly affects females in the fourth to fifth decades (80%). Approximately 5–10% of patients with FMD experience arterial dissections because of the disease. There are about 150 cases of FMD with arterial dissection reported in the literature, but angiographic studies suggest an incidence of 0.04%. Unlike the average patient with FMD, these patients are predominantly male and in their third to fifth decade. The cause of the disease is still unclear, but it is believed that mural hematomas develop within the media and rupture through the intima, allowing a dissection plane to develop. The dissections can occur wherever the FMD is present, and have been reported in the renal arteries, carotid arteries, iliac arteries, and even in the aorta.

Patients who present with renal artery dissection with parenchymal ischemia generally complain of flank pain on the affected side. The renal parenchymal infarction can result in fevers, nausea, and vomiting. Hypertension can be caused by renal infarction, but patients with renal artery dissections may also have a component of renal artery stenosis; both mechanisms are felt to be renin-mediated. Laboratory findings generally include an elevated lactate dehydrogenase, trace to extensive proteinuria, and either microscopic or gross hematuria. These tests were not obtained in this patient on presentation.

Most patients with spontaneous renal artery dissections have a stable course, often requiring antihypertensive therapy. Approximately 10% of these patients have recurring episodes of dissection with worsening hypertension and renal function.

The key to this diagnosis is recognizing the connection between the acute onset of hypertension, flank pain, and the laboratory findings in this relatively young man. The symptoms often mimic those of kidney stones, and an intravenous urogram is usually obtained but rarely helpful. An abdominal CT scan with intravenous contrast is very sensitive at detecting areas of renal parenchymal infarction (see figure, page 235). Even if there is no renal infarction, it is often possible to detect pathology within the main renal arteries (such as dissections or aneurysms) on a quality high-resolution CT scan. The gold standard for detecting and characterizing renal artery dissections is **angiography**. It is possible to discern irregularities in the renal arteries from the main branch to the intra-parenchymal vessels (see top figures, page 236). This patient had evidence of chronic dissections in both the right and left renal arteries that extended to the distal branch vessels. Dissections also were noted within his external iliac arteries (70% on right, 50% on left; see bottom figure, page 236).

The treatment of patients with spontaneous renal artery dissections depends on the severity of their hypertension, the extent of the dissection, and the amount of renal parenchyma at risk. Most patients described in the literature have had hypertension controllable with one or two agents along with normal or only mildly decreased renal function. In young patients with severe hypertension or evidence of severely decreased blood flow to a kidney, an aggressive approach to surgical repair has been advocated. In patients with dissections that extend to the peripheral vessels of the kidney, a nephrectomy is the only surgical option and will restore normotension. If the lesions are limited to the main renal artery, an *in situ* repair can often be performed. For lesions that extend into the first or second order branches of the renal artery, an *ex vivo* repair may be possible. This entails removing the affected kidney, perfusing it with cold preservation fluid, reconstructing the vessels on the backtable, and autotransplantation. This is not performed frequently and requires a surgeon with considerable experience.

In the present patient, dissections extended throughout both renal arteries to the parenchyma, and thus he was not a candidate for surgical repair. He had hypertension that was well controlled on enalapril, and had only a slightly elevated creatinine. He has done well since his initial presentation and has had no further symptoms.

Clinical Pearls

1. Spontaneous renal artery dissection is an uncommon but important cause of new onset hypertension and flank pain in young patients, especially men.

2. A CT scan with intravenous contrast can diagnose renal infarction, renal artery disease stenoses, occlusions, segmental perfusion defects, and even urolithiasis.

3. The gold standard for evaluation of renal artery pathology is angiography; however, MRA is becoming more accurate in defining renal artery anatomy.

REFERENCES

1. Hare WS: Dynamic CT diagnosis of primary dissecting aneurysm of the renal artery. Urol Radiol 1985; 7(2):106–108.
2. Mokri B, Stanson AW, Houser OW: Spontaneous dissections of the renal arteries in a patient with previous spontaneous dissections of the internal carotid arteries. Stroke 1985; 16(6):959–963.
3. Beroniade V, Roy P, Froment D, Pison C: Primary renal artery dissection. Presentation of two cases and brief review of the literature. Am J Nephrol 1987;7:382–389.
4. Reilly LM, Cunningham CG, Maggisano R, et al: The role of arterial reconstruction in spontaneous renal artery dissection. J Vasc Surg 1991;14(4): 468–477; discussion 477–479.
5. Gatalica Z, Gibas Z, Martinez-Hernandez A: Dissecting aortic aneurysm as a complication of generalized fibromuscular dysplasia [see comments]. Hum Pathol 1992;23:586–588.
6. Martin X, Salas M, Bouvier R, et al: Extracorporeal repair of primary renal artery dissection. Eur Urol 1993;24:424-427.
7. Alamir A, Middendorf DF, Baker P, et al: Renal artery dissection causing renal infarction in otherwise healthy men. Am J Kidney Dis 1997;30:851-855.

David H. Ingbar, MD

PATIENT 79

A 25-year-old woman with cystic fibrosis and hemoptysis

A 25-year-old woman with a long history of cystic fibrosis presents with increasing dyspnea and hemoptysis. She was doing well until 6 months ago, when she required systemic corticosteroids for deteriorating pulmonary function. Her most recent FEV_1 and PCO_2 were 0.8 L and 60 mmHg, respectively. She recently was treated for increasing cough and sputum purulence with home intravenous antibiotics, which included ticarcillin and ceftazidime. Her usual regimen includes home oxygen, tube feeding by gastrostomy, frequent inhaled bronchodilators, and chest physiotherapy. She requires insulin for diabetes and uses pancreatic enzyme replacement.

Physical Examination: Temperature 37, pulse 100, respirations 20, blood pressure 100/60. General: cushingoid. Chest: crackles bilaterally, increased resonance. Cardiac: 2/6 systolic murmur with increased P2. Abdomen: normal. Extremities: clubbing.

Laboratory Findings: Hct 33%, WBC 2100/μl, platelets 178,000/μl; INR 1.2; fibrinogen 387; magnesium 1.8 mg/dl; calcium 7.6 mg/dl; phosphate 3.1 mg/dl. Chest radiograph: diffuse cystic and interstitial abnormalities.

Hospital Course: The patient developed worsening chest pain, dyspnea, and fever despite intravenous high-dose solumedrol and expansion of her antibiotic coverage. She suddenly coughed up 200 ml of blood and became severely short of breath. She was initially managed with noninvasive ventilation and red cell transfusions. Within hours, she coughed up 500 ml of blood and became severely short of breath.

Questions: What is the likely anatomic source of the hemoptysis? How should this patient be managed?

Diagnosis: Massive hemoptysis with respiratory failure due to bronchiectasis related to underlying cystic fibrosis.

Discussion: Patients with cystic fibrosis (CF) demonstrate severe bronchiectasis in a diffuse distribution, accompanied by proliferation of bronchial artery vessels in regions of persistent airway inflammation. When bleeding occurs, the source of hemorrhage is usually the bronchial circulation, although vascular ingrowth from the systemic arterial circulation into regions of lung inflammation also occurs in CF patients. Consequently, airway bleeding is supplied from high-pressure vascular systems, which increases the risk for massive hemoptysis. Localizing the exact site of hemorrhage is difficult because of the **diffuse nature of bronchiectasis** in CF. Contrast injected during angiography rarely extravasates from bleeding vessels to allow detection of a site of bleeding.

The first priority in patients with massive hemoptysis is stabilization of the airway and promotion of airway secretion clearance. Patients with massive hemoptysis more commonly die of asphyxiation than exsanguination. Thus, urgent intubation with a large-diameter endotracheal tube is indicated in unstable patients. A double-lumen endotracheal tube to allow suctioning of the bleeding lung and ventilation of the unaffected lung is technically difficult to perform and usually only delays the institution of adequate airway support. The second priority of management is hemodynamic stabilization with infusion of intravenous fluids. The third priority is reversal of any coagulopathy and repletion of red blood cells.

After patient stabilization, the first diagnostic goal is to determine if the bleeding is localized or diffuse in origin by performing fiberoptic bronchoscopy through an endotracheal tube. Extensive collections of airway blood in actively bleeding patients, however, compromise visual inspection of the airways and complicate detection of the source of bleeding. The bronchoscopist cannot establish the likely source of bleeding by determining the location of endobronchial collections of pooled blood, because this is an unreliable finding. Brisk bleeding from a bronchial orifice that continues after it is suctioned clear is stronger evidence of the source of bleeding. Radiographic evidence of airspace opacities or findings on physical examination cannot accurately determine the site of bleeding.

Patients with localized or indeterminate but non-diffuse sites of bleeding are best managed with **angiography with embolization**. Because the bronchial arterial circulation is the source of most large-volume hemorrhages in patients with CF, bronchial artery embolization is initially performed. Embolization of pulmonary or systemic arteries may have additional value if these vessels provide significant vascular supply to the region of hemorrhage or if the bronchial circulation appears relatively normal. Inadequate embolization of bronchial vessels and failure to embolize contributing systemic vessels are the primary reasons for failure of embolization therapy to arrest bleeding. Late recurrence of hemoptysis usually results from recanalization of embolized vessels or further proliferation of vessels in the region of inflammation.

Occlusion of the anterior spinal artery with resulting paraplegia represents the major complication of embolization therapy. Fortunately, this complication is rare and occurs in significantly less than 1% of patients managed by experienced angiographers.

The present patient was intubated emergently because of her poor respiratory reserve, the severity of her dyspnea, and the large volume of hemoptysis. Bedside fiberoptic bronchoscopy was performed, and large amounts of blood were suctioned from her airways. The source of bleeding was established to be in her right upper lobe. Angiography demonstrated bilateral tortuous and aneurysmal bronchial arteries in the right upper lobe; systemic arteries branching from the thyrocervical arteries also supplied this region of the lung. All of these vessels were embolized, which successfully stopped the airway hemorrhage. The patient was successfully weaned from the ventilator several days later.

Clinical Pearls

1. Patients with cystic fibrosis demonstrate proliferation of bronchial arteries and arteries from the systemic circulation in regions of lung inflammation.

2. Massive hemoptysis requires establishment of a secure airway as the first priority.

3. Early bronchoscopy is indicated to identify the source of bleeding.

4. Because lung resection is not an option in patients with poor respiratory reserve, embolotherapy is the primary therapeutic approach to control hemmorhage.

5. Some patients may require embolization of systemic blood vessels, which may be the source of hemoptysis in patients with severe bronchiectasis.

REFERENCES

1. Cahill BC, Ingbar DH: Massive hemoptysis. Clin Chest Med 1994; 15:146–168.
2. Brinson GM, Noone PG, Muro MA, et al: Bronchial artery embolization for the treatment of hemoptysis in patients with cystic fibrosis. Am J Respir Crit Care Med 1998; 157:1951–1958.
3. Mal H, Rullon I, Mellot F, et al: Immediate and long-term results of bronchial artery embolization for life-threatening hemoptysis. Chest 1999; 115:996–1001.
4. White RI: Bronchial artery embolotherapy for control of acute hemoptysis. Analysis of outcome. Chest 1999; 115:912–915.

John E. Heffner, MD

PATIENT 80

A 26-year-old woman with fever after a near-drowning

A 26-year-old woman is brought to the emergency department (ED) after she failed to resurface after diving into a small lake. Her swimming companions found her submerged near the muddy lake bottom apparently unconscious. The patient was brought to the surface within 1 minute of her dive. She aroused after several minutes of mouth-to-mouth and began coughing vigorously and complaining of a sore head. Paramedics transported her to the medical center where she denied previous medical illnesses.

Physical Examination: Vital signs: normal. Head: no trauma; mud around her face. Eyes: normal fundi. Neck: neck collar in place. Chest: scattered rhonchi, clearing with cough. Cardiac: normal. Neurologic: alert; normal motor and sensory examination.

Laboratory Findings: Hemogram and blood chemistries: normal. Chest and cervical radiographs: normal.

Clinical Course: The patient was discharged after overnight observation with a diagnosis of near-drowning after hitting her head on the shallow lake bottom. One week after discharge, she noticed a cough, low-grade fever, and progressive shortness of breath. Two days after the onset of symptoms, she presented to the ED with the following laboratory results: Hct 32%, WBC 15,000/μl with 85% neutrophils and 10% bands, and normal electrolytes and renal indices. Sputum Gram stain: branching fungal elements. Chest radiograph: see below.

Question: What are the possible diagnoses for the delayed onset of respiratory symptoms?

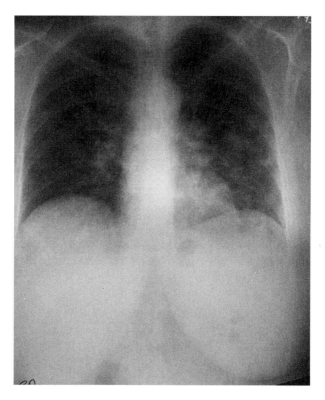

Diagnosis: Aspiration pneumonia due to *Pseudallescheria boydii* after near-drowning.

Discussion: Any episode of near-drowning represents a potentially life-threatening event. By definition, *drownings* cause death by asphyxia while victims are submerged, or from complications within 24 hours of submersion. In contrast, *near-drownings* are any submersions of sufficient severity to warrant medical attention. Near-drownings can produce complications immediately after submersion, or days to weeks after apparent clinical stabilization and recovery. In either event, the complications of near-drowning can progress to death or permanent disabilities.

Organ dysfunction related to prolonged hypoxia, ischemia, and acidosis are the most common immediate complications of near-drowning. Neurologic damage represents the most catastrophic of these hypoxia-related events. Noncardiogenic pulmonary edema, renal failure, cardiovascular instability, and disseminated intravascular coagulation can also occur.

Delayed complications are most often **infectious in etiology** and develop as a complication of aspiration. Prolonged submersion initiates voluntary breath-holding that is eventually followed by involuntary efforts to breath as $PaCO_2$ increases above a threshold level. Initial aspiration of water often produces laryngospasm that subsequently remits in 90% of near-drowning victims, causing large-volume aspiration. Aspiration of gastric contents may also occur. Autopsy series indicate that 25% of drowning victims have gastric contents in their lungs.

Aspiration due to near-drowning can contaminate the lower respiratory tract with oral flora, causing an aspiration pneumonia. Aspiration of contaminated environmental water may further increase the risk of pulmonary infection. Many bodies of water are contaminated with human pathogens. Aspirated particulates of mud, sand, and fragments of aquatic vegetation are additional sources of pathogens—many of which are unusual causes of pneumonia. It is stated that victims of near-drowning in shallow natural bodies of water have a high risk of aspirating such pathogen-laden particulates; more than 60% of drowning victims have autopsy evidence of particulate aspiration.

A variety of bacterial and fungal pathogens have been reported to cause pneumonia after near-drownings. *Streptococcus pneumoniae*, *Staphylococcus aureus*, and a spectrum of aerobic gram-negative and anaerobic pathogens have been reported. Pneumonia caused by these bacteria may result from aspiration of pathogens from the mouth or from contaminated water.

Certain causes of pneumonia related to near-drowning require special mention. Aeromonas species are aerobic, gram-negative bacteria that typically cause pneumonia in the setting of liver disease or hematologic malignancies. They can also cause pneumonia, however, in previously healthy victims of near-drowning. *Aeromonas hydrophila* is the most frequently isolated species in this setting, which produces a bacteremic pneumonia in 70% of near-drowning patients with this infection. *Chromobacterium violaceum* is an unusual human pathogen found in soil and freshwater in the southeastern United States that has been reported to cause pneumonia after near-drowning. *Francisella philomiragia* and non-*cholera Vibrio* species are additional unusual pathogens causing pneumonia after aspiration of contaminated water during submersion.

Fungal pathogens can also cause pneumonia in victims of near-drowning. Aspergillus species are common contaminants of natural bodies of water, especially those polluted with sewage. Rare reports exist of invasive aspergillus pneumonia after accidental submersion. *P. boydii* represents the most common fungal pathogen associated with near-drowning. This ubiquitous pathogen has been isolated from freshwater lakes and coastal waters, as well as polluted streams. Onset of symptoms generally is delayed, occurring from 1 week to 4–6 months later. Radiographic manifestations may be focal or diffuse, with evidence of varying degrees of tissue necrosis. Because of the ability of this pathogen to invade blood vessels, early hematogenous dissemination is the rule. Most patients with *P. boydii* pneumonia have spread to the CNS with complications that include brain abscesses, meningitis, and endophthalmitis.

P. boydii pneumonia is difficult to treat. This fungus is often resistant to amphotericin B. Reports exist of successful outcomes after therapy with itraconazole, miconazole, and ketoconazole. Many experts consider **itraconazole** the agent of choice for this infection.

The present patient presented with bilateral, patchy pulmonary opacities and fungal elements in her sputum. She was initially treated with amphotericin B, which was changed to itraconazole when her sputum cultures grew *P. boydii*. Her pulmonary infection progressed despite therapy, and she expired on the seventh day of hospitalization 17 days after her near-drowning event.

Clinical Pearls

1. Near-drownings are defined as any submersion that is sufficiently severe to warrant a medical evaluation. Drownings are defined by the occurrence of death by asphyxia during submersion or within the first 24 hours.

2. Only 10% of near-drowning victims avoid aspiration during submersion. Many patients aspirate particulates laden with human pathogens that can cause pneumonia.

3. Pneumonia caused by near-drowning is often delayed in onset. Aspirated fungal pathogens may have a slow initial course, with patients presenting with pulmonary infections several months after submersion.

4. Pneumonia due to *Pseudallescheria boydii* is an especially serious complication of near-drowning. This pathogen is often resistant to amphotericin B and disseminates widely to involve the CNS.

REFERENCES

1. Levin LL, Morriss FC, Toro LO, et al: Drowning and near-drowning. Ped Clin North Am 1993;40:321–336.
2. Modell JH: Drowning. N Engl J Med 1993;328:253–256.
3. Weinstein MD, Grieger BP: Near-drowning: Epidemiology, pathophysiology, and initial treatment. J Emerg Med 1996;14: 461–467.
4. Wilichowski E, Christen HJ, Schiffman H, et al: Fatal *Pseudoallescheria boydii* panencephalitis in a child after near-drowning. Pediatr Infect Dis J 1996;15:365–370.
5. Ender PT, Dolan MJ: Pneumonia associated with near-drowning. Clin Infect Dis 1997;25:896–907.

Acknowledgement: This case has been modified from Heffner JE: What caused fever in this 26-year-old woman after a near-drowning? J Crit Illness 1998;13:629–631.

INDEX